Oxford University Press, Walton Street, Oxford OX2 6DP

Oxford New York Toronto Melbourne Auckland
Delhi Bombay Calcutta Madras Karachi
Petaling Jaya Singapore Hong Kong Tokyo
Nairobi Dar es Salaam Cape Town

Associated companies in Beirut Berlin Ibadan Nicosia

OXFORD *is a trade mark of Oxford University Press*

Published in the United States
by Oxford University Press, New York

British Library Cataloguing in Publication Data
Loudon, Irvine
Medical care and the general practitioner,
1750–1850.
1. Physicians (General practice)—
Great Britain—History
I. Title
362.1'72'0941   R729.5.G4
ISBN 0-19-822793-0

Library of Congress Cataloging in Publication Data
Loudon, Irvine.
Medical care and the general practitioner, 1750–1850.
Bibliography: p.
Includes index.
1. Family medicine—Great Britain—History—18th
century.   2. Family medicine—Great Britain—History—
19th century.   3. Medicine—Great Britain—History—18th
century.   4. Medicine—Great Britain—History—19th
century.   I. Title.
R487.L68   1987   305.9'616'0941   86-14172
ISBN 0-19-822793-0

Printed in Great Britain
by Butler & Tanner Ltd,
Frome and London

Medical Care and the General Practitioner 1750–1850

IRVINE LOUDON

CLARENDON PRESS · OXFORD

1986

Preface

IN February 1773, Gibbon confessed he was 'soon disgusted with the modest practice of reading the manuscript [of *Decline and Fall*] to my friends. Of such friends some will praise from politeness, and some will criticise from vanity. The author himself is the best judge of his own performance. ...'[1] It is an opinion we can respect from the giants of historical authorship, but one that most of us would be foolish to adopt. For my part, I am deeply in debt to many people for their assistance, most of all to colleagues in the Wellcome Unit in Oxford, and especially to Charles Webster and Margaret Pelling. Jonathan Barry's assistance has been invaluable. His breadth of historical knowledge and sharply critical eye resulted in numerous (and invariably useful) criticisms of the draft manuscript. Paul Laxton, Joan Lane, David van Zwanenberg, and Jonathan Barry have all generously allowed me to utilize data from their own research; their specific contributions are acknowledged in the text or footnotes. Richard Palmer and William Schupbach of the Wellcome Institute in London have provided valuable material, and I am grateful to many librarians and archivists in Oxford (especially the staff of the Lankester room in the Radcliffe Science Library), in London and in the many County Record Offices which I visited during the course of my research. I am grateful to Adrian Wilson for permission to quote from his thesis on Childbirth in Seventeenth- and Eighteenth-Century England. Dr Dick Maurice of Marlborough, Mr Philip Awdrey of Oxford, and Mr Simon Beadles of Stoke-sub-Hamden, have allowed me free access to valuable manuscripts in their private possession. Dr John Ford of Tonbridge allowed me to use his typescript copies of the important Weekes correspondence held by St Thomas's Hospital Medical School, whom I thank for permission to publish.

For anyone working on the history of medicine in the late eighteenth and nineteenth century, few publications are as important as W.R. LeFanu's *British Periodicals of Medicine, 1640–1899*, rev. edn., ed. Jean Loudon (Wellcome Unit for the History of Medicine, Oxford, 1984). My debt to this is obvious; not only is it an essential guide through a jungle, but it is a revelation to anyone who believed that the *Lancet* and

---

[1] Edward Gibbon, *Memoirs of my Life*, Penguin English Library edn. (Harmondsworth, 1984).

the *British Medical Journal* (numbers 78 and 263 respectively in the chronological list) were the earliest British medical periodicals. During her work on periodicals, Jean Loudon found numerous important references to general practitioners and medical reform which would otherwise have escaped me. I am deeply grateful to her for this, and for her continual support and encouragement through the four years in which I was occupied with this study. Mrs Greta Ilott and Mrs Ann Cheales typed the manuscript with speed and efficiency; to both I am indebted. My greatest debt is to the Wellcome Trustees. Without their generous support in the form of a Wellcome Fellowship, this study would not have been possible.

I.L.

October 1985

Contents

List of Tables, Figure, and Appendices

TABLES

FIGURE

APPENDICES

Abbreviations

AMJ	*Association Medical Journal*
BFMCR	*British and Foreign Medico-Chirurgical Review*
BFMR	*British and Foreign Medical Review*
BIBM	Bristol Infirmary Biographical Memoirs. The papers of Richard Smith junior, surgeon of Bristol
BMA	British Medical Association
BMJ	*British Medical Journal*
CRO	County Record Office
EMSJ	*Edinburgh Medical and Surgical Journal*
DNB	*Dictionary of National Biography*
LMG	*London Medical Gazette*
LMPJ	*London Medical and Physical Journal*
MCR	*Medico-Chirurgical Review (and Journal of Medical Science)*
MPJ	*Medical and Physical Journal*
NS	new series
PMSA	Provincial Medical and Surgical Association
PMSJ	*Provincial Medical and Surgical Journal*
PP	Parliamentary Papers
PRO	Public Record Office
RO	Record Office
SCME	*Report of the Select Committee on Medical Education,* PP 1834, XIII
SCMR	*Report of the Select Committee on Medical Registration,* PP 1847, IX, and pp 1847–48, XV
Wellcome MS	Manuscript from the collection held by the Wellcome Institute for the History of Medicine, London

Introduction

It is neither easy, nor particularly important, to be quite certain when the term 'general practitioner' was first used in its modern sense. Certainly it was the early nineteenth century, and the earliest example I have found was published in 1809.[1] The occasional appearances of 'general practice' in medical works of the eighteenth century can be dismissed as red herrings; in these, 'general practice' is simply used in the sense of 'usual' or 'broadly based' and the authors were not describing a specific type or division of medical practice.[2] It is therefore anachronistic to describe any practitioner in or before the eighteenth century as a general practitioner.

Whenever the term was introduced, however, it is certain that it came into common usage in the second and third decades of the nineteenth century. Even so, its initial use was confined to the medical profession. The public was slow to recognize and adopt the new designation. Most early Victorian novelists, even in the 1850s, labelled the family doctors of the villages and market towns as 'apothecary' or 'surgeon'. The slow acceptance of 'general practitioner' by the public as a whole may have been due in part to the fact that it was a term with no statutory definition or recognition. Consequently, it seldom appears in legal documents or state papers in the first half of the nineteenth century. Moreover, the term was not universally popular within the profession. G. J. Guthrie, President of the Royal College of Surgeons, and Thomas Wakley, editor of the *Lancet*, both irascible men but politically at opposite poles, treated

---

[1] Writing on 9 Feb. 1809 about the troubles of young practitioners, 'H' opened the second paragraph of his letter with: 'If he is destined to follow his profession as a *general practitioner of medicine* in the country ...' (my italics), *MPJ* 21 (1809), 382–5, p. 382. Four years later 'C.W.S.' wrote of the proposals of a Bill for medical reform: 'I think the bill might with a great deal of propriety be termed that of the general practitioner in medicine, surgery and midwifery in which the apothecary would be included ... the character of the general practitioner was always respectable, whilst the regular apothecary of the present day retains little else than the name of his predecessor.' *MPJ* 30 (1813), 478–81, p. 479.

[2] As, for instance, when John Bellars in *An Essay on the Improvement of Physick* ... (London, 1714) referred to certain physicians who were 'General Practitioners in Physick'. Or when T. Champney in *Medical and Chirurgical Reform* ... (London, 1797) referred to 'general education and general practice' on p. 73.

the term with scorn long after it was in common use.[3] Some general practitioners, by virtue of holding the diploma of the Royal College of Surgeons (MRCS) as well as the licence of the Society of Apothecaries (LSA) preferred the more prestigious term 'surgeon'. Wakley, briefly a general practitioner himself, believed that 'surgeon' was correct. Nevertheless, as we know, the term has stuck fast in Britain with its colloquial twin, 'family doctor'. More recent fashions such as 'family physician' and 'primary care doctor' have also been seen but they are unlikely replacements.[4]

In Britain, at least, the general practitioner was not a sudden creation. He evolved from the surgeon-apothecary and man-midwife of the eighteenth century. Nevertheless, the new term was more than just a change in fashion. It came into use amongst the largest group of practitioners, the rank and file, because of the development of a new sense of common purpose—of corporate identity—which was combined with self-confidence and optimism. They believed they had advanced beyond their predecessors to become respectable, scientific, professional men.

In many ways it was a remarkable change, and many have assumed that the change and the new title were both creations of the well-known Apothecaries Act of 1815. Instead, of course, the change and the title preceded the Act, and were products of the upheavals between the late eighteenth and mid-nineteenth century that have earned that period the sobriquet 'The Period of Medical Reform'.[5] It is not the most apt of descriptions. The word reform has inescapable associations with improvement and progress, in this case with improvement in medical education, skill and, by inference, in the medical care of the population. Popular belief tends to support this view, seeing the rank-and-file practitioner of the eighteenth century as uneducated, poor, and unskilled, while the nineteenth-century equivalent was properly trained in scientific principles. This story of steady upward progress is far from the truth.

The period of medical reform was not a coherent movement dedicated

---

[3] Thus Guthrie in 1847 professed not to know what the term meant unless it was 'general practitioner in nothing' (*SCMR*, Q. 122 and 135) although he had defined the term clearly and correctly in 1834 (*SCME*, Part II, Q. 4901.) Wakley's diatribe against 'general practitioner' appeared in the *Lancet* (1829–30), ii, 690–3.

[4] Not at any rate in Britain although they have been adopted in North America together with the term 'primary care specialties'.

[5] Conventionally the limits of the period of medical reform are 1794–1858 (see chapter 6). There are good arguments, however, for extending the period from the beginning of the last third of the eighteenth century to the Medical Act Amendment Act of 1886.

to the improvement of medical education and medical care; rather, it consisted of a bitter struggle between various groups of medical men, and also between medical men and those who were stigmatized as 'quacks' or irregulars (a group which included druggists and midwives), in an attempt to achieve a monopoly of all forms of medical care. In theory, the introduction of formal medical education, examination, and licensing should have produced a corpus of much better educated and competent doctors for the mass of the people. In practice it is difficult to point with confidence to many improvements in medical care in the first half of the nineteenth century at the level of the general practitioner. It is even doubtful whether he occupied a higher status in society than his predecessors, and it seems certain that he was less rather than more prosperous. But there can be no doubt that extensive changes in the organization of medical practice occurred between the mid-eighteenth and the mid-nineteenth century. There is only a faint resemblance between the structure of medical practice in 1750 and the one with which we are familiar today. Indeed, it is doubtful whether one could justify the use of 'the medical profession' to describe the relatively fragmented groups of practitioners that existed in the first half of the eighteenth century. By 1850, however, the main structure of the present medical profession had been created. The only major changes in professional structure in the last 130 years have been a consequence of the multiplication of specialties and sub-specialties with their attendant programmes of training and examinations, all of which have occurred within the broad framework of physicians, surgeons, and general practitioners; a structure with which practitioners in the 1850s would have been entirely familiar.

Much of this is common ground. Historians of the medical profession in the eighteenth and nineteenth centuries are in general agreement that a period of transition occurred in which a disunited, pluralistic, or even non-existent medical profession changed to a unified one. Most would agree that this change was associated with the increasing dominance of the teaching hospitals and the growth of university departments of medicine. There are, however, wide differences of opinion about the true extent of change and the time when it occurred. The group which changed least of all were the physicians—the graduate practitioners—and this may be true of most European countries during this period.[6] It was amongst the non-graduate practitioners that the

---

[6] Graduate practitioners were not necessarily physicians throughout Europe. In Holland it was possible to graduate in either physic or surgery or the *ars obstetricae.*

major transition occurred. To put it at its simplest, it is usually suggested that the rank-and-file practitioners advanced from the position of a tradesman of lowly status, or at best a craftsman, occupying a social world which was totally different from the graduate physician, to membership of a unified profession in which they were, albeit at a lower level, professional doctors.

This suggestion, however, is far from simple, since it begs so many questions. What, for example, is meant by 'lowly status'? To place the eighteenth-century non-graduate practitioner neatly into a pigeon hole labelled tradesman or craftsman is to do no more than categorize him conveniently. It leaves open the question of the position granted to him by his contemporaries, and the relative importance in the past of various trades and crafts in the social hierarchy. It is easy to assume, incorrectly, that our present tendency to value brain over hand was shared in the eighteenth and early nineteenth century by all levels of society. And the assumed upward progress of the rank-and-file practitioner always leads in the end to the criteria by which we decide whether or not an occupation was, or was in the process of becoming, a profession.[7] Moreover, when the nature of the transition of the rank-and-file practitioners has been settled, how do we decide whether the change is of such magnitude that there is a discontinuity between the old and the new, or alternatively, that there was no more than a gradual evolution? This may be the hardest question of all. In measuring the change, how many points should be awarded for state licensing *per se*? How many for a formal system of medical education in university or hospital, a judgement that should surely take into account the quality of the syllabus and the teaching? How many for the raised social status of the practitioner? How many for changes in income? And, not least, how many for the standard of care provided for the population as a whole?

Gelfand has addressed some of these questions with clarity and concludes there was a substantial difference—a discontinuity—between the lowly grades of the medical professions of the eighteenth century and the general practitioner in the nineteenth.[8] The conclusion is based on the modest origins, status, and aspirations, the limited activities,

---

[7] For a recent, wide-ranging, and illuminating contribution to the trade *v.* profession debate with regard to medicine, see M. Pelling, 'Medical Practice in the Early Modern Period: Trade or Profession?' in W. Prest (ed.), *Professions in Early Modern England* (Croom Helm, London, in press).

[8] T. Gelfand, 'The Decline of the Ordinary Practitioner and the Rise of the Modern Medical Profession' in S. Statum and D. E. Larson, *Doctors, Patients and Society: Power and Authority in Medical Care* (Ontario, 1981).

and the apprenticeship-only-training of the former, compared with the 'proper' training of the general practitioner within the context of a unified profession whose members shared a common basic medical education. His model, however, is the medical profession in France and his conclusions cannot be applied to England without important reservations. For example, it seems that the care provided by the barber-surgeon, the lower order practitioner in France in the mid- to late eighteenth century, was much more restricted than in England; that the general opinion of the effectiveness of care that was provided was poor; and that the social origin and education of the French provincial barber-surgeon was lower than that of his English counterparts. Moreover, the French revolution precipitated a sudden transformation in the organization of medical care compared to the slower changes in England which were almost entirely unaffected by political events. Work such as Gelfand's suggests that a comprehensive comparative study of the evolution of the medical professions throughout Europe would be a valuable contribution not just to the history of medicine but also to the history of professions in general. It has not been attempted here, not even at an elementary level, for two reasons—space and ignorance.

As far as the medical profession in England is concerned, Waddington's recent book tends to support Gelfand's thesis of a substantial change in the rank-and-file practitioners associated with the process of professionalization.[9] Both Gelfand and Waddington are impressed by Jewson's sociological analyses which suggest that medicine was client-dominated in the eighteenth century and doctor-dominated in the nineteenth, and that this change in the practitioner/patient relationship was important, affecting the ideology of medicine and the very nature of the transition.[10] Holmes places the transition much earlier. He believes that the 'doctor' for the mass of the people arrived in English society during the period between 1680 and 1730. This is not to deny the importance of changes a century later; but it elevates the practitioner of the eighteenth century to a higher level than others have suggested. Holloway, on the other hand, sees 1830 to 1858 as a crucial period in which medicine became more scientific, medical education more systematic, and the medical profession more unified.[11] Peterson, in her

---

[9] I. Waddington, *The Medical Profession in the Industrial Revolution* (Dublin, 1984).

[10] N. Jewson, 'Medical Knowledge and the Patronage System in 18th-century England', *Sociology*, 8 (1974), 369–85.

[11] S.W.F. Holloway, 'Medical Education in England, 1830–1858: A Sociological Analysis', *History*, 49 (1964), 299–324.

book on the medical profession in mid-Victorian London, suggests that the vital period of unification was between the Medical Act of 1858 and the Medical Act Amendment Act of 1886.[12] There is certainly logic in this view, since it was only after 1886 that examination in all three main branches of medicine—medicine, surgery, and midwifery—was made compulsory for registration.

The views of these authors, which are merely paraphrased here but will be considered in more detail later in the text, are mentioned in order to emphasize the complexity and the fascination of this period of transition in the medical profession. It can be seen that historians do not agree with one another, not only in points of detail which are of no more than minor academic importance, but also in quite major assessments of the clinical activities and the social and economic status of the rank-and-file practitioners. The differences of opinion might be explained by the scarcity of source material. Data on the daily lives of surgeon-apothecaries and general practitioners throughout the period from 1750 to 1850 are far from plentiful, although such difficulties are not nearly as great as they are for earlier periods. Often, however, disagreement hinges on the criteria adopted by different authors for the definition of concepts such as professionalization and the meaning of unification in the context of the evolution of the medical profession. For example, the introduction of a formal system of medical education which was the same for all branches of medicine and the move towards compulsory registration of all medical practitioners are clear evidence of unification; the simultaneous existence of vicious and widespread dissension between different groups of practitioners is evidence to the contrary.

It is against the background of such matters that this study of the rank-and-file practitioners has been written. Throughout, the emphasis is on the social and economic aspects of medical practice. The appearance of the term 'general practitioner' is used to divide the book into two parts. Part 1 is concerned with the predecessors of the general practitioner in the second half of the eighteenth century and the first decade of the nineteenth; part 2 with the transitional period of medical reform and the early phase of the general practitioner up to 1850. Although the practitioner occupies centre stage, the diseases he treated, methods of treatment, and the relationship of the practitioner to his

---

[12] M.J. Peterson, *The Medical Profession in Mid-Victorian London*, (Berkeley, Calif., 1978).

patients, to society, and to other members of the profession, are important themes.

Part 1 begins with the whole spectrum of medical care—regular and irregular—in the eighteenth century, and with the rise of the surgeon-apothecary. This is followed in chapter 2 by an account of the social origins and education (medical and general) of the eighteenth-century surgeon-apothecary. Clinical aspects follow in chapters 3 (physic and pharmacy) and 4 (surgery and obstetrics). In both, fees and income from various types of medical practice are considered. The economics of medical practice play a large part in this study, partly because of the nature of existing records. Practitioners (and patients) were more likely to preserve accounts and bills than letters, diaries, and clinical records. But the emphasis on money is justified on the grounds that throughout this period most practitioners thought of medical practice as a business as well as a profession. They were deeply concerned with money, judging, correctly, that their status in society as well as their personal comfort was closely attached to their income.

In chapter 5 the social and economic status of the eighteenth-century practitioner is considered in the context of the supply and demand for medical care. This chapter concludes with a brief account of a neglected but important subject—the practitioner and his transport. Part 2 begins in chapter 6 with the early phase of the period of medical reform and emphasizes the importance of the rise of the dispensing druggist which was seen as a major threat to the livelihood of the regular practitioners. This is followed by the most widely known part of the story: the establishment of the Association of Apothecaries and Surgeon-Apothecaries and the Apothecaries Act of 1815 (chapter 7); and an assessment of the qualities and consequences of the Act (chapter 8). Chapter 9 turns to the status of the general practitioner in the second quarter of the nineteenth century and the problem of the practice of pharmacy which, in so far as it mimicked the practice of the druggist, degraded the rank of the general practitioner.

One of the central themes of this study is the over-production of practitioners in the first half of the nineteenth century. There were continual complaints that the medical profession was overcrowded. To the public this was an asset, ensuring that fees were kept low; to the profession it was a source of excessive competition and, to many, of relative poverty. Much of chapter 10 consists of a statistical analysis of the number of medical men, their qualifications, and their appointments. It seems incontrovertible that the profession was overcrowded to an extent not seen before or since, and general practitioners competed desperately for patients not only with each other, but with physicians and surgeons. One of the purposes here is to emphasize the extent to which physicians, surgeons, and general practitioners overlapped each other in education, in the nature of their daily clinical practice, in their formal qualifications, and in honorary appointments to medical institutions.

The general practitioner derived his income and employed his skills in a number of different roles. Private practice came first, but club practice, dispensary practice, and poor law practice played a large and sometimes forgotten part. The role of the general practitioner as poor law medical officer before and after 1834 is the subject of chapter 11. Chapter 12 deals with his other roles and sources of income. The final chapter sees the general practitioner established. On the one hand he had become accepted by the public as the family doctor. On the other he had failed to achieve the aim of full and equal status with other medical practitioners, an aim which imbued him with optimism in the earlier part of the century. The failure is symbolized by the unsuccessful attempt to establish a College of General Practitioners. Defeat followed a three-year struggle, ending in 1850, which explains the reason for choosing this rather than 1858 (the date of the Medical Act) as the endpoint of this study. The Act of 1858 is reviewed briefly as a postscript (chapter 14).

In studies of the medical profession, irregular practice has sometimes received too little attention—not so much as a valid form of alternative medical care, but as a threat to regular practice and therefore as a generator of change and reform. It plays a major part in this study, but it proved in the end impossible to contain irregular practice neatly in a chapter of its own. Accounts of it therefore appear in various chapters, where appropriate. The subject is complex, and the choice of 'irregular' deliberate. Quackery is unnecessarily perjorative, empiricism is ambiguous. Unqualified practice is misleading in a period when many regular practitioners were not, in the modern sense, medically qualified. 'Irregular' is therefore the best of the alternatives although, as the first chapter will show, a clear division between the regular and the irregular practitioner was a feature of medicine which belonged to the period after, but not before, the middle of the nineteenth century.

PART 1

The Predecessors of the General Practitioners, 1750–1810

I

Practitioners, Regular and Irregular

The rank-and-file practitioners of the eighteenth century

OUR perception of medical men in the eighteenth century tends, perhaps inevitably, to be based on a small and highly literate élite of practitioners, most of whom practised in London. There is an obvious imbalance between the copious records of these men and the sparse records of the ordinary rank and file who, as the predecessors of the general practitioners, are our immediate concern. Who were the ordinary medical men of towns and villages in the provinces? What was the nature of their practice? What was their background and what was their standing in the community? Were they in general illiterate or educated, skilful within the context of their time, or crudely ignorant of even the rudiments of medical knowledge? Were they on familiar terms, professionally and socially, with the gentry and other professionals, or were they classed, by themselves and their neighbours, with the grocer, the draper, and the ironmonger? The questions are obvious, the answers are not. Anyone who has undertaken research in this field will confirm the difficulties. Little was published about the social state of the rank-and-file practitioner; still less about the clinical aspect of his work. One is dependent for most of the answers on manuscript sources either in libraries, county record offices, or in private possession; on the few published diaries of eighteenth-century practitioners; and a fairly small number of other sources such as Samuel Foart Simmons's valuable *Medical Register*,[1] and the county directories of the eighteenth and early nineteenth century.

Broadly speaking there are two contrasting views concerning the general level of medical practice in the eighteenth century. The traditional view of the rank-and-file provincial practitioners perceives them as 'the unpretentious apothecaries—the quasi-irregulars',[2] a group of ill-educated, near-illiterate tradesmen who kept a shop and sold groceries

---

[1] See J. Lane, 'The Medical Practitioners of Provincial England', *Medical History*, 28 (1984), 353–71, which is based on a discussion of the *Medical Register*.

[2] R. H. Shryock, *The Development of Modern Medicine* (Wisconsin, 1979), 52.

and articles of toilet as well as medicines. Their practice, it is suggested, was based on a primitive knowledge of physic and pharmacy coupled with a crude lack of skill in surgery. An immense gap, it is thought, separated the highest standards of the time as practised, for example, by Heberden, Percival, the Hunters, or Smellie, and the standards of the average provincial practitioner. Moreover, the tendency (not uncommon) for medical practitioners to combine medical practice with another occupation such as farming is cited as evidence of the poverty of orthodox practice; and the suggested poverty is attributed to public preference for the quack, further demonstrating the low regard for the orthodox practitioner.

For those who consider this an accurate picture of eighteenth-century practice, or at worst as a mildly Hogarthian caricature, it is clear that the evolution of such practitioners into respectable professional men could not, and did not, occur until the nineteenth century, following the Apothecaries Act of 1815 and the appearance of the general practitioner.

Recently, however, Holmes has proposed a very different thesis in which he suggests that the medical profession came into existence between 1680 and 1730.[3] It was then, he suggests, that for the first time 'the doctor truly arrives in English society'. He claims that this important and extensive change in medical practice in England was due to the breakdown of the tripartite system and the Rose case of 1704 (both of which are considered later in this chapter) leading to a new and broadly based form of medical practice signified by the emergence of the surgeon-apothecary. But his main thesis is that there was in this period a significant improvement in the education of medical practitioners through attendance at the hospitals. Through all these factors, medical men developed a sense of corporate identity and achieved public recognition as professionals. Thus Holmes sees the birth of a medical profession as taking place between 1680 and 1730 in stark contrast to the more conventional view that it took place a century later.

Is this contrast more apparent than real? It could be argued that, in the end, the difference consists of no more than a rehearsal of the familiar and fashionable arguments about the nature of professionalization, and the criteria on which such arguments hinge. But the difference is much greater than that, and its mere existence demonstrates how little is still

---

[3] G. Holmes, *Augustan England: Professions, State and Society, 1680–1730* (London, 1982).

known about the nature of medical practice as a whole in England in the eighteenth century.

The research on which this book is based suggests that Holmes's view is much nearer the truth than the traditional story. If I differ from Holmes it is on timing. My belief is that substantial changes in the extent of regular medical care and medical prosperity occurred after, not before, 1740. Certainly there is no evidence of any substantial change in the education of the rank-and-file practitioners before the mid-eighteenth century, and the chronology of the voluntary hospital movement rules out hospital training as a significant factor before the 1740s, at the earliest. Evidence concerning these points will be produced in subsequent chapters.

The diversity of practitioners

Quite apart from the scarcity of sources, there are two major difficulties in attempting a coherent picture of ordinary medical practice in the eighteenth century. First, there is the diversity of medical men, and second, the absence of a clear distinction between the orthodox or regular practitioner and the unorthodox irregular or quack. Only a moment's consideration is necessary to see that when there was no system of formal education, registration, and licensing, no sharp dividing lines could exist between the qualified and the unqualified. Some of the orthodox practitioners, of course, held university degrees or were members of the Company of Surgeons; others had acquired certificates of attendance at courses of lectures in London hospitals, while a large number had served a full apprenticeship. These were obvious criteria for identifying the orthodox practitioners. But in many cases nothing is known of the background, and it may be only an assumption that there was at least an apprenticeship. The 'grey area' of uncertainty is brought out by examples such as medical men who started as grocers, selling drugs as a sideline, who simply changed the board over their door to 'surgeon' or 'apothecary' if it suited them to do so. In the opposite direction, so to speak, practitioners whose background was impeccably orthodox, later appear in the flamboyant guise of the itinerant quack.[4] A clear distinction between the orthodox and unorthodox is often impossible: at each end of the spectrum the two are easily distinguished; in the centre they mingle imperceptibly.

---

[4] The most famous example being 'Chevalier' John Taylor (1703–72, MD Basle 1733, MD Liège and Cologne 1734), who trained at St Thomas's Hospital, London and was an **expert** oculist.

A useful approach to this problem is perhaps to adopt the criterion proposed by Pelling and Webster for an earlier period;[5] that is, to include under the heading 'medical practitioner' anyone whose living was derived largely or wholly from the treatment of the sick, regardless of title, background, or education. It is an approach which allows one to see the treatment of the sick as a whole and avoids the need to decide in certain instances whether a certain individual should be included as a 'proper' practitioner or excluded as a quack.

The traditional picture of the quack is that of an ignorant and unscrupulous pretender, often itinerant, who preyed on a credulous public for profit; a confidence-trickster, in fact, who, by taking away his rightful means of making his living, enraged the regular trained practitioner. Coltheart, a surgeon, was only one of a series of early eighteenth-century practitioners who exclaimed with venom against the 'Coal-Porter, Tinker, Taylor, Midwife, Nurse, etc. [who] spring up like Mushrooms in a night to be Physicians and Surgeons'.[6] Such quacks were easy to identify, easy to condemn. There were also, however, the educated men who 'took up' medicine as a hobby or as a means of helping their less fortunate neighbours. Profit was sometimes one of their motives, but usually it was a minor consideration. These people remind us of the extent to which medicine in the eighteenth century was not a subject largely confined to a closed professional group as it is today, but a subject for open and informed argument amongst educated men from all walks of life to be discussed like science, music, politics, or poetry.

The clergy especially, both Anglican and dissenting, were fond of treating their flock and anyone else who chose to consult them. Richard Wilkes (1690–1760, MA St John's College, Cambridge, 1715), for example, was deacon of Stowe by Chartley in Staffordshire. His only known connection with medicine was his brother John, who was a surgeon. Richard had no medical training, or licence, let alone a degree, but he practised physic widely and became a fashionable physician.[7]

But it was not only the clergy. George Winter, for instance, described himself as 'a practical farmer'. In his *Compendious System of Husbandry*,

---

[5] M. Pelling and C. Webster, 'Medical Practitioners' in C. Webster (ed.), *Health, Medicine and Mortality in the Sixteenth Century* (Cambridge, 1979).

[6] P. Coltheart, *The Quacks Unmasked* (London, 1727). See also F. Guybon, *An Essay concerning the Growth of Empiricism* (London, 1712).

[7] N. W. Tildesley, 'Richard Wilkes of Willenhall, Staffs: An Eighteenth-century Doctor', *Transactions of the South Staffordshire Archaeological and Historical Society*, 7 (1965–6), 1–10.

containing ... the Elements of Agriculture (2nd edn., London, 1797), of all unlikely places, one finds a preface devoted to medicine. Here he tells the reader that in 1782 'the author became possessed of his uncle's [who was a physician] most invaluable manuscripts and books' which were 'so pleasing and instructive' that he treated himself and succeeded in a cure. 'He next practised physic on his servants, and the poor of the neighbourhood, upwards of fourteen years ago; and for the last ten years, appropriated a certain number of hours, three days in a week, to attend the poor people'. This is followed in the preface by a summary of his cases. To George Winter medicine was a hobby, 'As he [the author] does not spend his evenings at coffee-houses or taverns, he is never happy at his leisure hours, without perusing some favourite medical author ...' There is no reason to believe that the author, or his friends and neighbours, lay or medical, thought this farmer's excursion into medical practice unusual, improper, or unethical.

Irregular practice was undertaken by men and women, the midwives being an example of a large and important group of female practitioners. Few had any formal training or licence, but they undertook nearly all the normal deliveries before 1740 and many abnormal ones as well. Some were highly regarded by regular practitioners. Dr Allen of Bridgewater, for example, wrote in glowing terms of the skill of Sarah Stone, a midwife whose practice started in that town and ended in London. Her mother Mrs Holmes was described by Dr Allen as 'the best midwife that ever I knew'.[8] Nevertheless, the midwife was usually classed by regular practitioners as one of the group of irregulars. Probably wisewomen or self-styled nurses were also numerous, but little is known about them. A passing glimpse is provided in the ledger of a Somerset surgeon in the 1740s who employed a nurse on occasions to carry out routine dressings of a leg ulcer in the manner of a district nurse.[9] The relative rarity of sick babies and children in the records of regular practitioners suggests that in the eighteenth century this branch of medical practice was very much in the hands of local irregulars, an impression which is reinforced by the virtual exclusion of children from the care of the hospitals and dispensaries of the eighteenth century.[10]

---

[8] Sarah Stone, *A Complete Practice of Midwifery* (London, 1737), pp. xxi–xxiv.

[9] Somerset CRO, Taunton. 'Doctor's Journal: ?Benjamin Pulsford', DD/FS Box 48. For further details of this important manuscript, see chapter 4.

[10] The foundation of the Dispensary for the Infant Poor by George Armstrong in 1767, and of the Universal Dispensary for Children by John Bunnell Davis in 1816 were a response to the neglect of sick children by orthodox practitioners. Davis remarked that parents would not take children to infirmaries or dispensaries, believing 'they would be

The probability that women combined the roles of healers (especially of babies and children), nurse, midwife, and layer-out of the dead, is suggested obliquely by a number of sources, including Wilson's comment that midwives in the early part of the century were seldom fully employed in midwifery alone.[11] There were also, of course, the herbalists. One, a Mrs Halton, was said to have drawn Withering's attention to the therapeutic value of the foxglove, although it is doubtful if the two of them ever met and the existence of Mrs Halton is by no means firmly established.[12] Home treatment, family care, and care by neighbours and local men or women who were known as healers in the broadest sense, obviously formed a large part of total care, although little is known about this aspect of medicine.

The itinerants are much better known, partly because they were the target of polemical attacks by regulars and partly because of their habit of advertising as they travelled from one town to another 'quacking' their wares and skills by posters and bills.[13] An anonymous pamphlet published in 1676 complained of the quack: 'Such impudent ostentious [*sic*] Decoy-papers he dayly spreads about the Streets, as if he had undertaken to serve the whole City with Bum-fodder, and plaisters with his quackeries every Pissing-post ...'[14] In the eighteenth century, such irregulars proclaimed in their posters that certain diseases were their special province and that cure was invariably guaranteed. Venereal disease, usually described by some euphemism such as 'a certain condition however inveterate', was the most prominent. But eye diseases, cancers (cured without incision), ruptures or 'broken bellies' (cured usually by some special new apparatus), and deafness ('if the drum of the ear is intact') were common in the lists of the quacks.

In August 1783 a certain Mr Farland advertised in the Bristol press

neglected where grown-up persons were attended to'. J. B. Davis, *Annals, Historical and Medical ... of the Universal Dispensary for Children* (London, 1821), 10.

[11] Adrian Wilson, 'Childbirth in Seventeenth- and Eighteenth-century England' (Sussex University, Ph.D. thesis, 1984).

[12] J. K. Aronson, *An Account of the Foxglove and its Medical Uses, 1785–1895* (Oxford, 1985); and personal communication, J. K. Aronson.

[13] The word 'quack' is usually attributed to 'quacksalver', a 'salve' being an ointment whose virtues were 'quacked' in the market place. T. Horn, in *Important Hints connected with the Present Medical Practice or Real Quackery* (London, 1834), suggested, however, that the derivation of quack was from the old German 'Quacksalber' meaning quicksilver or mercury, used in the treatment of venereal disease, one of the main specialties of the irregular.

[14] Anon., *The Character of a Quack Doctor or the Abusive Practices of Impudent Illiterate Pretenders to Physick Exposed* (London, 1676).

that he had arrived from his house in 'Temple Bar, London' and he claimed to cure:

Broken bodies ... in six weeks without trusses; Cancers ... without incision; Gravel and Stone ... in a short time; Palsy, if under the age of seventy; All Diseases of the eye even when blind; Hardness of hearing if the drum of the ear is not broken; Consumptive cases if the lungs are not ulcerated; Dropsy; Wens; Hare-lip in eight days; venereal disease of ever so long standing.[15]

Such advertisements were very common. A similar one in 1784 informed the public that 'Doctor and Oculist Goergslenner from his house, No 34 in Queen Square in Bristol, is arrived in the City of Exeter, where he intends to stay a considerable time and from thence he shall come to Plymouth.' The diseases 'he most perfectly cures' consisted of a list similar to the above, with venereal disease implied by the sentence 'all the degrees and symptoms of a certain disorder, whether inveterate or recent, or ever so bad, [cured] in a short time.'[16]

More bizarre was Ann Stanley. Through a large and ornate poster she advertised in 1784 that she had returned from Philadelphia to which, she claimed, her father, once an eminent physician in Hampshire, had emigrated. Although born deaf and dumb, Ann Stanley 'by divine favour had naturally an extraordinary Genious and Conception' and could cure

most curable distempers belonging to the eyes. She also cures deafness and thickness of Hearing if the Drum of the Ear be not hurt or broke; can cure broken Bellies in Old and Young; Gravel, Scald Heads, Rickets in Children ... and has a peculiar method in curing most Calamities incident to Women and Children, for which she is famous. ... She is Honest and Prosperous and knows People's Diseases at First Sight and takes none in hand for any Reward but those she does good to.[17]

The range of irregulars was, as indicated, very wide, and they shaded off imperceptibly into the regulars. Indeed, one of the complaints of some irregulars was their condemnation by the 'self-styled regular-bred physician' for using the very same remedies used by the regulars themselves.[18] The irregulars can not be simply dismissed as a group of fraudulent opportunists. Nor can they be defended *en masse* as providers of a form of alternative care which was safer, cheaper, no less effective,

[15] BIBM 3, 184.
[16] *The Sherbourne Mercury*, 20 Sept. 1784.
[17] Gloucestershire CRO, Gloucester, ref. PC 1159.
[18] F. Spilsbury, *Free Thoughts on Quackery* (London, 1776).

and available to the poor. There is an obvious banality in both extreme views, although each has its advocates. Whatever one's views of alternative medicine, however, it is certain that the irregulars played a large part in the history of medical practice between 1750 and 1850. Further accounts of who the irregulars were and how they practised are included in chapters 6 and 10. Here it is only necessary to stress that their importance went beyond the simple facts of economic competition for medical care. To regular practitioners the irregulars were always the enemy, injuring the health of the people and the pockets of the regular faculty. But the extent to which the regulars complained of irregular practice was often related to periods of professional anxiety about the status and rewards of medical practice. In the late seventeenth and early eighteenth century the physicians were angered by the encroachment of the apothecaries on the practice of physic, and it is notable that they turned their anger not only on the apothecaries but also on the irregulars. In the late eighteenth and early nineteenth century it was the turn of the rank-and-file practitioners to feel their livelihood threatened. This time it was they, not the physicians, who complained stridently about the scandal of quackery. The irregular was both a genuine source of competition and a scapegoat when the practice of any section of the profession was threatened. Statements by regular practitioners in any period to the effect that quackery 'is becoming rampant', 'is increasing', or 'is getting out of control' can not therefore be trusted as evidence of true changes in the extent of irregular practice.

It was, in other words, the perception of quackery which mattered rather than the true extent of irregular practice or the true extent to which the irregulars were depriving the regulars of income. In later chapters it will be shown that when that perception was quickened by the belief that quackery was on the increase and either was becoming, or had already become, a serious threat to their livelihood, regular practitioners united in their demands for reform and state intervention. They pressed for systems of formal medical education, examination, and licensing. Through such systems it was believed the public would be able to tell the true from the false, the irregulars would be rejected and either go out of practice or be outlawed.

The divisions of regular practitioners

Orthodox medicine before 1850 fell into the four well-known categories of physic, surgery, pharmacy, and midwifery. Only from the mid-nineteenth century was there, to any significant extent, an increasing multiplication of specialties. The practice of physic was concerned with the treatment of internal diseases by medical means. Diagnosis was based on the detailed history of the illness, including the patient's constitution and way of life, by observation of the patient and his urine (uroscopy), and by feeling the pulse. The routine of physical examination appeared around the mid-nineteenth century.

Surgery consisted of the treatment of external disorders (including skin,[19] eye, and dental disorders) and surgeons obtained a monopoly in the treatment of venereal disease. All disorders which required 'manual interference'—the dressing of wounds and ulcers, the setting of fractures and the reduction of dislocations, as well as operations which required incision— were, of course, part of surgery. Until the very end of the eighteenth century druggists were almost exclusively wholesalers so that the practice of pharmacy, that is the compounding and dispensing of drugs, was an integral part of medicine. Midwifery was in an anomalous position, and remained so well into the nineteenth century. Traditionally it had belonged to midwives and some practitioners believed that medical men should only be involved in rare cases of difficulty, if at all. But the eighteenth century saw a growing number of medical men who attended not only when summoned to the late complications of neglected labours, but also to attend the normal cases for which they were often 'booked' or 'bespoken' by the patient early in pregnancy.

Corresponding to the three main divisions of medicine were the three kinds of medical men—the so-called tripartite profession consisting of physicians, surgeons, and apothecaries. Peterson refers to these as the three 'estates' using this term to denote the characteristic form of stratification of pre-industrial society.[20] Each estate, in this sense, possessed legal rights, duties, and claims to legitimacy, as well as exclusiveness of membership and function; and each, through its exclusiveness, was firmly demarcated within the hierarchical system.

Physicians possessed a university degree in medicine (but not necessarily a university education since MDs could be bought) and those practising in London were required to be members of the London College of Physicians.[21] The position of physicians as the highest of the three

---

[19] Largely through the work of Robert Willan (1757–1812) and Thomas Bateman (1778–1821), physicians to the Public Dispensary, London, who are sometimes called the fathers of modern dermatology, skin disorders were recognized as part of medicine rather than surgery.

[20] M. J. Peterson, *The Medical Profession in Mid-Victorian London* (Berkeley, 1978), 6.

[21] The ranks of the College were licentiate, candidate, elect, and fellow. Membership with a capital 'M' was introduced in the second half of the nineteenth century when the

orders or estates demanded that they undertook no form of manual operation and that they prescribed but did not dispense medicines. Indeed, they scarcely touched their patients, keeping their distance both literally and metaphorically.[22] But their superior education was, nevertheless, supposed to embrace the whole of surgery and pharmacy conferring on the physicians the right to oversee the work of the surgeons and apothecaries.

The surgeons formally severed their links with the barbers when the Company of Surgeons was established in 1745. The first attempt to turn the Company into a College in 1797 was unsuccessful. But a direct appeal to the throne led to the establishment of the Royal College of Surgeons of London in 1800. This in turn led to a new charter in 1843 (which established the Fellowship of the College) when the College became the Royal College of Surgeons of England. One point is worth mentioning in connection with surgery in the eighteenth century. Few provincial surgeons—not even those with appointments at the voluntary hospitals—were members of the Company or felt that the Company was relevant to their work or their status as surgeons. It was not until the early nineteenth century that the newly founded College of Surgeons began to play an important part in the lives of students, provincial surgeons, and the rank-and-file practitioners.

The apothecaries, who corresponded most closely to the category of tradesmen, originated as members of the Company of Grocers but separated to found their own Society in 1615.[23] Their role, in legal terms, consisted of dispensing the prescriptions written by physicians, and the latter had the power to inspect the apothecaries' shops and destroy impure drugs. If the apothecary undertook the direct treatment of patients—if he listened to their complaints, decided on the nature of their maladies, and then sold them the appropriate medicine—he was guilty of encroaching on the monopoly of the practice of physic possessed by the physicians, and risked prosecution. This applied even to the patients who visited the shop and were treated 'over the counter'; but the sin was more blatant if the apothecary left his shop to visit

licentiate became one of the standard qualifications of the general practitioner and one half of the conjoint diploma.

[22] The introduction of the techniques of physical examination, especially percussion and auscultation, which required a new and threateningly intimate contact with the patient, was delayed in England by this tradition amongst physicians. See S. J. Reiser, *Medicine and the Reign of Technology* (Cambridge, 1978), 20–1.

[23] C. Wall, H. C. Cameron, and E. A. Underwood, *A History of the Worshipful Society of Apothecaries of London* (London, 1963).

patients in their homes. Nevertheless, apothecaries expanded their activities and risked prosecution to an increasing extent by visiting and treating patients from the middle of the seventeenth century. Christopher Merrett complained in 1670 of

the ways of the *Apothecaries* creeping into practice ... of late years some *Physicians* took them along with them on their Visits whereby they acquired a little smattering of diseases ... until these 10 years last past [they] kept themselves within some bounds and limits; but since that time have daily more and more incroached upon our Profession.[24]

In truth, the apothecaries had little choice. As a writer pointed out in 1702, one apothecary could dispense for at least three physicians; yet 'there were near a thousand apothecaries in London'.[25] Compared to this there were at that time just over a hundred fellows, candidates, and licentiates in the London College of Physicians.[26] In the provinces it was claimed that every market town contained two or three apothecaries, all dispensing medicine to 'hundreds of patients a week'. In this, England was unique, and in 'regulated cities abroad [they] allow no more than can readily make up the *Physician*'s Directions, in the ... proportion of one in ten'.[27] Hamburg, it was said, had one apothecary, Stockholm and Copenhagen four to five each, and Paris only 150.[28] In England, however, 'the apothecaries destroy themselves by their Numbers, multiplying from a Thousand to as many more in the space of Eight Years'.[29] Even with allowance for exaggeration, the excess of apothecaries over all other forms of medical practitioner was striking and the huge excess over the physicians cannot be doubted. At the beginning of the eighteenth century apothecaries outnumbered the physicians by about ten to one in London and at least as many in the provinces.

Thus the apothecaries had two choices. Either they could reduce their numbers suddenly and drastically and remain the obedient servants of the physicians, imitating the practice of the Continent; or they could defy the law, practise physic, and continue to increase in numbers. The

---

[24] C. Merrett, *A Short History of the Frauds and Abuses committed by the Apothecaries* (London, 1670).

[25] Anon., *The Present State of the Practice of Physick* (London, 1702).

[26] Sir George Clark, *A History of the Royal College of Physicians of London*, vol. ii (Oxford, 1966), appendix.

[27] Anon., *The Present State of Physick and Surgery in London* (London, 1701).

[28] R. Pitt, *The Calamities of the English in Sickness* (London, 1707).

[29] Anon., *The Present State of Physick and Surgery in London* (1701).

fact that they chose the latter course was decisive in shaping the divisions of medical practitioners in England. It was against this background that matters were brought to a head by the case of the Royal College of Physicians *v.* Rose.

The Rose case

In brief, Rose was a London apothecary who, between 1700 and 1701, treated William Seale, a butcher at Hungerford market.[30] William Seale, who felt no better, was understandably annoyed when presented with a bill for fifty pounds. He sought redress through the College of Physicians and Rose was prosecuted. At the trial the foreman of the jury, asked by the Lord Chief Justice why they hesitated over the verdict, replied that the defendant had done no more than all apothecaries. The verdict against Rose, although inevitable, was given with reluctance. Lord Chief Justice Holt termed the action 'extravagant' although he felt obliged to support the College on a point of law, and the attorney-general recommended to the Society of Apothecaries an application to the House of Lords for a 'writ in error', giving his opinion that a reversal of judgment would follow. Their Lordships heard the case on 15 March 1704. For Rose it was argued that the consequence of the judgment would be the ruin of the apothecaries, that customary practice should be a paramount consideration, and that physicians, by insistence on an outdated Act, would lay a heavy burden on the nobility and gentry who would always have to fee a physician for themselves and their servants. The poor, unable to afford physicians, would be oppressed, and so would sick persons, who 'in case of sudden accidents or new symptoms appearing in the night time, generally send for an apothecary', knowing that a physician would not attend 'if at dinner or abed'. If the judgment stood, no apothecary would risk attendance. The House of Lords reversed the judgment, but from the practical point of view the situation of the apothecary remained as it always had been before; he could practise physic, but only charge a fee for his medicines, not for his advice or for visiting.

This decision, which remained unchallenged until 1830, has been seen as having very important implications for the development of general practice, reaching even into the twentieth century. The decision, it is said, perpetuated the inferior status of the apothecary by underlining

---

[30] For a full account of the Rose case see Sir George Clark, *History of the Royal College of Physicians* (1966), ii, 476–9, and Wall, Cameron, and Underwood, *History of the Society of Apothecaries* (1963), 389–402.

his financial dependence on the sale of goods rather than his expert knowledge and advice. More than that, however, it has been said that the decision was responsible for a habit of over-prescribing, the results of which are with us yet. But if these were the undesirable consequences of the case, the desirable result was the freedom of the apothecaries to practise physic freely and thus become the 'doctors' of the lower classes.

There are good reasons for believing that the implications of the Rose case have been exaggerated. For example, the extent of alleged over-prescribing in twentieth-century Britain is a highly complex subject. Many factors are involved in the demand for medicines in general practice and the response to that demand. The decision in the Rose case in 1704 contributed little if anything to the problems of prescribing today. Moreover, the extent of prescribing in other countries, where the history of medical practitioners was quite different, often exceeds that of Britain.[31] At the time, the effect of the Rose case was to do no more than confirm, rather than confer, the freedom of the apothecary to practise physic. Had the case never occurred it is doubtful if the habits of the apothecaries would have been different. It can not even be said that the proviso concerning fees prevented the apothecaries from charging for visits. The study of a large number of medical practitioners' bills dating from the eighteenth century shows that some practitioners charged for medicines only, a few printed 'for attention/advice/journey what you please' so that any payment under this head would be a gift rather than a fee, but a majority of practitioners charged their patients regularly and often substantially for visits and journeys and did so with impunity. If the Rose case, as often suggested, had dominated the practice of the rank-and-file practitioners, its reversal in 1830 should have led to a new level of prosperity. No such change occurred.[32] Nevertheless, the case, and its consequences, were often quoted in the context of medical reform in the first half of the nineteenth century.

The nature of regular medical practice in the eighteenth century

The decision in the Rose case in 1704 gave legal confirmation to the role of the apothecary as a medical practitioner rather than a tradesman. It was followed by an increasing tendency for the old tripartite division

---

[31] A recent publication has shown that the number of prescriptions per head of population and the number per diagnosis is substantially higher in West Germany, France, Italy, and Spain than it is in Britain. *Patterns of European Diagnoses and Prescribing* (Office of Health Economics, London, 1983).

[32] See chapter 12.

to give way to a merging of physic, surgery, and pharmacy in the practice of most practitioners. Indeed, the three 'estates' of the tripartite model, as Roberts has shown, were much less rigidly applied in the provinces than previously supposed, even in Tudor and Stuart England.[33] The tendency for medical practitioners to practise broadly was underlined by the growth of the description 'surgeon-apothecary'. Table 1 shows the distribution of medical men in provincial England in 1783. It can be seen that the plain 'apothecary' and 'surgeon' (together 6.1 per cent of the total) was vastly outnumbered by 'surgeon-apothecary' (over 80 per cent of the total). The additional term 'man-midwife' was often implicit in the description 'surgeon-apothecary' after the middle of the century; but, as 'man-midwifery' became to an increasing extent part of the routine of practice, and thereby earned new respectability, the triple description 'surgeon-apothecary and man-midwife' became increasingly common.

Usually the one category of medical practitioner which remained clearly demarcated was the physician, by virtue of his medical degree. But even here there is room for confusion. As we have seen, some called themselves 'physician' but had no degree; others who were fully fledged physicians in the provinces sometimes dispensed medicines, although refusal to dispense was one of the features which typically distinguished the physician from the apothecary and the surgeon-apothecary.

A study of medical practitioners which was based solely on legal documents and state papers would suggest that the tripartite division was a reality in theory and practice throughout the eighteenth and early nineteenth century. A study of the records of practitioners, however, shows this to be false. Even the traditional superiority of the physician within the hierarchy of medicine disappeared with the spectacular rise in surgery during the eighteenth century: a rise due in part to the advances in anatomy and surgery as academic disciplines and in part to the rise of the voluntary hospitals in which, by the early nineteenth century, the surgeons were dominant.[34] 'There was a time',

[33] R. S. Roberts, 'The Personnel and Practice of Medicine in Tudor and Stuart England', Part 1: 'The Provinces', *Medical History*, 6 (1962), 363–82; Part 2: 'London', *Medical History*, 8 (1964), 217–34.

[34] A. M. Carr-Saunders and P. A. Wilson, in *The Professions* (London, 1964), 74, for example, remark that 'Few episodes in Medical History are more remarkable than the rapid rise of the surgeons in the latter half of the eighteenth century'. Thomas Short in 1750 commented that 'The Improvements in Surgery in General have far out stripped those in Physick . . . Reasoning on Facts [being] much better and surer than from Theories'. Surgery depended on the 'Dexterity of Hand directed by a Good judgement . . . We find that Men of the Greatest Merit in Surgery, though they may have less Learning, yet they

said Abernethy in 1812, 'when surgeons were considered as mere appendages of physicians, the mere operators to be put in motion by their directors; but times are changed and surgeons are changed too . . . and in consequence have got a kind of information which puts them on a par with others of the profession.'[35] The rise of both the surgeon and the apothecary in the second half of the eighteenth century earned them the tacit right to practise as they pleased. John Gregory of Edinburgh justified this new state of affairs in 1772.

If a surgeon or apothecary has had the education, and acquired the knowledge of a physician, he is a physician to all intents and purposes, whether he has a degree or not, and ought to be treated and respected accordingly. In Great Britain surgery is a liberal profession. In many parts of it, surgeons or apothecaries are the physicians in ordinary to most families, for which trust they are often well qualified by their education and knowledge; and a physician is only called in where a case is difficult, or attended with danger.[36]

Similarly, Jeremiah Jenkins in 1810 wrote that

The apothecary of this country is qualified by education to attend at the bedside of the sick, and, being in general better acquainted with pharmacy than the physicians of English Universities . . . is often the most successful practitioner. The most laborious part of practice falls upon him, while the physician, although he has no pretention to superiority of judgement or skill, reaps the emolument, and assumes the merit of the cure.[37]

In Britain today the newly qualified doctor, having passed through a training common to all members of the profession, chooses his future specialty. Having undertaken further training and examination he practises within clearly defined limits in the specialty of his choice. Moving from one part of medical practice to another in mid-career is possible but unusual, and requires further training and examination. Medical practice in the eighteenth century was quite different. There was no common basic medical training, and changing from one branch to another was common and usually easy. The title by which a practitioner was known was seldom a certain indication of the nature of his practice, which was usually determined by such factors as family background,

---

often compensate that by a closer Application to the Study of their own Profession.' T. Short, *New Observations . . . in City, Town and Country Bills of Mortality* (London, 1759).

[35] Royal Society of Medicine, London, the notebooks of John Greene Crosse of Norwich, MS 285,g,11.

[36] J. Gregory, *Lectures on the Duties and Qualifications of a Physician* (London, 1772).

[37] J. Jenkins, *Observations on the Present State of the Profession and Trade of Medicine* (London, 1810).

Table 1 *The distribution of medical practitioners in England 1783, based on Samuel Foart Simmons's* Medical Register *for 1783*

County	Surgeon-apothecaries	Physicians	Surgeons only	Apothecaries only
Bedfordshire	17	2		
Berkshire	44	11 (2)[b]	1	
Buckinghamshire	27	3		
Cambridgeshire[a]	20	3	4	
Cheshire[a]	48	5	5	1
Cornwall	71	6		
Cumberland	60	11 (1)		
Derbyshire	35	6		
Devonshire[a]	117	11	8 (1)	17
Dorset	59	9	1	
Durham	52	8		
Essex	112	13 (1)		
Gloucestershire[a]	60	6	2	
Hampshire[a]	86	6		
Herefordshire[a]	33	5	3	1
Hertfordshire	37	7		
Huntingdonshire	17	4		
Kent	161 (1)	12 (1)		
Lancashire[b]	102	26	14 (1)	6
Leicestershire[a]	43	6		
Lincolnshire[a]	94	18	1	2
Middlesex	68	3		
Norfolk[a]	129	14	1	1
Northamptonshire[a]	46	9	1	
Northumberland[a]	66	13		2
Nottinghamshire[a]	38	5		
Oxfordshire[a]	54	9	4	1
Rutland	5	1		
Shropshire[a]	84	4		1
Somerset[ab]	93	29	18	53 [+ 2 men-midwives]
Staffordshire[a]	70	7		1
Suffolk	70 (1)	10	2	
Surrey	63	8		
Sussex	81	5	3	3
Warwickshire[a]	54	9	10	4
Westmorland	13	2		
Wiltshire[a]	78	9	3	1
Worcestershire[a]	67	5		
Yorkshire[ab]	233	42	8	11
TOTALS	2607	363	89	105 + 2
PERCENTAGE	82.3	11.4	2.8	3.3

[a] a hospital building in existence in 1783
[b] retired practitioner included in total

Source: Joan Lane, 'The Medical Practitioners of Provincial England', *Medical History,* 28 (4) (1984), 353–71. I am grateful to the author and the editors of *Medical History* for their kind permission to reproduce this table.

apprenticeship, and other forms of training if any, but most of all by commercial opportunity. It was possible in the eighteenth century to practise fully in all branches of medicine—physic, surgery, pharmacy, and man-midwifery. Richard Kay of Baldingstone in Lancashire (1716– 51) did so to the fullest extent on the basis of an apprenticeship to his father, a pupilship to Mr Steade, the apothecary to Guy's Hospital, and attendance while in London at a course of surgical lectures and two courses of midwifery under Mr Smellie. Kay referred to himself in his diary as a physician on one occasion and as a surgeon and physician on another.[38]

The openings for different kinds of practice varied from one district to another, as John Barr discovered when he arrived in Birmingham from Scotland in the 1780s with a 'medical diploma in one pocket and a surgical in the other'. Finding an excessive number of physicians in the town he 'kept his higher diploma *in retentis*' and made a fortune as a general practitioner amongst the Unitarians, becoming, incidentally, the general practitioner and friend of James Watt.[39]

Thomas Shute, born in Iron Acton in 1750, practised surgery briefly in Winterbourne before moving to Bristol in 1790. There he continued as a surgeon until 1803 when he 'took out a diploma from St Andrew's and led a successful career as a physician, making the same if not greater annual income at about half the trouble.'[40] Joseph Shapland (1727–1801), also of Bristol, had a highly successful career as an apothecary treating 'all the first families in the City and the Suburbs' and visiting more patients than most of the physicians of his day. In 1783 he 'procured a diploma from Aberdeen', a self-awarded promotion to the rank of physician, and virtually retired on his considerable earnings doing little more in the way of medical practice.[41] Other examples appear in later chapters.

On the one hand the breaking down of the tripartite division was leading to a much greater breadth of practice; on the other, the hospitals, dispensaries, and medical corporations tended to perpetuate the old divisions and the social values and prestige attached to them. A surgeon with an honorary appointment to a voluntary hospital would confine his hospital activities to the practice of surgery. Outside the hospital,

[38] W. Brockbank and F. Kenworthy (eds.), 'The Diary of Richard Kay (1716–1751) of Baldingstone near Bury', *The Chetham Society*, 16 (1968).
[39] Birmingham RO, notes and queries, 15, 22, and 29 June 1870.
[40] BIBM 2, 860.
[41] Ibid. 1, 435.

however, he often undertook the treatment of medical and midwifery cases as well as acting in a consultant capacity to other practitioners in surgical cases.

The failure of medical men in the eighteenth century to confine their practice to one or other branch of medicine is apt to cause confusion. Historians sometimes search for the appropriate description of a medical man, uncertain whether to describe him as a physician, surgeon, a surgeon-apothecary, or even as 'an early general practitioner'. The search is seldom productive because it is based on the fallacy of clear divisions of practice within a medical profession such as those which exist today. The broadly descriptive term 'medical practitioner' is often preferable to a fruitless attempt to find the 'right' designation for a medical man.

Change and diversity of practice, with the ability of practitioners to move easily from one branch of medicine to another, were therefore characteristics of medical practice in the second half of the eighteenth century. It was a period of increasing commercial opportunities in medical practice and of major changes in the education and prosperity of medical practitioners. Medicine was both a business and a profession, both terms appearing frequently in the writings of eighteenth-century medical men. In the next chapter the background and the education of medical men is considered.

2

Background and Education

Social and family background

MEDICAL practitioners in the eighteenth century came from a very wide background; but, as might be anticipated, a large number were the sons or nephews of medical men. There were substantial advantages in following in the footsteps of a father or an uncle. The apprenticeship premium was usually nil or a token amount such as £5. An even greater advantage was the introduction to an established practice without the expense of buying a partnership. The early years of a single-handed practitioner who settled in an area where he was a stranger could be very difficult. A new, young practitioner was often distrusted and faced back-biting competition from established practitioners. It was far better, if possible, to join a medical relation first as apprentice, then as partner, and finally as his successor. It was a painless entrance to a prosperous occupation, and it was frequently done.

The range of paternal occupations is shown in tables 2, 3, and 4. The first of these tables, which covers the period from 1760 to 1830, is based on the biographies recorded by the Bristol surgeon, Richard Smith junior. Most of the practitioners in this table practised either in Bristol or in some other part of the south-west of England. The father's occupation is recorded for two groups of medical men, physicians and all other practitioners.

Table 3 is based on the records of the Society of Apothecaries. Between 1764 and the end of 1781 (but not before or afterwards) all the entries in the apprentice bindings book contained details of the father's occupation, his address, whether he had died, and the 'consideration' (premium) paid, as well as the name and address of the apothecary to whom the apprentice was indentured. Nearly all the apothecaries lived in London; a few lived in the home counties. Of the apprentices, eighty came from London or the county of Middlesex, sixty-four came from the provinces—almost all from the south of England from Essex to Cornwall—two came from Wales, and one each from Newfoundland,

Table 2   *The occupation of the fathers of medical practitioners in Bristol and the West of England, 1760–1830*

Father's occupation	Surgeons, apothecaries, general practitioners		Physicians
Surgeon, apothecary, or surgeon-apothecary	19		4
Clergy: established church	8		2
dissenting	3		1
Barrister/attorney	2	62%	
Naval and Army officers	2		
'Esq.', landed proprietors, 'gentlemen', 'of independent means'	8		4
Farmer	3		
Bank employee	2		
Clothier	2		
Master, merchant navy	1		
Schoolmaster	1		1
Musician	1		
Brewer	1		
Ironmaster	1		
Linen merchant	1		
Raffia merchant	1		
Vinegar merchant	1		
Tobacco merchant			1
Wine merchant	1		
'In employment'	1		
Coast waiter: HM Customs	1		
Land waiter: HM Customs	1		
Sailmaker	1		
Dyer and cleaner of feathers	1		
Malster	1		
Liquor dealer	1		
Grocer			1
Sugar baker			1
Wine cooper	1		
Carrier	1		
Mealman	1		
TOTAL		83	

Source: Bristol Infirmary Biographical Memoirs, Bristol Record Office, The Council House, Bristol.

Jamaica, and St Christopher's Island. The total number thus recorded, 149, provides a uniquely valuable source on the cost of apprenticeship and the background of medical men in the second half of the eighteenth century.

The data recorded in these tables are representative of what might

Table 3   *The occupation of the fathers of 149 apothecaries' apprentices in London, 1764–81*

Apothecary	28	
Surgeon	2	
Clergy	7	
'Doctor in Divinity'	1	
'Doctor of Musick'	1	64%
'Esq.'	3	
'Gentleman'	53	
'Late Governor, S. Carolina'	1	
Mercer	1	
Merchant	1	
Clerk	9	
Grocer	3	
Victualler	3	
Unspecified	3	
Farmer	2	
Yeoman	2	
Tea Dealer	2	
Mariner	2	
and one each of: ship's purser, mathematical instrument maker, tailor, butcher, distiller, vintner, sugar refiner, vinegar merchant, malster, carver, upholsterer, innkeeper, coachman, tobacconist, coal merchant, painter, tinman, foundling from the Foundling Hospital, glover, ironmonger, poulterer, stationer, watchmaker, builder, and silversmith	25	
TOTAL	149	

Source: Records of the Society of Apothecaries, apprentice bindings book, MS 8207, Guildhall Library, London.

be called the upper crust of the ordinary rank-and-file practitioners. Most of those in table 2 had some connection with the Bristol Infirmary as pupils, apprentices, or members of the hospital staff. Premiums for a hospital pupilship or apprenticeship were relatively high[1] and, expense apart, those who sought such posts were probably the more ambitious, literate, and energetic. The same may have been true of those who chose to travel to London to serve their apprenticeship to a London apothecary, such as those included in table 3.

It is clear that there was, below this level of medical practitioners, another group who, although illiterate and uneducated, carried on a business under the names of 'surgeon' or 'apothecary' and were seen as such by the public. In 1815 John Yeatman, a well-known practitioner in Frome in Somerset, denounced such men as the 'surreptitious mul-

[1] Numerous entries in the BIBM show that the premium for apprenticeship to a surgeon at Bristol Infirmary in the late eighteenth and early nineteenth century was in the range of £200 to £350.

titude' of irregulars and ignorant practitioners. In a memorable paper he instanced the

surgeon with whom I was intimate requesting 'the loan of a pear of phorcepts' in a difficult case of labour.... A man in the lower part of this county unrivalled for swearing and effrontery, professed to know every disease by examining the urine of the afflicted—and, dying, the words 'eminent apothecary' were inscribed on his monument. Near Kingswood Gloucestershire, I was not a little amused with a sign embellished with a pestle and mortar, on which were the following words:

I Popjay, Surgeon, Apothecary and Midwife, etc.
draws teeth and bleeds on the lowest terms.
Confectionary, Tobacco, Snuff, Tea, Coffee, Sugar
and all sorts of Perfumery sold here. NB New
laid eggs every morning by Mrs Popjay.[2]

The existence of such as these, who were probably as common, if not more so, in the eighteenth century as in the early nineteenth, underlines the diversity of practitioners and, as mentioned in the previous chapter, the borderland in which the orthodox and irregular practitioners merged with each other.

At the upper and literate level, however, there is close agreement between the data shown in tables 2 and 3. If the parental occupations that can be described broadly as the professions, gentlemen, and men 'of independent means' are placed together in one group and the tradesmen and craftsmen in the other, the first group amounted to 62 per cent of the total in table 2 and 64 per cent in table 3. How does this compare with the occupation or status of the physicians who were licentiates or fellows of the London College of Physicians? The answer is provided, albeit imperfectly, in table 4 which is based on Munk's *Roll* of the College for 1701–1800. In contrast to the previous two tables it shows a higher proportion of professional and upper-class backgrounds. This is the result that would have been expected, but it should be accepted with caution because of the large number of instances in which the father's occupation was not recorded. It is unlikely that the recorded paternal occupations were a representative sample; information was conspicuously lacking in the case of provincial physicians holding the extra-licence of the College. Table 2 suggests that the social background of provincial physicians was no different from that of other medical men, but the numbers are too small for confidence.

---

[2] J. Yeatman, 'Remarks on the Profession of Medicine', *MPJ* 34 (1815), 187–93.

Table 4   *The occupation or status of fathers of members of the Royal College of Physicians of London in the eighteenth century*

Occupation or status of father	Licentiates and extra-licentiates	Fellows	Total
Not recorded	317	115	432
Physician	13	21	34
Surgeon	9	—	9
Apothecary	3	—	3
TOTAL (medical profession)	(25)	(21)	(46)
Minister—Established Church	10	16	26
Church of Scotland	3	4	7
Dissenting Ministry	7	2	9
TOTAL ('The Ministry')	(20)	(22)	(42)
Lord Chief Justice	—	1	1
Barrister	1	1	2
Lawyer/attorney	2	2	4
Naval officer	—	1	1
Army officer	2	1	3
Baronet	2	—	2
'Esq.'	9	15	24
Gentleman	14	13	27
'Historian'	1	1	2
Banker	1	2	3
Merchant taylor	1	—	1
Wine merchant	—	1	1
Malster	1	—	1
Farmer	1	—	1
Druggist	—	1	1
Bookseller	1	—	1
Butcher	—	1	1
'Respectable tradesman'	—	1	1
'Humble parents'	1	—	1

Source: William Munk, *The Roll of the Royal College of Physicians of London* (London, 1878), Vol. ii, 1701–1800.

A study by Van Zwanenberg of the training and careers of three hundred apothecaries' apprentices in Suffolk provides a valuable comparison. This study covered the period between the Apothecaries Act of 1815 and the Medical Act of 1858. Here it was found that the range of occupations of the fathers of the apprentices was broadly similar to those shown in tables 2 and 3. The main difference is that an even larger proportion in Van Zwanenberg's study were the sons of medical men, while those who were the sons of craftsmen and tradesmen formed a smaller proportion of about one-quarter of the total instead of one-third. This study suggests that those recruited to the ranks of the general practitioners after 1815 came, broadly speaking, from the same social groups as the apothecaries and surgeon-apothecaries of the eighteenth and early nineteenth century.

Because of the well-recognized tendency for the sons and nephews of medical men to follow in their relatives' footsteps, medical dynasties in which successive members of the same family practised for at least a century were by no means uncommon. The Pulsfords of Wells in Somerset, for instance, and the Carrs of Leeds[3] are two examples of importance in this study because their records have survived. The Comperes of Stow in the Wold in Gloucestershire provide another example. Thomas Compere was an apothecary, a freeman of the London Society (March 1704), and Master of the Society from 1713 to 1714.[4] His brother (d. 1743) who was a country surgeon had three sons, two of whom became medical practitioners in Stow.[5] The Goldwyers of Bristol produced thirteen surgeons and two physicians in five generations, of whom seven, all surgeons, were—to the confusion of historians—christened William.[6] The Maurice family of Marlborough has been in family practice without interruption for six generations from the time that Thelwall Maurice (1767–1830) settled there in 1792 to the present day.[7] First prize in the competition for length of dynasties probably goes to the Beadles who, in successive generations from the late seventeenth century to the mid-twentieth, always produced one medical practitioner and often several. They, however, moved around, mainly in the south Midlands and the West Country.[8]

Thus medical practice at the level of the surgeon-apothecary was open to men from a wide social background; but very few were the sons of the aristocracy or the richer landed gentry. Most were the sons of medical practitioners, non-medical professionals, and the minor gentry.

Education, general and medical

Hans, in his study of education in the eighteenth century includes a sample of 120 medical practitioners.[9] Thirty-four were educated at

---

[3] Notebooks of William Carr, Wellcome MS 5203–7.

[4] Records of the Society of Apothecaries, MS 8206 (vol. 1), Guildhall Library, London.

[5] Gloucestershire CRO, Gloucester, ref. E.N./Miss Stewart, 1982.

[6] BIBM 4, 54, and G. Munro Smith, *History of the Bristol Royal Infirmary* (Bristol, 1917), 257.

[7] Dick Maurice, 'Six Generations in Wiltshire', *BMJ* 284 (1982), 1756.

[8] I am grateful to Mr Simon Beadles for permission to publish details of his family history.

[9] N. Hans, *New Trends in Education in the Eighteenth Century* (London, 1951), table 3.

home, thirty-four at the 'great public schools', twenty-nine at grammar schools, seventeen at private schools, and six at dissenting academies. The distribution was similar to that of the clergy (Anglican and dissenting) but many more of the group of 'peers, baronets, squires, and gentlemen of independent means' attended the public schools or received private tuition. Hans's group of medical men, however, were mainly the élite of the profession, drawn from the *Dictionary of National Biography*. It is uncommon to find that the rank-and-file practitioners attended the public schools, although some were educated at home or privately.

The typical surgeon or surgeon-apothecary was a grammar school boy, and his success at school was measured in terms of the extent of his reading in the classics. He left school between the ages of twelve and fifteen with at least some knowledge of Latin and often a smattering of Greek. Then he became an apprentice. In the first half of the eighteenth century this was, for the majority, the full extent of his general and medical education. But from mid-century an increasing number proceeded to a further period of medical instruction which could, for example, include a year or more at a provincial hospital as a pupil of one of the surgeons, followed by a further year in London attending lectures and 'walking the wards' of the hospitals as well as attending private courses on various medical subjects. Such instruction was apt to be haphazard. There was no official syllabus and no examination. Only rarely was the diploma of the Company of Surgeons acquired. Instead, the student returned home with certificates of attendance at lectures, often large and impressive documents which he could hang on his wall if he chose to.

Some examples will illustrate the general pattern of education of provincial practitioners in the eighteenth and early nineteenth century before the Apothecaries Act. Richard Smith senior, surgeon of Bristol,[10] was born in 1748 the son of a brewer and malster of whom his grandson, Richard Smith junior wrote: 'No one could be more unfit for trade. Elegant in his manners and person, delighting in books and hating the bustle of the world he spent whole days in his study, leaving to his active and intelligent wife the care of his ledger and the general management of his business.' This placid and delightful man sent his son to Warminster grammar school, but the boy ran away because of the severity of the discipline. He was found 'with a hod of mortar upon

---

[10] BIBM 2, 558–66. This is the father of Richard Smith whose biographical memoirs have been used extensively in this study.

his head at some masons' and sent to Winchester. In 1763, aged fifteen, he was apprenticed to a surgeon in Bristol but, being a bit of a wild lad, he returned home late one night, was locked out, quarrelled with his master, and left for London. There he studied surgery under Joseph Else and midwifery under Colin Mackenzie.[11] He returned to Bristol, set up as a surgeon, and was elected to the Infirmary at the age of twenty-six.[12]

John Padmore Noble followed a similar path. Born in Taunton in 1755, the son of a wine merchant, he was educated at Tiverton grammar school. In 1770, aged fifteen, he was apprenticed to Abraham Ludlow who had been elected surgeon to the Infirmary three years before. In 1776 he went to London, 'dissected under Cruickshank—attended Dr Jon Fordyce upon the Materia Medica—and learnt midwifery from Denman and Osborne'. Returning to Bristol he 'put his name upon a door in the old Market ... as a "Surgeon and Man-Midwife"'. In 1777, when he was twenty-two, he was elected surgeon to the Infirmary. A previous apprenticeship to an Infirmary surgeon conferred a clear advantage at such elections.[13]

Edward Phillips, born c.1776, the son of a surgeon, was educated privately before attending the grammar school at Monmouth. After apprenticeship to an apothecary and a year as a pupil at Bristol Infirmary he attended the Borough Hospitals in London and returned home to Pontypool where he became the coroner and, with two others, 'divided the Usk-Monmouth-Pontypool area between them'.[14]

Francis Newberry, born in 1798, whose father was 'in employment', was educated at Mr Johnson's Academy at Kingsdown where he read Virgil, Horace, Cicero, Homer, and Demosthenes. After an apprenticeship of five years to Thomas Shute, surgeon at Bristol Infirmary, he spent a year at the Borough Hospitals in London, travelled on the Continent and returned to practise in Bristol.[15]

---

[11] MacKenzie reproved Smith for going to a midwifery case 'in a scarlet cloak with a sword, which was then the mode of students, saying it was "inapproprate to be going to bring a person into the world with a weapon intended to send a person out of it"'. BIBM 2, 558–66.

[12] Election at such an early age was by no means uncommon for surgeons; physicians were, on average, older when elected to Bristol Infirmary. Smith took the unusual precaution on this occasion of soliciting the vote of lady subscribers, something that had never been done before. In the event, however, he was elected without the need to produce them. BIBM 2, 564–6.

[13] BIBM 2, 832.

[14] Ibid. 6, 564.

[15] Ibid. 9, 428.

Trevor Morris, born in 1796, the son of a sailmaker in Chepstow, was another pupil at Monmouth grammar school who, after apprenticeship to the apothecary of Bristol Infirmary, sailed to Leith to go to Edinburgh for further education and ultimately returned, as so many did, to his home town and a successful career as a general practitioner.[16] Thomas Jackson, born in 1797, the son of a mealman, was educated privately and read Virgil and Horace. He was indentured to a surgeon at Chew Magna for 200 guineas (indoor), went to the Middlesex Hospital, and ended in practice in 'Tredaga' (Tredegar, Monmouth).[17]

Frederick Granger, born in 1799, a 'hooper's son', was placed under the tuition of the Revd Samuel Seyer for three years, read Ovid, Virgil, and the Greek Testament, as an outdoor apprentice to a Bristol surgeon, and then went to St Bartholomew's Hospital.[18]

Henry Goldwyer, who became a surgeon/oculist, was born in 1795, the son of a surgeon and one of the dynasty of medical practitioners mentioned above, was educated at Bristol and Reading, where he read Horace, Virgil, Cicero, Homer, and Sophocles. He spent five years as the pupil of Richard Smith (he was the 'star pupil' of the hospital) and travelled to Leith with Trevor Morris (see above) when they were shipwrecked *en route* and nearly drowned. In Edinburgh he obtained the MD.[19]

Edward Day, born in 1795, the son of a clergyman, read Horace, Virgil, and Homer under the tuition of the Revd Dr Johnstones of Montagu Hall, was indentured to Mr Daniel, surgeon at Bristol (indoor, for 200 guineas), and studied under Abernethy, Clutterbuck, and Gooch in London before practising in Brisol as a general practitioner.[20]

These examples show that there was already in the late eighteenth and early nineteenth century a well-trodden path, a recognized system of general and medical education not only for the intending élite of hospital physicians and surgeons, but also for the surgeon-apothecaries of this period. What is more, the medical practitioner, having followed the usual path of general and medical education typical of the second

---

[16] Ibid. 9, 468.
[17] Ibid. 12, 442.
[18] Ibid. 12, 546.
[19] Ibid. 9,4.
[20] Ibid. 9, 248. For other examples from this period see BIBM: James Monday (12, 206); Thos. Wade Smith (9, 320); George F. Burroughs (8, 299); Henry Jefferies (8, 457); John Bishop Estlin (7, 315); James Thomas (6, 296); Richard Chaflin Edgell (6, 350) and William Jefferies (6, 410), all of whom followed a similar educational path to become established in general medical practice.

half of the eighteenth century, could, after a spell in practice, progress to the highest positions in the profession. Edward Jenner provides an obvious example. There was nothing in his early years as schoolboy, student, and surgeon-apothecary that would have led anyone to guess his ultimate fame, unless they had been so unusually perceptive as to recognize the potential of his interest in natural history.

Edward Jenner, born in 1749, the youngest child of the vicar of Berkeley in Gloucestershire, received his schooling at Cirencester grammar school and at a small private school near his home at Wootton-under-Edge.[21] He left school at the age of twelve and was apprenticed to Mr Ludlow, a surgeon at Sodbury. At the age of twenty-one he went to London to become John Hunter's first pupil for the comparatively small sum of £100 including bed, board, and hospital fees. He stayed there for two years and returned to Berkeley with certificates in the practice of physic, chemistry, and midwifery. For twenty years he practised as a local surgeon-apothecary until, in 1792 (and reputedly because he found the work too heavy) he decided to practise as a physician and bought a St Andrews MD, sponsored by Dr J. H. Hicks of Gloucester and Caleb Hillier Parry, MD, of Bath. Parry had been his near contemporary at Cirencester grammar school. Jenner's first vaccination with cowpox was carried out in 1796, four years after he became a physician.

Jenner illustrates the ease with which a provincial practitioner could raise himself to the status of a physician through the MDs of Aberdeen or St Andrew's without ever setting foot in Scotland. All that was required was a modest fee and the recommendation of two colleagues for the MD to come back through the post. It is, of course, easy to pour scorn on such paper qualifications, as indeed many did in the nineteenth century. But in Jenner's day there was something to be said for a system which, in theory at least, believed that proven clinical ability was the important criterion. In contrast, the London College of Physicians placed all the weight on Latin and a knowledge of the classical authors, and none on practical experience.

Jenner is often given as a famous example of an early nineteenth-century physician. It should be remembered, however, that in family background, education, and his first twenty years of practice, he was no more nor less than a typical country rank-and-file practitioner with

[21] D. Fisk, *Dr Jenner of Berkeley* (London, 1959); J. Baron, *The Life of Edward Jenner*, 2 vols. (London, 1827–38). There are differences in these two accounts of the details of Jenner's schooling, but not important differences.

a passion for natural history. Like most of his contemporaries, the foundation of his medical training was an apprenticeship in his youth to an established and respected local practitioner.

The medical apprentice

Views on apprenticeship as the basis of medical training altered profoundly between 1750 and 1850. When the Apothecaries Act was introduced in 1815 it was accompanied by increasing criticism of the system, and this will be discussed in due course in chapter 8. Here we are concerned with the practical details of apprenticeship for rank-and-file practitioners before 1815.[22]

Apprenticeship was the appropriate method of training for the apothecary of the seventeenth century whose business consisted mainly of the 'shop'. It provided practical knowledge of drugs and their preparation and how to run a business. When, in the eighteenth century, the apothecary evolved into the surgeon-apothecary and man-midwife, and spent most of his time out of the shop visiting patients, apprenticeship as a system became increasingly inappropriate in its traditional form; but the apprentice became increasingly important to his master who relied on him to look after the shop, dispense medicines, and take messages. Until the mid-eighteenth century, however, when hospital teaching began on a significant scale, it was still the only formal method of training for all medical practitioners except physicians. Apprenticeship, therefore, persisted but needed to be modified. A more or less systematic course of reading was recommended by those who wrote on medical apprenticeship together with adequate opportunities for visiting the sick in their homes. These opportunities, however, were limited. Private patients were unlikely to be happy with being visited by an apprentice, and might even object to his visiting with his master. Often the apprentice was only sent to visit the poor. However, when the master took the trouble to ensure that his apprentice obtained adequate clinical experience, apprenticeship had advantages over the hospital form of education.

In hospitals the greatest emphasis was laid on surgery. James Makittrick remarked in 1772

A young lad goes from the country to London to attend lectures and hospitals. He enters himself as a surgeon's pupil, where he learns to dress an ulcer or forms an imperfect idea of performing an operation. He never considers that as

[22] 'Report of the Progress of Medical Science', *London Medical Repository and Review*, 5 (1816), 60–1.

he is to practise as an apothecary he must in the course of his practice have twenty medical cases for one that is chirurgical; yet returns to the country with an ostentatious display of hospital certificates; though in this trait he has been mispending both his time and his money.[23]

Physicians, if they took pupils at all, tended to select only those who intended to take a medical degree at a university, although Makittrick (himself an Edinburgh graduate) singled out Edinburgh as the exception where '... a man may attain more real knowledge in medical practice in one season than in any other hospital in the kingdom in seven years'.

J. L. Mann made the same criticism of hospital training some years later.

It may seem a fine thing to be able to operate for stone; but to many surgeons the occasion for such an operation, unassisted, never occurs in the course of their whole life ... for every case of surgery, even of the minor order, that claims your attention, you will have twenty cases of fever, and twenty or forty of other forms of bodily disease ... I would earnestly advise ... study medicine at the bedside.[24]

In Mann's opinion, the common disorders of general practice were 'best pursued in country practice' where the apprentice 'can best see the *ultimate results* of treatment. In the country he can study *men* as well as *patients*.' Apprenticeship was also the ideal for learning 'the method of book-keeping generally adopted, the proper economy of time, including all the commercial part, down to the proper receiving and attending messages at the door'.[25]

Apprenticeship, therefore, was potentially a good method of training, and it was one of the means of an introduction to a career. To have served under a master with a good reputation was a great advantage. Today one hears of craftsmen—builders, stonemasons, bricklayers, or carpenters—who are recommended because they 'served their time' with a good firm; and this may be enough to earn them the accolade of being 'real professionals' at their trade. Clearly, the same applied to medicine in the eighteenth century. Service under a master of good

---

[23] James Makittrick, preface: 'On the Education and Duties of Medical Men' in *Commentaries on the Principle and Practice of Physick* (London, 1772). James Makittrick (1728–1802), MD Edin. 1766, adopted the surname of Adair (possibly his mother's surname). He was a lively author but a disagreeable man. Wherever he went he provoked animosity (*DNB*).

[24] J. L. Mann, *Recollections of my Early and Professional Life* (London, 1887), 95–6.

[25] W. H. O. Sankey, *LMG*, NS 2 (1842–3), 394–6.

repute was, from the public's point of view, almost a guarantee of reliability.

Perhaps the most important aspect of apprenticeship was the continuing contact between the apprentice and his former master. Richard Smith records that James Goodeve, who started work in a bank with his father, 'was apprenticed to a Clifton surgeon for the huge sum of 700 Gns'. Subsequently he was a pupil at Bristol Infirmary (1817–18) and at the Borough Hospitals and St Bartholomew's in London (1818–19). He failed in the MRCS examination, although Smith says he was a good pupil, having the misfortune to be examined by the bad-tempered Sir Everard Home. Nevertheless, Goodeve returned to Bristol and set up as a private lecturer in anatomy and physiology, and then he 'settled comfortably in practice in Clifton, having entered into partnership with his former master. He did well, and the 700 Gns turned out a good investment.'[26]

A good master would keep an eye on his ex-apprentices and see them established, if possible, in good practice. Mr Hetling, clearly a man of influence in the south-west, found such an opening for practice in Chipping Sodbury for his ex-pupil, Poyntz Adams, who appears later in this chapter. Medicine in the eighteenth century was a small world with a network of masters, pupils, and apprentices keeping in touch to their mutual advantage. Apprenticeship was often the only way a young man could achieve a medical identity, and be identified as a well-trained and respectable young practitioner by a judicious choice of a practitioner under whom to serve his apprenticeship. With the rise of the teaching hospital, this disappeared. Then, the fledgling doctor introduced himself not as someone who had served his time with Mr So-and-So, but as a 'Bart's man' or a 'Guy's man', and apprenticeship was left out. Nevertheless, well into the nineteenth century apprenticeship premiums were often a good investment; and for the master the premium was often an important addition to his income.

In family apprenticeships, as we have seen, the premium was often waived, and it was also common to find that 'nil' or very low premiums were charged if the apprentice's father had died, or if the apprentice was the son of a medical man although not a relative of the master.[27] Usually a lower premium was charged for the sons of tradesmen than for the sons of gentlemen and professional men, but the correlation was

[26] BIBM 12, 26.

[27] This is evident from the entries in the apprentice binding book in the Records of the Society of Apothecaries, Guildhall Library, London.

not particularly close. The most important factors which influenced the size of the premium were the status of the master and whether the apprenticeship was served in London or the country. J. L. Mann, writing of the 1820s when, under the Apothecaries Act of 1815, apprenticeship was compulsory, stated that 'general practitioners in London received from five hundred to two hundred pounds, and in the country from two hundred to one hundred'.[28] During the eighteenth century the increasing prosperity of the provincial practitioners enabled them to raise the apprenticeship premiums. This can be seen in table 5 which is based on data from the apprentice books of Bristol. As the surgeons rose, so the barber-surgeons declined. The formal separation between the two took place in 1745, and some of those who persisted after 1745 with the title 'barber-surgeon' were primarily barbers or peruke-makers.

In table 6 the premiums required by provincial practitioners between 1710 and 1760 are compared to those paid to London practitioners between 1764 and 1773. The latter are generally in agreement with the quantities quoted in *A General Description of All Trades* (London, 1747) where apothecaries were quoted as charging between £20 and £300, and surgeons between £50 and £500.

The importance of the apprentice in running the day to day practice has been mentioned. G. J. Guthrie described this in his evidence to the Select Committee on Medical Education in 1834, and what he had to say applied as much to the eighteenth as to the first half of the nineteenth century.

A Gentleman, after having been duly educated ... goes back to establish himself ... in his native town. As he must probably visit patients six, eight or ten miles around the country, there must be somebody at home to give an answer, or to give out a dose of medicine, if the master sends home for it. The first thing he does, therefore, is to take an apprentice. Now a student of my own came to me two years ago, and said 'I have settled myself in the City.' I said, 'I hope you will succeed.' 'Yes', said he, 'I have nothing to do at present, but I hope I soon shall: but I want an apprentice.' So I said, 'What do you want with an apprentice, if you have got nothing to do yourself?' 'But I *may* have,' he replied, 'and then I should want somebody to answer the door, and receive messages that may be sent to me; and if I have anything to do, to make up medicines, and in fact to answer any purpose which may be desired of him.' ... The original gentleman, having got a little more practice, takes a second and a third [apprentice], and great is the manufacture in this way, of young doctors, who

[28] J. L. Mann, *Recollections* (1887).

Table 5 *Bristol apprenticeship premiums in the eighteenth century*[a]

Date and type of apprenticeship	Premiums (£)								Totals	
	Nil	1–9	10–19	20–49	50–74	75–99	100–199	200+	Number	Average premium[b] (£)
Apothecary										
1711–20	11	—	—	9	21	2	1	—	44	53.61
1731–40	6	—	1	6	9	8	20	—	50	77.88
1741–50	3	—	—	6	5	2	12	—	28	78.30
1767–75	4	—	3	2	—	1	16	—	26	85.77
TOTAL	24	—	4	23	35	13	49	—	148	
Barber-surgeons										
1711–20	16	2	23	52	7	1	—	—	101	28.26
1731–40	11	14	25	15	12	3	5	—	85	32.21
1741–50	14	8	26	7	1	1	2	—	59	18.87
1767–75	7	6	12	—	—	—	—	—	25	8.84
TOTAL	48	30	86	74	20	5	7	—	270	
Surgeons										
1711–20	—	—	—	—	—	—	—	1	0	
1731–40	—	—	—	2	1	1	4	7	9	103.94
1741–50	2	—	—	2	1	1	7	4	20	132.43
1765–75	2	—	—	—	—	—	—	—	6	205.00
TOTAL	4	—	—	4	2	2	11	12	35	

[a] Data for this table were kindly provided by Jonathan Barry.
[b] Nil premiums excluded from this calculation.
Source: Apprentices' books, Bristol Record Office.

Table 6 *Apprenticeship premiums of medical practitioners in the eighteenth century*

Surgeon-apothecaries in Surrey, Sussex, Warwickshire and Wiltshire (1710–60)		Apothecaries in London (1764–81)	
£	No. of examples	£	No. of examples
		Nil	54
1–12	4	0–19	1
20–35	17	20–49	10
40–48	13	50–99	19
50–55	23	100–149	45
60–63	34	150–199	6
70–84	18	200–249	10
86–90	2	250+ [a]	4
100–107	17	TOTAL	149
140–150	2		
210	2		
TOTAL	132		

Source: The data for the above table were kindly supplied by Dr Joan Lane.

[a] The two highest premiums were £315 and £840.
Source: Records of the Society of Apothecaries, apprentice bindings book, MS 8207, Guildhall Library, London.

are, for the most part, in regard to their preliminary education, unqualified people.[29]

A tyrannical master could exploit his apprentice shamelessly. Indeed the most common image of the medical apprentice was a downtrodden, aproned lad whose life was spent behind the counter of the shop or in a backroom, washing bottles and making up the stocks of medicine, working late into the night. The apprentice, bound by his indentures, had no redress, for the indentures required him to serve his master faithfully. Denman complained that only too often masters of apprentices were 'selfish and negligent in the performance of that share of the duty, which they undertake; ... having received the gratuity usually paid' they failed to instruct them properly and left them 'ignorant of many things which they ought to know, to their own misfortune and disgrace, and to the prejudice of society'.[30] But there are signs towards the end of the eighteenth century of masters regarding their duties more seriously than before. Makittrick recommended a syllabus of training. First, the apprentice should be taught about drugs, and then proceed to 'chymistry and anatomy'. He should be taught scepticism because 'a moderate degree of scepticism is in no profession so necessary as in

[29] Evidence of G. J. Guthrie, *SCME*, part II, Q. 4902.
[30] T. Denman, preface in *An Introduction to the Practice of Midwifery*, 5th edn. (London, 1805), xxvii.

physic'; and 'the young man, if he has the capacity, may at the end of the third year, be able to attend his master to the patient's bedside' where he should make notes of

the patient's mode of life, his profession, the situation of his dwelling, the season of the year and preceding and present state of the weather; together with an accurate account of his former state of health, the probable cause of the disease, and his habit of body. He should then enter into an inquiry on the symptoms, and this he ought to do with some regularity, beginning generally with the vital functions, proceeding to the natural, and from thence to the animal functions and qualities.[31]

The apprentice must also be taught to have humanity towards his patients and look after the poor, especially 'the honest and industrious, who are just a remove beyond absolute want, but are not able to support those expenses that necessarily attend want of health and consequently of employment'. The apprentice should cultivate 'prudence, decency of manners, candour and circumspection'—the absence of which were conspicuous in the author himself; and finally, 'a medical man should spend the principal part of the time he can spare from business at home and in his study'. Whether the author practised what he preached is immaterial; the sentiments of this essay were a sign of a new awareness of the responsibilities of medical education.

James Lucas, surgeon of Leeds, published a book on apprenticeship in 1800.[32] It emphasized the duties of the apprentice laying special emphasis on caring for 'the shop' and arranging the drugs on the shelves in accordance with his instructions. In common with other authors he underlined the need for moral instruction and discipline. Apprentices were regarded as potentially dangerous animals who could easily lapse into indolence or rebellion or both at the same time; but they could generally be brought to heel if the master was vigilant. Lucas was no exception in holding this view, and his dull and uninspiring little book at least had the virtue of stimulating William Chamberlaine, a London surgeon-apothecary, to publish in 1813 a much livelier account of apprenticeship.[33] Chamberlaine shared Lucas's view that apprentices were always a potential source of trouble, and both books

---

[31] J. K. Makittrick, *Commentaries* (1772). An apprentice's case-book in the Wellcome Institute Library, London (MS 4958), provides evidence of such notes.

[32] J. Lucas, *A Candid Inquiry into the Education, Qualifications and Offices of a Surgeon-Apothecary* (Bath, 1800).

[33] W. Chamberlaine, *Tirocinium Medicum: Or a Dissertation on the Duties of Youth apprenticed to the Medical Profession* (London, 1813).

place great emphasis on the apprentice's behaviour. The difficulty sometimes lay in the delicate position of the apprentice, somewhere between
the family and the servants. He was not to assume he was an equal of
the master and his family, even if his own social background was as
good or even better. Nor was he allowed to be familiar with the servants.
His evenings were to be lonely ones, spent in study. But first, he had to
be selected carefully. Parents, said Chamberlaine, were so dazzled by
the sight of medical men riding in their carriages that they set their
hearts on putting a son into the profession without considering whether
he had the qualities for it. The whole tenor of the book is one of warning,
like a sergeant-major faced with a group of raw and potentially unruly
recruits. Chamberlaine had no doubt that the first duty of the master
was to be stern, and of the apprentice to be obedient. The apprentice
had to see that the shop was at all times attended; 'it is the ruin of a
shop to have the name of being deserted'. Messages should be carefully
recorded in a book kept for the purpose. For example:

Wed 13th. Mrs Wright, 2 Red Lion Street.
           Mr Johnson, 63 Newgate Street, any time you go that way.
 Fri 15th. Mr Johnson, 63 Newgate Street. Call on him today. Wants to pay
           his bill.
           Lodger, back garret, Public House, corner. Would not give his
           name nor pay for Tinct Rhei: which he drank. Would you call on
           him (appears not worth powder or shot).
           Capt: Barry wants you to dine with [him] tomorrow at Hungerford
           Coffee-House at $\frac{1}{2}$p.4 [half-past four] and bring your bill.

Such details, particularly the financial details,were important. But there
were dangers in leaving the apprentice in charge of the shop. He could
'do business on his own ... using the drugs in the shop and entering
nothing in the book'. Or he could pocket the money if patients called in
at the shop to pay their bills 'without waiting for having them sent
out as usual at the year's end'. Dishonesty was not the only danger;
Chamberlaine hated the foppish and conceited apprentice:

To the dashing young men of fortune, who think they have learned enough
already; to those who (if there are Masters who will permit it) come down stairs
in the morning and lounge about the shop and surgery in a clean flannel gown,
silk stockings and red slippers ... to those who are never seen to wear a pair
of shoes, but pound their mortar, and roll their pills, in a pair of jockey boots,
with tops turned down to the ancles, in the hottest summer weather: to such
I do not address myself.

At night the apprentice was not to suppose he could sit sociably with the family. He had a 'little parlour' allotted to him for study. At all costs he must 'keep out of the kitchen. An apprentice or assistant has no manner of business in the kitchen ... one who is too fond of the kitchen is no good for anything ... [if] too great familiarity with the servants is manifest, THERE IS NO MORE GOOD TO BE EXPECTED ... [and] if the servant is too fond of being in the shop, the best way for a master to do, is to get clear of both as soon as he can.'

When it came to morning:

Be in the shop not later than SEVEN o'clock ever morning, summer and winter. If anything lies over from the previous day rise earlier.... Set the shop to rights ... sprinkle, sweep ... if your bed is in the shop, turn it up ... trim the lamps ... let this be done early, so as to be perfectly ready to come in to your breakfast with the family when called; combed hair, cleaned hands, clean face and clean shoes ... I have seen a young man make his first appearance in his employer's shop in a morning gown and red Morocco slippers; this foppishness ... ought by no means to be suffered.

The apprentice must be dressed so as to be ready for any emergency:

It is no time to be gathering up your stockings, tying the knees of your breeches, adjusting your neckcloth or hunting for your shoes when half a dozen messengers, one after another, are running into the shop breathless, to call you to a man that has fallen from a scaffold; to a child suddenly seized with alarming fits, a person apparently dead and just cut down or taken out of the water ... besides it is highly disrespectful to your employer to come into breakfast with your stockings about your heels.

Chamberlaine recalled how a lazy apprentice had 'lost a respectable and opulent family which did not pay less than from eighteen to thirty pounds per annum', and the author stressed how numerous calamities could be inflicted on patients by ignorant or lazy apprentices.

Chamberlaine was a sour man and probably a natural tyrant. With a sense of relief, one finds examples of practitioners who took a kindly and considerate view of their charges. Charles Brandon Trye, a surgeon to the Gloucester Infirmary was one, and it is revealed in a letter to a correspondent who had asked him to take his nephew into apprenticeship.

I will take your nephew as soon as you please, but I think the matter on your part deserves some consideration previous to your placing him with me. I have always been of the opinion that an apprenticeship is a bad mode of educating a young gentleman in any liberal employment. It is very rarely that two persons absolutely bound to each other for a term of five or seven years go on cordially together ... the young men who have been under my charge have entered into no articles or indentures and both parties have had it in their power to separate whenever the circumstances or inclination led them to do so, and that without any inconvenience or discredit ... and thus the youth has been accustomed to consider me not as his master, but as his tutor and instructor ... my terms are 100 Gns for the first year and 50 Gns for every subsequent year...[34]

The terms included hospital fees.

At one extreme apprenticeship could be a miserable period of slavery; at the other, an efficient and enjoyable introduction to medicine. A sensible master, if he wanted a continual supply of apprentices, would be careful to avoid a reputation for excessive severity, and many practitioners looked back on their apprenticeship with enjoyment and a deep affection for their old master and his family. J. L. Mann was one, when he recalled his time with Mr and Mrs Wells in Bourton-on-the-Water in Gloucestershire,[35] and the memoirs of Richard Smith junior contain many appreciative letters from ex-pupils and apprentices.[36] Medical apprenticeship probably reached its peak in the final years of the eighteenth and early years of the nineteenth century. At best it was an appropriate system of training the general practitioner and his predecessors, and it carried little of the stigma that soon became attached to it. But the end of apprenticeship was inevitable with the rise of the voluntary hospitals and the dominance of the teaching hospitals of London.

Medical education and the hospitals: a thriving industry

By 1800, with the increasing emphasis on hospital training, medical education was a thriving, expanding industry. Even in the mid-eighteenth century it often paid well. James Ford, a Bristol Infirmary surgeon, earned £950 between 1744 and 1757 from his pupils and apprentices.[37] During the late eighteenth and early nineteenth century a wide range of courses in the form of lectures, demonstrations, dissections, and 'walking the wards' became available in London, where well-known

---

[34] Gloucestershire CRO, Gloucester, ref. D 303. C.2. Letter undated, but probably written c.1808.

[35] J. L. Mann, *Recollections* (1887).

[36] See also a warmly appreciative letter from an ex-apprentice to his previous master, G. W. Charleton, in Gloucestershire CRO, Gloucester, ref. D 4432. 33.

[37] BIBM 1, 54.

lecturers could earn hundreds of pounds a year, and sometimes thousands, from teaching. As medical education expanded, private medical schools reached their zenith in the third decade of the nineteenth century and at least ten medical schools were established in the provinces between 1824 and 1834.[38]

With the rapid expansion of hospital training, the image of medicine improved and parents were increasingly tempted to put their sons through a medical training in spite of the considerable expense. The London teaching hospitals became the new powerful centres of English medicine, dominated in many cases by rich, influential, and flamboyant surgeons who produced the new breed of medical students, as proud of being a 'Guy's man' or a 'Thomas's man' as a subaltern was of being in the Guards or an undergraduate of being a 'Balliol' or 'Trinity' man. Bob Sawyer and Ben Allen were the traditional stereotypes of the medical student, coarse, ignorant, ill-mannered, and greedy. They were, however, a caricature. There were quiet, well-mannered, and serious students just as there were students and apprentices who were conceited, dandified men-about-town, with more than a touch of arrogance to them.

A vivid example of the latter is provided by the case of John Thorp who claimed to be the son of a clergyman. In 1779, in answer to an advertisement, he came to Essex fresh from St Thomas's Hospital to buy the practice of Richard Paxton. Paxton, kindly, gentle, but weak-willed and ill after forty-two years of continuous medical practice in Maldon, accepted Thorp's offer and took him into his house to introduce him to the practice. Thorp's promises of payment were continually postponed, but he installed himself in the house, behaved with outrageous arrogance, and monopolized Paxton's man-servant.

At breakfast it was his custom to place himself on the opposite side of the fireplace to Mrs Paxton, whence, stretching his limbs across, almost engrossed the benefit of the warmth to himself; in the midst of a meal he would exclaim aloud for the man 'Jo-Jo—bring my boots'; these were drawn on not by turning himself with decency to one side, but rudely by raising his feet across, almost to the very face and nose of Mrs P— and how disagreeable that must be, may be imagined when it is known that his feet, when not in the slipper, were palpably offensive, even to those who were at a distance.

[38] J. A. Shepherd, 'The Evolution of the Provincial Medical Schools in England', *Transactions of the Liverpool Medical Institution* (1981–2), 14–39.

Thorp had brought from London a horse 'slim and delicate of the half-breed kind, agreeable to his own taste, but totally unfit for the work of a country apothecary; but this horse must be clothed up and all day stand up to his belly in clean straw and his own and the servant's attendance upon him ten times a day'.[39] John Thorp thus provides an authentic example of the less attractive side of the London medical student at the turn of the century.

The importance of the teaching hospitals as powerful institutions comes out clearly in a remarkable collection of family letters dated 1801-2.[40] The father of the family, Richard Weekes (1751-1823), was a surgeon-apothecary at Hurstpierpoint with a busy practice in which he was assisted by his younger son and apprentice, Dick Weekes. The older son, Hampton Weekes, was a medical student in London when Cline was the London surgeon of the day. Hampton was encouraged by his father to cultivate his acquaintance with Cline; it would pay off in the future. Much of the correspondence consists of Hampton describing his life as a student to his father and younger brother. In October 1801 he wrote: 'Today has been our taking-in day. The number of patients taken in amounted to 63 men and women, it is my place to write down the medicine the physician prescribes, I have done it today, also to enter all their names—Mr Cline operates to-morrow.' The male clubbable atmosphere comes out clearly, with the sense of pride and excitement at being at the centre and hearing the latest views on medicine and surgery directly from the towering figures of London medicine.

To strengthen the club/regiment/college type of loyalty there was the initiation of the dissecting room and the operating theatre. At first, Hampton fainted away at the horrors he saw; but soon he was able to write: 'I have seen several operations since I last wrote and mind *nothing* about it, the more the poor devils cry the more I laugh with the rest of them'. A chilling comment, although it must have been laughter to keep up one's courage. Later still, he wrote that he attended several lectures each day, as well as dissections, did not go to plays but slept near the hospital, and, eager for practical experience, attended every accident: 'My mates and I are there as soon as anybody.' As to operations, he was soon acclimatized: 'As to fainting away, I have

---

[39] Notebooks of Richard Paxton of Maldon, Essex, Wellcome Ms 3820.

[40] These letters are in the possession of St Thomas's Hospital Medical School library. Dr John Ford of Tonbridge is planning to publish them in full. I am grateful to Dr Ford for allowing me to see his transcripts of the correspondence and for his and St Thomas's Hospital's permission to use some of this material in this chapter. Ref. St Thomas's Hospital Medical School Library, H1/ST/MS/H15.

entirely done that away, I take no Brandy now' and he was able to laugh at the newcomers: '2, 3 or 4 young fellows who are uncommonly sick, obliged to leave the theatre'. As a full-blooded student he joined the Clinical Society 'a dozen or 14 young men, almost all Cleaver Fellows (old dressers most of them) we have a Secretary and a President—meet every Tuesday night—fined 6d. if they do not turn up'. As for midwifery, attended at the nearby lying-in hospital, the students ('half a dozen together' at each delivery) called it 'the groanings'.

The process of training and initiation into the world of medicine was the same for the future physician, surgeon, or general practitioner. All were branded deeply with the mark of their teaching hospital. Being a Guy's, Bart's, Thomas's, or Middlesex man produced powerful emotional ties, glueing the profession together and sometimes even transcending subsequent differences in status, income, or position. The old-style apprenticeship, even at its strongest, had none of this element of tribal or institutional loyalty. The point that needs to be stressed is the chronology. By 1800, an essentially modern type of medical education centred on the hospital, was firmly established. It is therefore nonsense to talk of this as a product of the Apothecaries Act of 1815. Long before that, the system existed and was already expensive. Hampton Weekes spent £61 as soon as he arrived in London: £26. 6s. 0d. for hospital pupil fees, 12 guineas for Babington, Curry, and Roberts's lectures, 9 guineas for two courses under Mr Cline, 6 guineas for dissections, and the rest on instruments, books, stationery, and a desk. (Two lists of books bought by medical students can be found in Appendices I and II.)

A further example of the life of a medical student and near contemporary of Hampton Weekes was Mr Poyntz Adams who was supported as a student by his uncle, the Revd Mr Thomas of Farndon near Market Harborough. He had been a pupil of Mr Hetling, a surgeon at Bristol Infirmary, before going to London to study medicine in 1810. His letters to his uncle, usually requests for more money, have survived,[41] and one describes in detail his routine of study.

Every morning from 7.45–9.00 he attended Mr Haighton on midwifery, and from 10–11 Dr Babington, Dr Curry, Dr Marcet, or Mr Allen on medicine or chemistry.

Every afternoon from 2–3.30 he had Cline or Astley Cooper on anatomy.

On Monday and Wednesday evening he attended Mr Haighton on physiology from 7–8 p.m., and at 8, Mr Astley Cooper on surgery. On Tuesday and Friday

[41] Northampton CRO, Letters of Mr Poyntz Adams, Box X 5508, ZA 6277–6293.

evenings he attended Dr Curry or Dr Cholmeley on theory of medicine and every Tuesday at 6.30, Mr Allen on experimental philosophy.

Lectures were crowded. Adams estimated that Astley Cooper's lectures on surgery were attended by 'upwards of 230'.[42] From the fees he recorded, it seems that Astley Cooper was earning atout £700 a term for his surgical lectures and more than £1,000 for his lectures and demonstrations of anatomy. Entrance to the lectures was controlled by tickets 'printed in ink in various colours with appropriate Latin mottoes'. With all these fees for attendance an innocent new student soon found 'he had now disbursed almost the whole sum with which he was supplied on leaving the parental house'.[43] If the surgical lectures were best attended it was because of the well-known eccentricities of men like Abernethy who would ' indulge his disposition and propensities to an extent which occasioned the pupils frequently to regard it as an exhibition and called it "Abernethy at Home"'. He entered the lecture room, 'his hands buried deep in his breeches pockets, his body bent slouchingly forward, blowing or whistling, his eyes twinkling beneath their arches and his lower jaw thrown considerably beneath his upper. Then he would cast himself into a chair, swing one of his legs over an arm of it and commence his lecture in the most *outré* manner.'[44]

Medical life in London was attractive because of such people like Abernethy. It was a small world where the student could meet, or at least see, many of the famous medical names of the time. In some respects, however, the clinical facilities available to students were better in the provincial hospitals than in London. Adams claimed that more casualties could be seen in a year at Bristol Infirmary than in any hospital in London, or more than any practitioner could expect to see in a lifetime of practice; but the provincial hospitals suffered the disadvantage of not being recognized for teaching purposes by the Royal College of Surgeons.[45] In 1811 Adams left London to set up as a general practitioner in Sodbury. His career was typical of his time. Compared to his predecessors of fifty years earlier he considered himself to be a well-trained practitioner, fully prepared for a career as a country practitioner, and he bought a set of instruments to take with him.

---

[42] Northampton CRO, Letters of Mr Poyntz Adams, Box X 5508, ZA letter 6278.
[43] 'Licentiate of the Royal College of Physicians', *Observations on the Present System of Medical Education* (London, 1834).
[44] 'Medical Portrait Gallery', *MCR* 30 (1839), 527.
[45] Northampton CRO, Letters of Mr Poyntz Adams, letter 6278.

Summary: background and education
The typical young man who entered on a career in medicine in the eighteenth and early nineteenth century was a grammar school boy and, more often than not, the son of a professional man especially a surgeon, an apothecary, or a clergyman, or the son of minor gentry. In the early part of the eighteenth century his training was almost entirely in the form of an apprenticeship, usually of five years. Apprenticeship continued as a form of 'training' until the middle of the nineteenth century, but the emphasis on training rather than mere servitude became noticeable only towards the end of the eighteenth century. From the mid-eighteenth century, however, the number who sought additional training in London or in provincial hospitals, and often at both, increased steadily, and such training was supplemented by the opening of private medical schools. By the end of the eighteenth century hospital training, with its comprehensive and organized syllabuses of lectures and demonstrations, became the dominant feature of medical education. The voluntary hospitals achieved a new and increasingly important status as the main centres of medical education in England. Medical education was already a thriving industry before the Apothecaries Act of 1815—expensive for the student and his family, but very well paid for the teachers. Thus, the main features of medical education in England, which continued into the twentieth century, were born in the mid-eighteenth century and were well developed by the beginning of the nineteenth.

3

Physic and Pharmacy

THE practice of physic in the eighteenth century was, in theory, the province of the physician. In reality, however, it formed the major part of the daily routine practice of all the rank-and-file practitioners. What, then, were the medical disorders they treated? What medical treatments were used? What were contemporary opinions and retrospective judgements on the effectiveness of medical care? And what were the profits derived from the practice of physic and pharmacy?

The predominant medical disorders

Comprehensive morbidity studies are of very recent origin. Hospital statistics are available from the eighteenth century but they show only the carefully selected cases admitted to hospital which were in no way representative of diseases outside the hospital walls, nor even of the most serious forms of illness.[1] Mortality statistics have been the main source from which historians have been trying to unravel the pattern of disease in the eighteenth and nineteenth centuries. There are, however, two obvious disadvantages of such an approach. First, the reliability of data on mortality, especially before the introduction of death registration in 1838, was hotly debated by contemporaries and still is by historians. Secondly, morbidity can not be inferred accurately from mortality data. The attempt to do so may be due to the belief that there is no choice—that they are the only statistics available, or that morbidity data are too few, too inaccurate, or obscure to be of any use. It would be inappropriate here to argue at length on the relative merits of sources on mortality and morbidity. Both are important and both have difficulties and limitations. But data on morbidity do exist, in some instances carefully compiled by able physicians, and they provide our

---

[1] The rules of most voluntary hospitals excluded the admission of patients with 'infectious distempers' (including the continued fevers), smallpox, phthisis, venereal disease, the itch, and those in a 'dying condition or judged incurable'. Although not always obeyed, these rules kept the hospitals remarkably free of serious medical cases in the eighteenth and early nineteenth century.

most valuable source for the understanding of the whole spectrum of medical disorders treated by medical practitioners. Some accounts of morbidity, varying in their completeness, were recorded by private practitioners. An approximation to a morbidity survey based on the diaries of James Clegg (1679–1755) is summarized in table 7. But the most valuable of all morbidity studies are the 'lists of diseases' compiled by the physicians at the dispensaries. Tables 8 and 9 provide examples; the latter showing the complete list from Newcastle-upon-Tyne dispensary between 1777 and 1790, and the former the ten most common diseases at six dispensaries at various periods between 1777 and 1801.

The diseases of the rich and those of the poor were not identical. 'A fashionable physician attending on the rich, and another in the same district and at the same time, visiting the sick poor, would present lists of diseases widely different: gout and hysteria might stand foremost in the one; contagious fever and dysentery in the other.'[2] Dispensary physicians visiting the sick at their own homes were often astounded by the degree of poverty and the extent of disease amongst the urban poor. Indeed, it needed persistence to convince those colleagues who moved only amongst the well-to-do, of the truth of what they described.[3] The dispensary physicians, shocked by their experience, were partly responsible for opening the eyes of the medical profession as a whole to the connection between poverty and disease. Reports by men like Lettsom, Willan, and Bateman in London, Currie of Liverpool, Clark of Newcastle, and Campbell of Lancaster had a powerful and sometimes forgotten influence on measures designed to improve the public health in the nineteenth century. It would be a mistake, however, to exaggerate the differences between the diseases of the rich and the poor.[4] They were differences of degree rather than kind, and the spectrum of disease treated by the surgeon-apothecaries (who treated all classes of the community) would correspond broadly to that seen at the dispensaries.

[2] J. Reid, 'Report of the Diseases admitted to the Finsbury Dispensary', *Monthly Magazine* (1 April 1800), 287.

[3] For example, J. C. Lettsom, *Medical Memoirs of the General Dispensary in London for part of the years 1773–1774* (London, 1774); R. Willan, *Reports on the Diseases of London* (London, 1801); T. Bateman, *Reports on the Diseases of London* (London, 1819); J. Currie, *Medical Reports on the Effects of Water as a Remedy for Fevers* (London, 1805); J. Ferriar, *Medical Histories and Medical Reflections*, Vol. i (London, 1810); J. Clark, *A Collection of Papers* (Newcastle, 1802), and his reports of the Newcastle Dispensary in the Tyne and Wear archives department in Newcastle-upon-Tyne.

[4] Gilbert Blane, *Select Dissertations* (London, 1822) provides an opportunity to compare his cases in private practice with those admitted under his care to St Thomas's Hospital in London (esp. pp. 150 and 152). Continued fever and diarrhoeal diseases, classically the diseases of the poor, ranked high in the diseases of his private patients.

Table 7   *The most common illnesses recorded by James Clegg, physician of Chapel-en-Frith, early eighteenth century*

Infectious diseases		*Respiratory disorders*	
Fever	101	Consumption and phthisis	19
Smallpox	81	Pleurisy and pleuritic fever	51
Ague	39	Quinsy	35
Measles	12	Chincough	12
Scarlet Fever	3	Empyema	5
		Peripneumony	3
Gastro-intestinal		Catarrh/cold	2
Colic	44		
Diarrhoea	16		
Dysentery	2	*Surgical disorders*	
Hypochondriac colic	6	Injuries	13
Cholera	3	bones broken	11
Iliac passion	6	bruised	8
Jaundice	3	to head	1
Worms	2	industrial accidents	3
		Cancer	15
Genito-urinary		Toothache	6
Gravel	9	Fistula-in-ano	3
Nephritic pain	7	Tumor	3
Stone	5	Gangrene	2
Strangury	9	Ulcers	2
		Abscess	1
Mental disorders		Rupture	1
Melancholy	16	Piles	6
Hysterick fit	9		
Mental disorder	6	Accidents (general),	49
Idiot, treatment of	4	some of which are included in the injuries above	
Other frequent illnesses			
Convulsions	26		
Common disorder	10	Accidents concerning horses,	26
Rheumatism	16	some of which are included in injuries above	
Palsy/paralysis	15		

Source: Vanessa S. Doe, ed., 'The Diary of James Clegg of Chapel-en-Frith, 1708–55', *Derbyshire Record Society*, 3 vols., (1978, 1979, 1981).

Table 8 *The most common disease categories reported by six dispensaries, 1773–1801*

Newcastle Dispensary (John Clark, MD, 1777–90)[a]

	No.
Putrid fevers	1,992
Diarrhoeal diseases	700
Consumption	690
Stomach complaints	660
Rheumatism	581
Catarrh	537
Pleurisy: inflammation of the lungs	490
Intermittent fevers	362
Venereal diseases	347
Skin eruptions	326
TOTAL	9,830

The General Dispensary, London (J. C. Lettsom, MD, 1773–4)[b]

	No.
Febris putrida	192
Rheumatisms and sciatica	128
Febris hectica	86
Asthma and Dyspnoea	84
Febris remittens	82
Tussis and catarrhus	80
Diarrhoea and dysentriae	72
Febris nervosa	62
Phthisis pulmonalis	56
Tussis convulsiva vel pertussis	47
TOTAL	1,662

The Public Dispensary, London (R. Willan, MD, 1799–1800)[c]

	No.
Cough and Dyspnoea	203
Epidemic catarrh	144
Skin eruptions	140
Contagious Malignant Fever	112
Asthenia	94
Consumption	79
Dyspepsia	66
Febris infanta	54
Chronic rheumatism	50
Diarrhoea	48
TOTAL	1,740

Westminster General Dispensary, London (John Millar, MD, 1775–6)[d]

	No.
Consumption	303
Remitting fever	202
Epidemic catarrh	113
Stomach complaints	103
Rheumatism	97
Scurvy	65
Venereal disease	62
Dysentry and diarrhoea	29
Palsy	24
Uterine disorders	21
TOTAL	1,320

Liverpool Dispensary (Anon. 1800–01)[e]

	No.
Fevers	2,603
Skin eruptions	2,287
Diarrhoea, dysentry and cholera	1,593
Dyspnoea and cough	1,523
Stomach complaints	658
Syphilis	511
Catarrh	434
Debility	356
Amenorrhea	320
Diseases of the eyes	283
TOTAL	13,012

The Finsbury Dispensary, London (J. Reid, MD, and W. Webb, MD, 1800–01)[f]

	No.
Typhus/continued fever	431
Diarrhoeal diseases	278
Cough and Dyspnoea	229
Asthenia	189
Infantile fever	152
Amenorrhea and Chlorosis	128
Consumption	123
Pulmonary complaints	107
Dyspepsia	105
Menorrhagia	74
TOTAL	2,771

[a] *Source*: Annual reports of the Newcastle Dispensary, Tyne and Wear County Record Office, Newcastle-upon-Tyne.
[b] *Source*: J. C. Lettsom, *Medical Memoirs of the General Dispensary* (London, 1774).
[c] *Source*: R. Willan, *Reports on the Diseases of London* (London, 1801).
[d] *Source*: J. Millar, *Observations on the Practice in the Medical Department of the Westminster General Dispensary* (London, 1777).
[e] *Source*: 'Reports of the Diseases seen at the Liverpool Dispensary', *Medical and Physical Journal*, 5 (1801), 118.
[f] *Source*: J. Reid and W. Webb, reports from the Finsbury Dispensary published in *The Monthly Magazine* for 1800 and 1801.

Table 9   *Diseases reported by the Newcastle Dispensary, 1777–90*

	Admitted	Died		Admitted	Died
I Febrile Diseases			*II Nervous Diseases*		
Intermitting fevers	362	0	Apoplexy	5	4
Putrid fevers	1,992	128	Palsy	75	6
External inflammation with fever	53	0	Stomach Complaints	660	3
			Convulsions	47	12
Inflammation of the eyes	124	0	Epilepsy	33	3
			Asthma	316	211
Inflammation of the brain	1	0	Hooping Cough	99	14
			Colic	192	21
Quinsey	129	0	Hysterics	163	1
Catarrh	537	3	Insanity	13	0
Influenza of 1782	53	1	Obstinate Headache	94	1
Pleurisy: inflammation of the lungs	490	39	*III Diseases of the Habit*		
			Dropsy	205	51
Inflammation of the Liver	22	6	Water in the brain	27	24
Inflammation of the Kidneys	86	2	Scrophula	64	1
			Cutaneous eruptions	325	0
Rheumatism	581	2	Venereal disease	347	7
Gout	6	0	Jaundice	62	2
Erysipelas	72	2	Rickets	11	1
Smallpox	232	59	Worms	160	2
Chickenpox	2	0			
Measles	108	11	*IV Local Diseases*		
Scarlet fever and ulcerated sore throat	203	26	Dentition	45	3
			Uterine diseases	222	2
Nettle-rash	2	0	Suppression of urine	28	3
Haemorrhage from the nose	7	0	Abdominal obstructions	37	4
Spitting of blood	92	5			
Consumptive and afflicted with hectic fever	690	151	Incontinence of urine	8	0
			Schirrhus: and cancer	20	7
Haemorrhoides	18	0	Diseased bladder	3	0
Cholera morbus	23	0	Blindness	4	0
Diarrhoea: and obstinate fluxes	349	28	Stricture of the gullet	2	0
Epidemic dysentry of 1783 and 1785	328	17	Surgical cases	1,036	16
			TOTAL	10,866	688

Source: Annual reports of the Newcastle Dispensary, Tyne and Wear County Record Office, Newcastle-upon-Tyne.

For private and dispensary practitioners, it was the fevers which dominated the practice of physic, and they were classified into three main groups: the continued fevers, the intermittent and remittent, and the eruptive.[5] The distinction was never quite hard and fast, but this classification provided a useful framework from the eighteenth century to the mid-nineteenth. There is, of course, only a loose correlation between these categories and modern descriptions of infective disorders. Some cases of intermittent fever were undoubtedly cases of malaria, which was prevalent during the eighteenth and nineteenth century in the marshland of Kent and Essex, the fens of Cambridgeshire and Lincolnshire, south of the Thames in London, on the Somerset levels, and around Morecambe Bay in Lancashire.[6] While there is no doubt that in these particular areas malaria existed, the tendency may well have been to label a large number of different feverish illnesses as varieties of intermittent fever. Certainly it is unwise to assume that cases recorded as intermittent fever in other areas were also malarial. It was a popular rather than a precise diagnosis.

The specific infections in the eruptive group—smallpox, chickenpox, measles, and scarlet fever—were often confused with each other, while others were often not recognized as specific disorders—mumps, for example. It was the continued fevers which tended to dominate the picture of fevers, and they are usually thought to have been a mixture of typhus and typhoid, together with relapsing fever amongst the Scots and colonies of immigrant Irish.[7] Probably typhus predominated until about 1820, and after that date typhus and typhoid may have coexisted to an approximately equal extent. The interpretation of the continued fever can be uncommonly confusing because of the large number of synonyms; Murchison described no less than eighty-eight. The terms most commonly used were 'fever' prefixed with one or more of the

[5] C. Murchison, *A Treatise on the Continued Fevers of Great Britain* (2nd edn., London, 1873), 2.

[6] M. J. Dobson, 'Marsh Fever: The Geography of Malaria in England', *Journal of Historical Geography*, 6 (4) (1980), 357–89. The diaries of Matthew Flinders (1750–1802), who practised in the Lincolnshire fens from 1770–1802, provide evidence of his own regular summer attacks of malaria described as 'the common complaint' of his area—'the bilious remittent fever'.

[7] See A. Hirsch (trans. C. Creighton), *Handbook of Geographical and Historical Pathology*, 3 vols. (London, New Sydenham Society, 1883), i. 545–92; C. Creighton, *A History of Epidemics in Britain*, (London, 1894), vol. ii; C. Murchison, *A Treatise on the Continued Fevers of Great Britain* (London, 1873). For recent views on typhoid and typhus and the 'sanitary revolution', see Bill Luckin, 'Evaluating the Sanitary Revolution: Typhus and Typhoid in London, 1851 to 1900', in R. Woods and J. Woodward (eds.), *Urban Disease and Mortality in Nineteenth-century England* (London, 1984), 102–19.

following terms: 'malignant', 'putrid', 'slow', 'nervous', 'contagious', 'spotted', 'gaol', 'army', and 'ship', as well as 'typhus', 'typhus mitior', and 'synochus', the last two indicating what was believed to be a mild form of continued fever.[8]

Nowadays, when deaths from epidemics of feverish illnesses are so rare in the West, it needs an effort of imagination to realize what typhus meant to the patient and his helpless medical attendant. Occasionally death was swift. More often the illness which started with a 'sense of weight and uneasiness' lasted two to three weeks. Fever, sweating and shivering, restlessness, and intolerable thirst with a parched black tongue, were associated with intense pains in the back, limbs, and head. The typical miliary rash was described as looking like flea-bites. As the disease progressed, retching and vomiting were followed by diarrhoea and incontinence. If the patient survived, improvement, starting about the end of the third week, was followed by slow and prolonged convalescence. Those who died lapsed into ravings, delirium, and finally coma with characteristic twitchings of the muscles sometimes seen in uraemia. Most victims were poor and endured this in unheated rooms with no help or nursing care beyond that supplied by the family; but the family, all too often, went down with the illness as well. Medical men were especially at risk of infection. Richard Kay had the misfortune to see his family die and to end his own life in an outbreak of what was almost certainly typhus. He recorded that in October 1747 and December 1749 two patients, both young men, died of 'miliary fever'. This miliary fever increased in February and March 1749/50 and in October his father died of it, followed by his two sisters later in the year. His own premature death, aged thirty-five, in 1751, was probably due to typhus and his mother died shortly afterwards. One of the most moving accounts of such deaths is that of Richard Kay's brother-in-law, Joseph Baron, in the summer of 1750. All accounts of eighteenth-century country practice contain frequent references to the fevers.[9]

Next to the fevers in terms of prevalence and deaths, were the diarrhoeal diseases, mostly amongst babies and small children, and phthisis amongst adolescents and young adults. Phthisis tended to be

---

[8] C. Murchison, *Continued Fevers* (1873), 22–5.

[9] W. Brockbank and F. Kenworthy, 'The Diary of Richard Kay', *Chetham Society*, 16 (1968). Some of the most vivid accounts of typhus amongst the poor are to be found in J. C. Lettsom, *Medical Memoirs of the General Dispensary in London for Part of the Years 1773–1774* (London, 1774) and, especially, *Hints Designed to Promote Beneficence, Temperance and Medical Science* (London, 1801); also R. Willan, *Reports on the Diseases of London* (London, 1801).

prolonged and accompanied by a grim process of slow wasting. One practitioner described his visit on 26 October 1726 to 'A boy ab^t ten years of age in ye last stage of phthisis'. It had begun almost two years earlier with a cough which gradually got worse: 'His cough is still very violent, he is now wasted to a Degree almost beyond imagination . . . and his belly is now swelled to a vast Bigness as in an Ascites. . . . He is weak as possible but yet, as is common in this Disease, he talks sometimes pretty briskly and doubts not of a Recovery. He hath tasted no meats but a Bit of Chicken or Pigeon without any Bread to it, nor will he drink anything but Beer. He continued thus till about ye 2nd November and then he died.[10]

If one looks for similarities between the practice of the eighteenth century and that of the second half of the twentieth, they are to be found in the fields of surgery and obstetrics, and in physic in the minor, less dangerous medical disorders such as colds, lumbago, rheumatism, menstrual disorders, and skin conditions. The outstanding differences which would be instantly noted by a modern practitioner are in the prevalence of the fevers—continued, intermittent, and eruptive—and in the severity and danger of chest and throat infections. These dominated the practice of medicine and the reality of such conditions was described in the following account:

A surgeon-apothecary is called up soon after retiring to bed, from a hard day's work, to attend a patient in an acute disease five or six miles off. Weary as he is, his necessities compel him to mount his jaded horse . . . and to make his way through the wind and the rain in the darkest night, over fields perhaps, to a farm house where he finds his patient labouring under a severe attack of inflammation of the lungs. He takes some active measures immediately and waits, probably, two or three hours, cold and shivering in his wet clothes [to see] the effect of the remedies employed. His first visit, at an early hour of the morning, is to this patient, who continues so ill as to require his attendance again in the evening; and these results are repeated twice a day . . .[11]

The practice of William Pulsford of Wells in Somerset between 1757 and the early 1760s was predominantly surgical and it occupies a prominent place in the next chapter; but 18 per cent of his cases were of a medical nature.[12] Most of these were sore and ulcerated throats

---

[10] Anon., extract from the case-book of a medical practitioner, probably a physician, 1726–8. Library of the Royal College of General Practitioners, ref. 711.
[11] 'Medico-chirurgus', *A Letter addressed to the Medical Profession on the Encroachments on the Practice of the Surgeon-Apothecary by a New Set of Physicians* (London, 1826).
[12] Somerset, CRO, Taunton, ledger of William Pulsford, DD/FS Box 48.

which occurred in an epidemic closely similar to that described at the same time by John Fothergill in London[13] and others in Plymouth, St Albans, and Kidderminster.[14] Many of these cases were mild, but the minority of severe cases caused William Pulsford more anxiety than any others recorded in his ledger. His blacksmith, Mr Vincent, was 'almost suffocated by a sore throat'; Farmer Hill of Hinton 'was near losing his life in a Quincy, swallowing nothing for five days and nights', and two other patients, young women, had 'excessive bad ulcere^d throats' and one, 'ye most alarming symptoms I ever saw in any Person who recovered ... there seemed but the least chance for Life, yet we recovered her'. One patient, a young woman, seven months pregnant, died suddenly in the night within a few hours of her first mild symptoms.[15]

Acute infective disorders therefore dominated the practice of the ordinary medical practitioners of the eighteenth and nineteenth century. In times of epidemics they usually outnumbered all other calls to medical disorders, but even when they did not they were always the cause of the greatest anxiety to patient, family, and practitioner.

The effectiveness of medical care

Amongst the questions most frequently asked about the practice of medicine in the eighteenth century are those concerning the effectiveness of treatment—the ability to cure—either from the modern point of view, or from the viewpoint of contemporary patients and practitioners. From a twentieth-century viewpoint the most important function of the eighteenth-century practitioner in medical disorders was to provide the comfort of his presence and exercise his skill in diagnosis and prognosis. This aspect should not be underrated, any more than his advice on 'regimen' or the 'non- naturals' defined as 'a term under which physicians comprehend air, meat and drink, sleep and watching, motion and rest, retention, excretion and the affections of the mind'[16] Advice under this head was, sometimes at least, sensible and effective.

As far as specific therapies are concerned, only four would pass the scrutiny of today— quinine, digitalis, fresh fruit and vegetables, and of

---

[13] J. Fothergill, *An Account of the Sore Throat attended with Ulcers* (London, 1748) and article in *Gentleman's Magazine*, 25 (1755), 343.

[14] See Creighton, *History of Epidemics*, ii. 696–706.

[15] Ledger of William Pulsford, f. 11.

[16] R. Morris and J. Kendrick, *Edinburgh Medical and Physical Dictionary*, 2 vols. (Edinburgh, 1807).

course, opium. Smallpox vaccination, although introduced at the very end of the eighteenth century properly belongs to the nineteenth. Quinine ('cortex' or 'the bark') was probably effective in cases of malaria. Digitalis, at least in the hands of Withering, was effective for dropsy but its usefulness was diminished by a tendency to use it as a panacea, in wrong dosage, and in conditions in which it was not indicated; in this way it fell into disrepute.[17] The importance of fresh fruit and vegetables for the prevention and treatment of scurvy was discovered (or, rediscovered) by James Lind in 1753 in his famous and beautifully designed clinical trial.[18] But appreciation of Lind's work, even in the Navy, was scandalously slow. Opium provided the means of relieving pain, but here again there were difficulties. Its analgesic properties were often forgotten in the lengthy and tedious arguments concerning its properties as either a nervous sedative or as a stimulant.[19] Two other measures which come to mind are more debatable: the effectiveness of smallpox inoculation and the use of mercury for syphilis. Were practitioners in the eighteenth century ever sceptical about their remedies? The answer is that a few were, but the degree of scepticism varied widely.

William Petty in the seventeenth century had asked 'whether of 1,000 patients to the best physicians, aged of any decade, there do not die as many as out of inhabitants of places where there dwell no physicians' and 'whether of 100 sick of acute diseases who use physicians, as many died and in misery, as where no art is used, or only chance'.[20] Dealing with the same general question, but specifically in the context of continued fever, Sir Gilbert Blane argued cogently in 1822:

Unless we can calculate with some degree of precision the extent of the powers of nature [to cure fever] we shall find it impossible to assign what is due to them, and what to the agency of medicine, in framing our experience with regard to the treatment of diseases; for, without such discrimination we may

[17] E. H. Ackernecht, 'Aspects of the History of Therapeutics', *Bulletin of the History of Medicine*, 36 (1962), 389–419.

[18] James Lind, *A Treatise on Scurvy* (London, 1753). A study of the 'Surgeon's Journals'— the accounts of sickness which all naval surgeons were required to keep—for the late eighteenth and early nineteenth century, shows not only the persistence of outbreaks of scurvy on board ship but a surprising ignorance of, or indifference to, the work of James Lind some fifty years earlier. These journals can be found in the Public Record Office at Kew, ADM 101.

[19] This point is dealt with by V. Berridge and G. Edwards in *Opium and the People* (London, 1981).

[20] The Petty Papers, 2, 169–70, quoted in R. Greenwood, *Medical Statistics from Graunt to Farr: The Fitzpatrick Lectures for 1941 and 1943* (Cambridge, 1948), 16.

not be able to satisfy ourselves whether recoveries have been affected by *virtue* of medicine or in *spite* of it ... and we run the risk of congratulating ourselves on a great *cure* where there may have only been a happy *escape*.[21]

It was an important, intelligent, and honest question to ask; but having asked it he answered it crassly by comparing his own experience with the mortality rates given by Hippocrates, convincing himself that they were more successful in 1822. But at least the question was asked.

Richard Smith of Bristol took a surgeon's view as far as medicines were concerned. In his opinion:

even the London and Edinburgh pharmacopoeias were loaded with a miserable farrago of useless trash ... three fourths of the medicines purchased of the Druggist were mere adulterations ... opium, antimony, mercury and many others when needful, of course, employed ... but the great bulk of bottles were mere placebos.[22]

Some physicians were 'regimen physicians' either because of their scepticism concerning the effectiveness of drugs, or because they wished to be free of being tied to the apothecary; but most practitioners probably shared the views expressed by Marryat in 1764, where he found it necessary to support the use of drugs even when their mode of action was obscure.

With respect to the mode of operation of medicines it must be confessed we are somewhat in the dark.... Nature is often very unmannerly to theories.... Would it not be more ingenious to acknowledge that medicines do generally produce effects, though we cannot satisfactorily account for the manner in which they act? ... it seems as novel for physicians to inveigh against the use of drugs, as for a man of learning to decry erudition.... When a person is ill, he naturally and justly looks for the restoration of his health from a physician, and the number of those who are disappointed is comparatively exceeding small.[23]

An almost total therapeutic nihilism, which present knowledge may suggest, was a luxury no practitioner could afford and no ill patient could face. Since the rank-and-file practitioner depended most of all on the provision of medicine for his living, he had the strongest reason for believing in the remedies he dispensed.

Some of the rank-and-file practitioners, following long-standing tra-

---

[21] Gilbert Blane, *Select Dissertations* (London, 1822).
[22] BIBM 1, 46.
[23] T. Marryat, *Therapeutics: Or the Art of Healing* (Birmingham, 1785, 7th edn.)

dition, charged their patients for medicine only. They were a minority, however. Most charged separately for journeys and for bleedings, issues, setons, and clysters; and most charged extra for night calls. Fees were usually met by the patient, but sometimes by sick clubs, or the parish. But in virtually all cases the main source of income was the dispensing of medicines.

One thing is certain: they were great medicine-takers in the eighteenth century, whether to combat illness, to improve 'the quality of the blood' (often taken for this purpose as a routine every spring), or to overcome melancholy, the effects of intemperance, or the common if vague feeling of being slightly under the weather. A common belief that unnecessary medicine-taking is a vice of patients and doctors in the twentieth century finds no support from historical evidence. Since his livelihood depended on it, the ordinary practitioner of the eighteenth and nineteenth century, however secretly sceptical of his own remedies, encouraged this welcome tendency on the part of the public. There was a mixture, draught, bolus, pill, or lotion for every disorder known to medicine.

The profits of pharmacy

It would be hard to find a better example of the profits from pharmacy than the bill presented to the family of Thomas Carew (1729–63) in Somerset.[24] This bill, presented early in 1755, covered treatment for this one family for the previous year. Closely written on twenty-three foolscap pages the bill listed two 'blisters', seven 'bleedings', and 687 items of medicine. Medicine was delivered almost every day of the year, Sundays included. The total cost amounted to £154. 5s. 7½d. of which £50 was outstanding from 1753. The medicines consisted largely of bland preparations—a 'pectoral linctus', gentle laxatives, and 'pacific' and 'nervous' draughts, the tranquillizers of the eighteenth century. There are no clinical details, but there is nothing to suggest that serious or chronic illness was being treated, except, possibly, some brief minor episodes amongst the children. No charge was made for visits by this practitioner, who must have regarded as a gold-mine a family that would pay for medicines alone the equivalent of between a third and a half of an average practitioner's income.

Other examples from the eighteenth century include a bill of

[24] Somerset CRB, Taunton, bill from Mr Bernard Baine, surgeon-apothecary to Thomas Carew, DD/TB box 14/20.

£93. 9s 6d. consisting of several hundred items dispensed to Mr Alexander Popham in 1735,[25] and a bill of over four hundred items presented to Mr Caleb Dickinson, a Bristol merchant, covering the years 1745–8 and costing £21. 9s. 1d.[26] Between 1772 and 1779 a surgeon-apothecary (Mr J. Bryant) attended a Mrs Sandford for two leg ulcers and a fractured arm. During this time she was bled three times, medicine was dispensed for her on fifty-one occasions, and fifty-two journeys were made. The total cost was £44. 3s. 0d.[27]

A great number of bills have survived, and it can be said with confidence that the above examples, although large, are by no means unrepresentative. There is evidence that the prices charged by medical practitioners in the eighteenth century rose significantly, often by as much as 100 per cent around 1740 to 1750 and then remained on the whole constant throughout the rest of the century. This evidence, which has been presented elsewhere, shows that the increase in medical charges could not be attributed to any general rise in prices or the cost of living.[28] It is, in fact, evidence of increasing demand for medicine and the increasing status of medical care from the ordinary rank-and-file practitioner.

The sale of medicines conformed to certain conventions. Bottles of medicine, either mixtures (usually of 6 fl. ozs with 1 fl. oz to be taken three or four times a day) or draughts (a single dose of 1 to 2 fl. ozs) were the most commonly dispensed. For each of these the charges, which before 1740–50 were usually 1s. to 1s. 6d.[29] sometimes rose in the second half of the eighteenth century to 2s. 6d. to 3s. Charges for visits and journeys also rose from about 1s. to 2s. to about 3s. to 5s. The art of pharmacy was to dispense medicine in such a way as to maximize profits. Containers and ingredients were cheap,[30] and patients were forced to pay much more for three small bottles, neatly labelled and wrapped, than for a single bottle three times the size. Medicines, whether they were dispensed as mixtures, draughts, decoctions, infusions, tinc-

---

[25] Somerset CRO. Taunton, Box 13/8.
[26] Ibid. DD/DN 206.
[27] Ibid. DD/DP 23. OB4.
[28] I. Loudon, 'The Nature of Provincial Medical Practice in Eighteenth-century England', *Medical History*, 29 (1985), 1–32.
[29] The records of an apothecary near Leeds from 1703 to 1710 showed even lower charges, in the region of a few pence for such items of medicine. Day-book of a medical practitioner, Library of the Royal College of General Practitioners, London.
[30] 'You might make a gallon of Elm Bark Decoction for twopence', wrote Richard Smith, BIBM 2, 153.

tures, pills, boluses, electuaries, or powders[31] were therefore supplied to the patient frequently but in small amounts. The single dose draught was a favourite form, and pills were often dispensed in ones or twos or, at most, half a dozen.[32] Sugar, honey, or cosmetic agents were added, and charged for, in medicine for the rich. The other charges, for surgical procedures, etc., were often substantial; but the increased prosperity of the mid-eighteenth-century practitioner was achieved mostly through the practice of pharmacy. Medical cases always outnumbered surgical in their practices.[33] It was hard on the poor. 'The apothecaries in the country', wrote a steward of a Bedfordshire estate in 1787, 'charge so high for their attention that a poor distressed working man (if he be a few weeks in illness) dreads the consequence of employing them, as if he survives the illness he knows it will be an additional drawback on his labour (for perhaps several years) to get clear of the apothecary.'[34]

It must, therefore, have been a delight to the apothecaries when Adam Smith leapt to their defence in a well-known passage in his *Wealth of Nations* (1776).

Apothecaries' profit is become a by-word, denoting something uncommonly extravagant. This great profit, however, is frequently no more than the reasonable wages of labour. The skill of an apothecary is a much nicer and more delicate matter than that of any artificer whatever; and the trust which is reposed in him is of much greater importance. He is the physician to the poor in all cases, and of the rich when the distress is not very great. His reward, therefore, ought to be suitable to his skill and trust, and it arises generally from the price at which he sells his drugs. But the whole drugs which the best employed apothecary, in a large market town, will sell in a year, may not perhaps cost him above thirty or forty pounds. Though he should sell them, therefore, for three or four hundred, or at a thouand per cent profit, this may frequently be no more than the reasonable wages of his labour charged, in the only way he can charge them, upon the price of his drugs. The greater part of the apparent profit is wages disguised in the garb of profit.[35]

[31] See appendix for explanation of terms used in pharmacy.
[32] 'I have known an apothecary make fifteen pounds of a patient in ten days, by rating boluses at 2s. 6d. a piece, and other medicines proportionately ... if a physician ordered an electuary of four ounces, the apothecary would divide it into twenty or thirty boluses, at 1s. 6d. each, and a quart azopem into four half-pint phials, each charged 3s. or 3s. 6d.' Thus a physician in 1702 quoted in *MPJ* 12 (1804), 428.
[33] Thomas Misters, surgeon of Shipton-on-Stour, Worcs., earned in the 1760s about three-quarters of his income from the sale of medicines. Visits and surgical procedures accounted for the remaining quarter. Wellcome MS 3584.
[34] Bedfordshire CRO. CRT 100/27/3 (11) 132.
[35] Adam Smith, *Wealth of Nations* (London, 1776).

The practitioner, maximizing his profits on the sale of medicines, was doing no more than other men of trades and businesses in eighteenth-century England. A number of historians have suggested that a 'consumer revolution' and the 'birth of the consumer society' took place in England during the latter half of the eighteenth century.[36] Sales were influenced by fashion in a rapidly expanding market economy and medical care was a commodity affected as much by fashion as necessity.

It would not be accurate, however, to describe the practice of medicine in the eighteenth century as a trade or business just like, for example, drapery, ironmongery or cabinet-making. As Adam Smith had emphasized, it was more than that. To be an apothecary needed a 'nicer and more delicate' skill than any other trade and the apothecary, who was 'the physician to the poor in all cases', was greatly trusted. There was, therefore, the hint of the qualities of a professional man. Two authors who, in 1747, published accounts of various trades, emphasized both the prosperity of the apothecary and his new enhanced status. One, R. Campbell, put it thus:

the Apothecary is esteemed both by Patient and Physician as a Man acting in a qualified Sphere.... There is no Branch of Business, in which a Man requires less Money to set him up than this very profitable Trade.... His Profits are unconceivable: Five Hundred *per cent* is the least he receives.[37]

The anonymous author of *A General Description of All Trades* confirmed the recent increase of the business of the apothecary, which was now

A very genteel business and has been in great vogue of late years ... [Apothecaries] especially in the country ... often become Men of large Practice and eminent in their way.[38]

John Gregory, referring to the passage quoted above, went even further in his assertion that the educated surgeon and apothecary were to all intents and purposes physicians as well.[39] But these affirmations of the rise in the status of the apothecary and surgeon-apothecary gave no hint at this stage of the dilemma which was to haunt the future general practitioner in his bid for full professional respectability. If, through a better education and a greater prosperity, the rank-and-file practitioners were to be accepted as gentlemen and the equal of the physicians, what

---

[36] N. McKendrick, J. Brewer, and J. H. Plumb, *The Birth of a Consumer Society* (London, 1982).

[37] R. Campbell, *The London Tradesman* (London, 1747).

[38] Anon, *A General Description of all Trades* (London, 1747).

[39] J. Gregory, *Lectures on the Duties and Qualifications of a Physician* (London, 1772).

were they doing keeping a shop? For there was the indelible stigma of trade attached to the practice of pharmacy. It had always been so. The whole apparatus of pharmacy—the shop, the stock of drugs, the rows of bottles on the shelves, the manufacture of medicines, and, after labelling and wrapping, their sale over the counter—all this was incontrovertible evidence of shopkeeping. And it was the element of the shop which stood in the way of the social advance of the rank-and-file practitioners. There was, however, at this time, no one else who possessed the skill and knowledge to compound medicines; and to abandon pharmacy, even if possible, would have been commercial suicide, just at the time when pharmacy had become a highly prosperous business. It might be imagined that, when 'profits were unconceivable', who cared about the stigma of trade in an era of bounding commercialism? The answer was that some surgeons did.

With a sound commercial instinct, Richard Smith junior of Bristol, when he started in practice in 1797, put 'Smith, Surgeon' over his front door and Smith, Surgeon and Apothecary' over the back door in Lamb Street and did a roaring trade in pharmacy. When, in 1803, as an established surgeon, he moved to No. 7, The Green, he dropped the 'Apothecary' at the door although he continued to treat all medical cases which came his way and to dispense medicines for his patients.[40] Mr Alland, a surgeon in Bristol who was senior to Smith, 'held himself very high and was very indignant of being otherwise than "A Surgeon"—yet he not only practised physic, but was actually known by the name of "Shop". He however, had his bills for medicine made out in the name of his apprentice and pretended it was a perquisite for the "young man"—but the fact was ... every shilling went into his pocket.' Alland was finally taken to court by a patient he had charged £100 for 'cutting for stone' and £80 for medicines. Alland had either to admit to practising as an apothecary and therefore to the right to charge for medicines or forfeit the £80. Cupidity won.[41]

Meanwhile, the unashamed apothecary made the most of what was, as it turned out, a short-lived monopoly in the practice of pharmacy. As Richard Smith described it, in addition to treating the sick

there were an abundance of people who, every spring and every fall, lost blood and were disciplined for a fortnight or three weeks and several who, occasionally, and especially previous to entering into the holy estate of

---

[40] BIBM 2, 152.
[41] Ibid. 2, 152–3.

Matrimony—though it might be well to clean off old scores by 'an alternative course of medicine' ... Decoction of Bark—infusion of Senna—Almond emulsion—saline mixture—decoction of Hart's Horn—these were the great stable commodities—an oz. and a half were charged fifteen to eighteen pence according to circumstances.... The powders were chiefly rhubarb and prepared chalk with two or three grams of pulvis antimonalis ... a packet of twelve cost 4 shillings—to Grandees or where a costly charge could be made, a drop or two of cinnamon was added and rubbed up and then the packet was six or seven shillings—it was a fashion in those days to give musk, where they could afford it, to patients in extremis, so that you could smell it even in the street as you opened the door ... the profits on these could not be much less than ten shillings a draught—but then this lasted only perhaps a few days.[42]

Practitioners tended to have their favourite remedies.[43] None was more successful in the drug trade than William Broderip of Bristol who practised in the last quarter of the eighteenth century and the early years of the nineteenth. He made no charge for attendance in the city and immediate surroundings, but at the bottom of the bill was written 'Attendance what you please'. In practice, 'some gave nothing, but in one instance where the bill was £30 the patient added £50'.[44] For journeys outside Bristol he charged 5s. but his staple commodity was medicines. One patient of his swallowed twelve draughts daily at the cost of 18s., and the assistants worked until '12 at night during the winter months, coughs and colds and one thing and another generally produced 40 patients to be ordered for daily, the average booking for which was £12.' During an influenza epidemic Broderip visited seventy patients in one day and his apprentices 'were obliged to make a firkin of saline mixture and from the cask it was bottled off'. 'There was a family at Clifton—the Greenlys—they were so wrapped up in him that they could not move without a regular supply of physic—they took with them to Weymouth 200 "tonic draughts"—and one thousand pills of various descriptions—Lassall [the apprentice] told me he was

[42] BIBM 2, 154.

[43] An analysis of the ledger for 1794 of Thelwall Maurice, surgeon-apothecary of Marlborough (retained in the private possession of Dr Dick Maurice of Marlborough), shows the limited variety of remedies used by country practitioners, for example: 'Mist. Stomach' (for indigestion); 'Pulv. Febris' (for fevers); 'Pulv. Emetic' (for a vomit); and 'Mist. Aper.' or 'Pulv. Jalap' (as purgatives). External applications included 'Lin. Oleos' (an oily linament), 'Ung. viride', 'Ung. Ophthalm', 'Ung. ad vesicator' (to raise a blister), 'Empl.' (a plaster), 'Gargarisma' (a gargle). These examples show the impossibility of determining the actual drugs or dosage used. None was a standard preparation. Each practitioner had his own formulae.

[44] BIBM 2, 156.

"sick to death with the rolling of them".[45] On one occasion Broderip was paid £350 by a patient for three years' supply of medicine.[46] He soon exhibited signs of his wealth: a carriage and coachman, a museum, pictures and elegant furniture, and a country residence 'where his wife and family lived two-thirds of the year.... It is true that people called it Gallypot's Hall but it was not the less splendid and elegant on that account.'

Broderip earned more than most of the physicians in Bristol and was hated for it. 'Dr Moncrieffe held him in the greatest contempt and, being one day called in and asked whether he would like to see Mr Broderip who had been in attendance, Moncrieffe opened his great eyes and exclaimed—"Hey—what, the Apothecary? No, show me the patient— what the devil have I to do with the Apothecary!"' But even when the physician was called, the prescription went to the family apothecary who 'called to inquire how the patient was going on, and thus the link continued unbroken, and in all minor affairs the old routine went on as before'.[47] As long as the apothecary had the monopoly in pharmacy he could, and often did, squeeze out the physician, even amongst the rich. Joseph Shapland (1727–1801), who took William Broderip as a partner in 1775, was 'a handsome gentlemanly pleasant man, extremely respected and visited by all the first families in the City and Suburbs ... he visited more patients than any four physicians of his days except Dr Rigge—the only gentleman who kept pace with him was Mr William Dyer of Bridge St.— these two almost divided the City between them.'[48]

One of the conventional pictures of medicine in the eighteenth century portrays the physician as the practitioner with a monopoly of practice amongst the rich and a monopoly of treatment of medical disorders. Beneath the well-heeled physician was the down-trodden apothecary, obediently dispensing the physician's prescriptions and eking out a miserable, poorly-paid practice amongst the lower orders of society. Clearly this picture is incorrect. The treatment of medical disorders in the eighteenth century formed a part or the whole of the practice of all practitioners except for the small minority, mostly in London, who were able to live by surgery or obstetrics alone. Most of that large majority, including some provincial physicians, practised pharmacy. If the outstanding feature of ordinary medical practice in the second half of the

[45] BIBM 2, 157–9.
[46] Ibid. 1, 46.
[47] Ibid. 2, 159–60.
[48] Ibid. 1, 43–5.

eighteenth century was its prosperity, it was largely due to the ability of practitioners in a thriving market economy to persuade their patients to accept and pay high charges for an astonishing quantity of medicine. It was, in the words of Richard Smith junior, 'The Golden Age of Physic'.

4

Surgery and Obstetrics

Surgical practice

FOR most people the image of surgery in the eighteenth century is one of a succession of brutal operations so agonizing and beyond our experience that we can only react by feeling profoundly thankful we live in an age of anaesthesia and advanced techniques of pain relief. There is, undeniably, some truth in this image. A letter from an 'old patient' to James Y. Simpson recalling the experience of a pre-anaesthetic amputation could scarcely be more eloquent.

Of the agony it occasioned I will say nothing. Suffering so great as I underwent cannot be expressed in words, and thus fortunately cannot be recorded. The particular pangs are now forgotten; but the black whirlwind of emotion, the horror of great darkness, and the sense of desertion by God and man, bordering close upon despair, which swept through my mind and overwhelmed my heart, I can never forget, however gladly I would do so.[1]

The horror of such images, however, dominates and distorts our perception of surgery at a time when major operations formed only a very small part of that branch of medicine. For the surgeons and surgeon-apothecaries of small towns and villages and even for surgeons at voluntary hospitals, the reality of surgical practice was more prosaic. The major operations, amputations, herniotomy, trephining, and lithotomy, were, as far as most of them were concerned, rare events. Most surgery consisted of dealing with relatively minor conditions sometimes treated manually, but more often by medical measures applied internally or externally. Even for surgeons holding an honorary appointment at a voluntary hospital, this was largely true. At Nottingham General Hospital the surgeon John Wright admitted 152 cases to the wards between 1795 and 1797. The large majority were suffering from leg ulcers, accidents, or a variety of abscesses and inflammations. Nearly all were treated by rest, diet, medicines, and external dressings. Only

[1] The letter is reproduced in full in V. Robinson, *Victory Over Pain: A History of Anaesthesia* (New York, 1946), 209–17.

four were subjected to a major operation. A man of thirty had an arm amputated for caries of the wrist; a man of twenty-five had an injured testicle removed; a woman of thirty-seven had a leg amputated for a 'carious ulcer' and died five weeks later; and a woman (age not specified) had an amputation of a breast.[2] (See Table 10.)

What, then, was the nature of ordinary surgical practice in the eighteenth century? Thomas Baynton of Bristol (1761–1820) provides an example of a successful surgeon in a provincial city. He insisted on the title of 'surgeon' but kept a shop in the old market like any apothecary, leaving it in the care of his apprentice (later his partner) Josias Hill.[3] Baynton himself cultivated a well-paid practice in physic, surgery, and especially man-midwifery amongst the well-to-do in Kingswood. Richard Smith, the least malicious of biographers, described Baynton as an unctuous, vain, and arrogant man noted for his meanness. Baynton was rich, but life in his house was described by his apprentice as 'penury itself' and 'Baynton so close-fisted that the pump-handle was troubled at meal times more than the beer cock'; but he has one genuine, if minor, claim to fame. In 1797 he published a treatise on leg ulcers, describing a technique based on the application of overlapping adhesive strips.[4] It was used and known as 'Baynton's method' a century later, as well as being the forerunner of a method still in use today. His interest in leg ulcers was unusual, but it formed only a minor part of his work. His prosperity came from practising all branches of medicine amongst a very wide section of the population. The poor were served by his shop while he assiduously cultivated the gentry at their houses. Through such practice he achieved an income of £3,000 a year and left £33,000 when he died.[5]

Another example of the provincial surgeon was William Pulsford, a member of a family whose practice in Wells, Somerset, stretched from the late seventeenth to the early nineteenth century.[6] The interest of this family lies in the survival of a single ledger[7] which provides an

<hr/>

[2] University of Nottingham library, patients' treatment book, Uhg. 01.

[3] BIBM 2, 1064.

[4] T. Baynton, *A Descriptive Account of a New Method of treating Old Ulcers of the Legs* (Bristol, 1797).

[5] BIBM 2, 1080.

[6] A detailed account of the practice of William Pulsford and of his family history can be found in I. Loudon, 'The Nature of Provincial Medical Practice in Eighteenth-Century England', *Medical History*, 29 (1985), 1–31.

[7] Somerset CRO, Taunton, catalogued as 'The ledger of Benjamin Pulsford 1757–1766', DD/FS Box 48. There is little doubt that this surviving ledger was used solely by William, nephew of Benjamin Pulsford, and not by Benjamin. (See footnote 6.)

Table 10   *Surgical cases admitted to Nottingham Hospital, 1795–7 under the care of Mr John Wright, Surgeon*

Nature of ailment	No. of cases
Ulcers	
Ulcerated legs	44
breast	1
arm	1
tongue	1
face	1
palate	1
Accidents and orthopaedic conditions	
Fractures and dislocations	14
Bruises, sprains, burns, etc.	13
Diseases of bone and joint	18
Spinal disorders	3
Abscesses and inflammations	
Simple abscesses	4
Scrofulous abscesses and probable psoas abscess	9
Sepsis and inflammations	4
Other diseases	
Uterine disorders	3
Cancers	3
Hernia (strangulated)	1
Painful or swollen testes	3
Ascites: paracentesis	2
Fistula-in-ano	2
Tumour: unspecified	3
Eye disorders	4
Skin disorders	6
Venereal disease	3
Miscellaneous minor conditions	6
No diagnosis recorded	2
TOTAL	152

Major operations:
Male aged 30: amputation of arm for caries of wrist
Male aged 25: removal of injured testicle
Female aged 37: amputation of leg for carious ulcer. Died after five weeks
Female, age not recorded: amputation of breast

Source: Records of Nottingham General Hospital, patients' treatment book, Uhg. 01 University of Nottingham library.

unusually detailed account of routine daily practice from 1757 to the early 1760s. William Pulsford, who died aged twenty-nine in 1765, was in partnership with his uncle, Benjamin Pulsford (1716–84). Their practice consisted largely of surgical cases. Owing to their habit of using several ledgers at the same time, the total number of 'new' cases recorded in the surviving ledger in 1757 (334 in all) is a representative sample but not the total workload for that year. An analysis of these 334 cases can be found in Tables 11, 12 and 13. Accidents formed 27 per cent of the total, the largest single category. Next came sore and ulcerated throats (many quite mild, but a few very severe including two who died) associated with an epidemic. The remaining cases consisted of a wide variety of surgical cases, most of a minor nature. In only two cases was a major operation performed. The remainder were treated by minor surgery, local applications, and medicine.

Accidents were common in rural life and included injuries from hay-knives, scythes and tenterhooks, guns, and falling objects. Injuries associated with horses were common and often serious and also appear frequently in the diaries of James Clegg and Richard Kay. Even more common were inflammations and abscesses, both pyogenic and tuber-cular, and leg ulcers, which appear in this as in every account of surgery in the eighteenth century. It is certain that leg ulcers were many times more common then than they are today, especially amongst the labouring classes where they occurred most often in young adults in contrast to their present peak incidence amongst the elderly. In 1785, Marryat remarked of ulcers of the legs: 'of all disorders incident to poor people this is the most common.'[8] A London surgeon in 1799 estimated that 'among the lower classes in the community nearly ... one out of five labour, and have for many years, under this severe affliction.'[9] The cause of these ulcers is something of a mystery, but it seems likely that they were due to a wide variety of factors including dietary deficiency in general and scurvy in particular (especially in the Navy where they were exceedingly common) as well as diseases which included chronic osteomyelitis, syphilis, and tuberculosis of bone and joint. The common venous ulcer of today was probably not a major contributor.[10] Then,

---

[8] T. Marryat, *Therapeutics: Or the Art of Healing*, 7th edn. (Birmingham, 1785), 336.

9 C. Brown 'On the Necessity of establishing an Hospital for the Treatment of Ulcerated Legs', *MPJ* 3 (1800), 135–6.

[10] See I. Loudon, 'Leg Ulcers in the Eighteenth and Early Nineteenth Century', *Journal of the Royal College of General Practitioners*, Part I, 31 (1981), 263–73; Part II, ibid. 32 (1982), 301–9.

as now, they were notoriously difficult to cure. John Bell in 1801 recalled meeting 'a man who flattered himself with the expectation of becoming the greatest surgeon in Europe, by finding a cure for ulcers, but he failed'. An enormous variety of medications were applied to ulcers but 'each application has in its turn been proclaimed an infallible cure but the methods which are extolled today are despised tomorrow.'[11]

Two features are prominent in the ledger of William Pulsford. One is the willingness of large numbers of patients such as tradesmen and shopkeepers to consult him and pay substantial fees for minor self-limiting conditions such as bruises, sprains, and minor sore throats. The other is the extreme chronicity of so many of the cases, attended at frequent intervals for months or even years. Leg ulcers and chronic infections were the staple commodities of the country and the town surgeon. Most of William Pulsford's time was spent going his rounds on horseback, his saddle bags filled with medicines, lotions, bandages, and dressings. Occasionally he employed a nurse, but usually he applied the dressings himself. The routine of surgery was unexciting and often a smelly and distasteful business, as Chamberlaine pointed out,[12] but the number of visits generated by chronic conditions ensured a steady supply of high fees. The unusual predominance of surgical over medical cases in William Pulsford's ledger is an illustration of the variety of practice of country surgeons and the effect of commercial opportunity. It seems that Wells probably had an excess of apothecaries and phys-icians in the 1750s who cared for the medical diseases of the population, leaving the surgical to the old-established surgical practice.

Richard Kay, practising in Lancashire about ten years earlier than Pulsford, provided a similar account of the details of daily practice. On a typical day he saw the usual mixture of major and minor cases. Medical diseases predominated numerically, but the diary describes a number of major operations such as an amputation carried out with the help of his father. There is also the memorable account of the time when, at the insistence of the patient, he removed some five hundred secondary tumours from the chest wall of a Mrs Danvers. This was on 7 June 1749. He had previously operated on her for a cancer of the breast, and further operations were carried out in July and August. The patient died early the following year.[13]

---

[11] John Bell, *Principles of Surgery*, 2 vols. (Edinburgh, 1801), vol. i.
[12] W. Chamberlaine, *Tirocinium Medicum* (London, 1813), chapter 2.
[13] W. Brockbank and F. Kenworthy, 'The Diary of Richard Kay' *Chetham Society*, 16 (1968).

Table 11   *Cases treated by William Pulsford, surgeon of Wells, Somerset, in 1757—diagnostic groups*

Nature of ailment	No. of cases
Accidents and injuries	91
(see tables 4 & 5)	
Sore throats, ulcerated throats, and ulcerated	
tonsils and quinsies	35
Erysipelas	5
Smallpox	3
Fever	2
Venereal disease	6
Skin eruptions	7
The itch	4
Herpes of the lip	3
Sore legs (mostly ulcers of the legs)	31
Boils and abscesses	25
Abscess of the ear	2
Soreness, induration, or abscess of the breast	7
Whitlow	3
Inflamed arm following venesection	3
Fistula-in-ano	1
Perianal abscess	2
Inflammatory swellings	11
Swellings of the neck including scrofula	9
Dental disorders	4
Ulcers of the mouth	12
Hernia	4
Phymosis and paraphymosis	2
Hydrocoele	1
Piles	1
Corns on the feet	1
Warts	1
Ganglion	1
Haematoma	2
Suppression of the urine	2
Sore eyes	14
Albugo	4
Pain in the limbs	9
Caries of bone	3
Incisted [sic] tumor of lip	1
Cancer of breast	2
Cancer of tongue	1
Nose bleed	2
Oedema, cause obscure	1
Inoculation against smallpox	9
Diagnosis obscure or uncertain	7
TOTAL	334

GLOSSARY: *The itch*—scabies; *Phymosis* and *paraphymosis*—inflammatory swelling of the foreskin; *Hydrocoele*—accumulation of fluid surrounding the testicle; *Ganglion*—cystic swelling arising from the tendon, usually on the back of the hand or wrist; *Haematoma*— a tumor consisting of an extravasation of blood; *Albugo*—a scar on the cornea following a corneal ulcer; smallpox was here a common cause.

Source: The Ledger of William Pulsford, Somerset County Record Office, Taunton, DD/FS Box 48.

Table 12   William Pulsford's cases—accidents and injuries

Bruises and sprains	
Slight	28
Severe	12
Wounds and lacerations	
Slight	8
Severe	10
Head injuries	8
(Definite fracturer skull)	(1)
Fractures and dislocations	18
Burns	4
Eye injuries	2
Wasp sting	1
TOTAL	91

Source: as for table 11.

Table 13   William Pulsford's cases—causes of accidents

Not recorded	42
Horses—falls while riding, or being kicked by horses	16
Falls (from ladders, trees, etc.)	10
Fighting	6
Accidents with guns or gun-powder	5
Dog-bite	2
Accidents with:	
Hatchet	2
Hayknife, scythe, tenterhook, millstone, fall of timber, glass, wasp sting, catgut flying into eye while mending musical instrument	1 each
TOTAL	91

Source: as for table 11.

Thelwall Maurice set up in practice as a surgeon in Marlborough, Wilts, towards the end of the eighteenth century. His ledger and prescription book show that the practice of physic and pharmacy overshadowed that of surgery, and that the latter consisted predominantly of the extraction of teeth, inoculation against smallpox, opening abscesses, and dressing wounds.[14] Similarly, the records of Thomas Misters, surgeon of Shipton-on-Stour in Worcestershire, which cover the years 1766–71, reveal a thriving practice based almost entirely on charges

[14] Records in the private possession of Dr Dick Maurice of Marlborough to whom the author is grateful for allowing access to his family practice records.

for visits and medicines. There is little evidence of surgical treatment apart from venesection.[15]

The records of two other provincial surgeons, Mr Sabin of Towcester in the latter part of the eighteenth century[16] and a practitioner from Odiham, Hants. (probably Mr Lee) for 1774–80,[17] also show an excess of medical cases. In the latter's records surgical cases consisted of dental extractions, accidents, abscesses, and the ubiquitous leg ulcers. On one occasion he prescribed a drench for a cow, charging sixpence. It was not uncommon for country surgeons to take on the treatment of animals and enter the charge in their ledgers. The notebooks of the Carr family in Yorkshire show a closely similar pattern of practice in which every kind of disorder was treated.[18]

The features which distinguish these surgeons from those most commonly the subject of medical histories is that they held no appointments at medical institutions and no position in the Company or College of Surgeons. Only rarely did they write or publish, and they contributed nothing to surgery as a discipline. None resembled the surgical specialist of the nineteenth and twentieth century, and all undertook the treatment of cases as they came, medical, surgical, or obstetric. In these respects they represented the very large majority of surgeons and surgeon-apothecaries of the eighteenth century. Occasionally—and often, to our surprise, only at the insistence of the patient—they were required to perform an amputation or other major operation. Their inevitable lack of experience, the danger to their reputation if the patient died, and their instinctive horror of the pain involved, were powerful disincentives unless operation was a last resort. Yet it was in surgical treatment that the rank-and-file practitioners were most likely to be effective. By simple procedures the eighteenth-century surgeon could relieve or cure many common complaints. His skills with fractures, dislocations, abscesses, and toothache achieved far more from the patient's point of view than could be achieved by the most wise and skilful physician. From the surgeon's point of view, surgery provided the satisfaction of producing, at least some of the time, effective care for his patients. Also, on many occasions it paid remarkably well.

    [15] Wellcome MS 3584.
    [16] Northamptonshire CRO, ledgers of Dr Sabin of Towcester, YZ 1770, misc. ledger 687.
    [17] Wellcome MS 3974. From the evidence of successive editions of the *Medical Register* it seems that these are the records of Mr Lee of Odiham who either died or retired in 1783.
    [18] Wellcome Institute for the History of Medicine, London. The diaries and notebooks of the Carr family, surgeons of Yorkshire, Wellcome MS 5203, 5204.

Surgical fees

There is reason to believe that patients and medical men in the eighteenth century recognized the greater effectiveness of surgical care.[19] The benefit of a physician in a fever was often a matter of doubt; the urgent need for a surgeon where it was a fracture, a dislocation, or a huge abscess was not. The difference may account for the surgeon's ability to charge high fees. It was widely known that London surgeons could command very high fees, measured in hundreds of pounds, which few if any could in the provinces. William Carr, for example, noted with mixed awe and envy that Mr Heaviside of London charged a Yorkshire family in 1814 700 guineas for operating on a child for a harelip, and visiting the child once afterwards at home.[20] While such London fees have often been recorded, little has been published on those of the country surgeon. Here, William Pulsford's ledger provides a wealth of information and one has to recall that he was only a young, relatively inexperienced and unknown surgeon, working in a country area.[21] His records, and similar evidence from other sources, tend to disprove a common assumption: that medical men graded their fees over a wide range according to the social circumstances of the patient. On the contrary, fees for medicine, for visits by day or night, for obstetric care, and for a whole series of surgical procedures tended to be the same whether the patient was a skilled labourer, a shopkeeper, a farmer, schoolteacher, merchant, miller, clergyman, or attorney. Only with the few country squires and the aristocracy was there a quantum jump in the size of fee, and not always then. Thus the Pulsfords routinely charged 10s. 6d. for smallpox inoculation but the wife of the Hon. George Hamilton Esq. was charged 4 guineas. Moreover, it is surprising how often the fees were similar for the same procedures whether it was a surgeon in Somerset, Gloucester, Lincolnshire, or Yorkshire. Whenever surgeons met each other, fees (or their horses) were the favourite subject of conversation, not surgery.[22] A network of financial information must have circulated amongst the medical men of England, mostly by word of mouth.

Pulsford's lowest fee was 5s. which was his charge for treating a hatmaker for a sore throat, a young woman with 'the itch', and for opening

[19] R. Campbell, *The London Tradesman* (London, 1747).
[20] The Carr diaries, Oct. 1814.
[21] Somerset CRO, Taunton, the Pulsford ledger, DD/FS Box 48.
[22] The Carr diaries in which page after page is concerned with fees, charges, and rumours of the fees of neighbouring practitioners, are a vivid illustration of this.

Table 14 *William Pulsford's cases—fees charged*

Nature of ailment and treatment	Fee
Accidents and Injuries	
Bruised arm from being kicked by a horse	5s.
Bruised head from a fall from a horse	10s. 6d.
A farmer treated for a fractured fibula	10s. 6d.
Reduction of a dislocated shoulder	11s. 6d.
Fractured clavicle from firing a gun	11s. 6d.
Farmer's wife: 'cut artery difficult to stop'	7s. 6d.
Fractured skull; perforater used on cranium	15s. 6d.
Bruised leg from a fall from a ladder	1 gn.
Child: dislocated wrist from a fall from a tree, necessitating three journeys	1½ gns.
'Ran nail into sole of foot: troublesome symptoms arose'	2 gns.
Millworker: 'Top of finger almost cut off: sewed back on'	5 gns.
Gunshot wound to hand	5 gns.
Wound of thigh from scythe: operation patient died	5 gns.
A shoemaker's sons: for one, the stitching back of a ripped open scrotum, and for the other, a broken thigh 'cured without lameness'. Charge for both:	10 gns.
Operations	
Child: haematoma of skull opened	5s.
Gardener's child; abscess of neck opened	7s. 6d.
Tumor in neck opened	10s. 6d.

Nature of ailment and treatment	Fee
'Ulcer on ankle'—treated and 'cured in 6 weeks'	2 gns.
Farmer treated for 4 months for a 'sore leg'	2 gns.
'Ulcer on ancle' treated for nearly 5 months	2½ gns.
'Sinuous ulcer on leg'; operation to 'cut integuments'; thirteen journeys	2½ gns.
Inflamed leg with ulceration, treated intermittently over 2 years and 6 months	14 gns.
Miscellaneous conditions	
Embrocation supplied to a farmer	5s.
'Strained shoulder' treated	5s.
Child treated for tonsillitis	7s. 6d.
Farmer's wife: inflammed breast 'numerous dressings'	8s.
Child treated for many small abscesses following smallpox	10s. 6d.
Albugo (corneal ulcer) following smallpox: treated with eye drops	10s. 6d.
Woman treated for pains in the neck	10s. 6d.
'Phymosis and a gleet'	10s. 6d.
Farmer treated (medically) for a hard tumor in the neck	1 gn.
A woman with gross oedema of the legs and abdomen. 'Treated by scarification'—and two gallons discharged	1½ gns.

Farmer: abscess in groin opened	10s. 6d.
Inoculation against smallpox: generally	10s. 6d.
Abscess of breast opened	1 gn.
Shoemaker's wife: removal of breast tumor	1½ gns.
Tumor (? TB glands) removed from neck	£1. 11s. 6d.
'Took an uncommon substance' from a child's side	5 gns.
Removal of breast tumor	5 gns.
An apprentice: fell, fractured skull, trephined, and 'ten pieces of bone removed'	5 gns.
Amputation of leg (paid by overseers of the poor)	7 gns.
A mason: 'mortification of the sacrum, dressed twice a day'	2 gns.
An innkeeper's wife treated for 'putrid mouth ulcers'	2 gns.
Peruke maker: 8 minor episodes of illness in the family over a period of 3 years	3. 16s. 0d.
An attorney: 12 minor episodes of illness in the family treated over a period of seven years	10 gns.
Treatment paid for by the overseers of various parishes	
Sore finger	5s.
Widow with 'violent pains in the limbs'	10s. 6d.
Quinsey opened and pus discharged	10s. 6d.
Treatment of multiple abscesses	1 gn.
Treatment of large wound in the leg from a hatchet	1½ gns.
Treatment of a fractured humerus	1½ gns.
Treatment of a fractured leg	3 gns.
Venereal disease treated by mercury	5 gns.
Amputation of leg	7 gns.
Leg ulcers and sore legs	
Venesection and dressings for an inflamed leg	7s. 6d.
Housemaid treated for leg ulcers	10s. 6d.
'Cured a sore on the foot'	10s. 6d.
Treatment of a 'foul ulcer on the leg from a dog-bite'	1 gn.

Source: As for table 11.

an abscess, or pulling a tooth. Other fees were graded upwards and a selection is shown in table 14. The most serious conditions and those requiring most skill were charged the highest, as one would have expected. But the chronic lesions which needed constant dressings, like leg ulcers and discharging abscesses and sinuses, could prove very expensive for their owners.

Now, what do these fees mean? Can we put them into context? It is, of course, well known that one cannot translate the prices of 1780 into those of 1980 by a simple standard multiplication. Nevertheless, one can take as an example Pulsford's minimum fee of 5s. The evidence of Arthur Young, who toured the southern counties of England and Wales recording wage levels in 1768, is well known.[23] He found that the average wage of a day labourer was 5s. 5d., varying from 4s. 6d. a week in the winter to 6s. in the summer, with a brief peak of 10s. in the harvest; and this level of wages varied little through the second half of the eighteenth century. A fee of 5s. in 1757 would be the rough equivalent of a fee of £30 in the 1970s. A farm labourer would not be able to call on the local surgeon at these rates, unless his employer paid. There is an example of this in the records of Mr Lee of Odiham. A farm girl, Sarah Stacey, was run over by a wagon in September 1774 and suffered 'an extremely bad compound fracture of the Os Humerus'. Mr Lee treated her almost daily for three months and effected a complete cure without resort to amputation. Her employer, paying the bill of £21. 9s. 2d., must have reflected that this was probably the equivalent of the girl's wages for at least a year.[24]

William Carr (entries undated but some time at the turn of the eighteenth century) noted the fees for certain surgical procedures. His list included 'Couching 5 Gns; hare-lip 2 Gns; inoculation in London 4 Gns, say 2 Gns [in Yorkshire]; extirpation of tumor of breast 5 Gns; tapping [hydrocoele] 2 Gns; Wen [sebaceous cyst] 1 Gn; venereal lues [syphilis] 2 Gns; Gonorrhea 1 Gn; compound fractures 6 to 10 Gns; simple fracture of leg 2 Gns, arm 1 Gn or £1. 11s. 6d. Consultation half a guinea, catheter 2/6d each time; abscess 2/6d; seton 2/6d; issue 2/6d'.[25] A standard fee for venesection in the second half of the eighteenth century was 10s. 6d., but a hospital surgeon treating the well-to-do might charge considerably more. These were not just the fees for the

---

[23] Arthur Young, *A Six Weeks' Tour through the Southern Counties of England and Wales* (London, 1768).
[24] Wellcome MS 3974.
[25] Carr diaries, undated entry, probably c.1788.

rich. They are found in the bills to the middling sort of people and there is evidence that similar fees were often paid by overseers of the parish for surgical treatment of the poor. In Somerset in 1776 a parish surgeon was paid 15s. 6d. for 'setting a lad's collar bone', the simplest of all fractures to deal with.[26] In 1771, also in Somerset, a parish surgeon was paid £8. 19s. 0d. for 'laying open and curing an imposthumation' [an abscess].[27] William Pulsford in his capacity as surgeon to the poor of the In-parish of Wells was paid 3 guineas for treating a fractured leg, 5 guineas for treating syphilis with mercury, and 7 guineas for an amputation of leg.[28] Similar fees were recorded by overseers in parishes in Bedfordshire, Wiltshire, Gloucestershire, and Dorset.[29]

There is always the possibility that surviving records are a self-selected sample of the more successful prosperous practitioners. No doubt there were poor surgeons in cities and villages whose fees were lower. Equally, we know that the hospital surgeons of provincial cities were able to charge higher fees than their colleagues in the small towns. James Ford, surgeon to the Bristol Infirmary, charged the Marquis of Granby 1 guinea for venesection, £21 for 'castrating Capt. Jefferies', and between £5 and £20 for inoculating children against smallpox. This was in the 1750s when he had a wide reputation for his skills as a lithotomist, operating on twenty-five cases and losing only two. In 1758, at the age of thirty-nine, his income was £1,762.[30] Hospital surgeons were a very small minority, but ordinary surgeons in town and country were nevertheless in a well-paid occupation. Provided that they could find enough cases they could make a comfortable living by practising quite simple surgical procedures. By the end of the century the majority undertook obstetric care as well, although the wisdom of doing so from the financial point of view was more debatable.

Obstetric practice

If there was one feature more than any other which distinguished the medical practitioner of the early eighteenth century from his successor at the end of the century it was the practice of midwifery. Broadly speaking, before about 1730, midwives had the monopoly of midwifery

[26] Somerset CRO, Taunton, DP Cad, S. 13/2/4.
[27] Ibid., DP Broo. 13/2/3.
[28] Ibid., ledger of William Pulsford, DD/FS Box 48.
[29] See for example Bedford CRO, DDP 35/12/2; Wiltshire CRO, Trowbridge, 1020/107; Gloucestershire CRO, Gloucester, P. 376 and OV. 7/4; Dorset CRO, Dorchester, P. 193/OU5 and P. 220/VE1.
[30] BIBM 1, 54.

in the provinces and a near monopoly in London. By 1800 that monopoly was broken; midwifery was a routine part of the practice of practically all the rank-and-file practitioners.[31]

This may seem too sweeping. After all, William Harvey (1578–1657) has been called 'the father of English midwifery' and Percival Willoughby (1596–1685) was one of a number of noted man-midwives in the seventeenth century. Moreover, Wilson has recently suggested that man-midwifery was probably much more common before 1700 than previously supposed. He believes it was such an integral part of the practice of most surgeons that, being taken as a matter of course, it was seldom mentioned as a separate entitity.[32] But the role of the man-midwife before and after 1730 was quite different. Before, it was confined to emergency intervention in complicated labours and the use of instruments. The surgeon-man-midwife had, therefore, little or none of the extensive experience of normal midwifery which is the basis of good obstetric practice. A few of the early practitioners with a wide reputation may have become highly skilled in the difficult and dangerous operations of craniotomy and internal version. For example, in a statement revealing both about the nature and the extent of man-midwifery in the seventeenth century, Peter Chamberlen complained that the 'burthen of all the midwives in and about London lay only on my shoulders'.[33] But the average surgeon in the provinces would probably be called so rarely that his experience must have been limited. Hence, as Chapman wrote in 1759, 'The Malicious but false Report that wherever a MAN comes, *the* MOTHER, or CHILD, *or* BOTH *must necessarily die.*'[34] The absence of man-midwifery in the country was emphasized in a letter written in 1724. In this, a father wrote to his daughter (Lady Drayton) congratulating her on her first pregnancy but imploring her not have her baby in Lincolnshire where she would 'run the hazard of a Country Midwife in a country place where upon extraordinary occasion, no other help could be had ... you should not think of lying in anywhere but in London'. As far as he was concerned,

---

[31] For general histories of midwifery in the eighteenth and nineteenth century, see especially Jean Donnison, *Midwives and Medical Men* (London, 1977); J. H. Aveling, *English Midwives* (London, 1872); J. Glaister, *Dr. William Smellie and his Contemporaries* (Glasgow, 1894); H. R. Spencer, *The History of British Midwifery from 1650–1800* (London, 1927); J. M. Munro Kerr, R. W. Johnstone and M. H. Phillips (eds.), *Historical Review of British Obstetrics and Gynaecology, 1800–1950* (London, 1954).

[32] Adrian Wilson, 'Childbirth in Seventeenth and Eighteenth-century England' (Sussex University, Ph.D. thesis, 1984).

[33] J. H. Aveling, *English Midwives* (London, 1872), 23.

[34] E. Chapman, *A Treatise on the Improvement of Midwifery* (London, 1759).

the provinces in the 1720s from the obstetric point of view might have been the jungle.[35]

Further evidence is provided by Sarah Stone, the midwife whose *Complete Practice of Midwifery* in 1737 tells us a great deal about the practice of her art in the provinces in the early eighteenth century. She was trained by her mother, Mrs Holmes, also a well-known midwife, and Sarah Stone in her turn trained others. She started her career in Bridgewater around 1702, moved to Taunton and then to Bristol in 1730 before going finally to London in 1736. While she was in Bridgewater and Taunton, both quite substantial towns in the eighteenth century, there were no men-midwives at all. If obstetric difficulties occurred it was Sarah Stone herself who was sent for. Only when she moved to Bristol did she witness something quite new which infuriated her. 'Every young MAN who had served his apprenticeship to a Barber-Surgeon, immediately sets up for a Man-Midwife, although as ignorant, and indeed, much ignoranter, than the meanest Woman of the Profession.' The war between midwives and medical men which grew into a bitter and prolonged state of mutual hatred and distrust had just begun.[36]

By the end of the eighteenth century, however, the man-midwife was no longer a novelty. John Blunt was certainly exaggerating when, in 1793, he wrote that 'there are 99 Men-Midwives for one Midwife ... five new ones (some men, some boys) have set up in one street near my house within 200 yards of each other within the last six months'.[37] It is most unlikely that there was ever a time when men-midwives outnumbered the female. Even by the end of the nineteenth century when general practitioner obstetrics was at its zenith, the majority of deliveries were by midwives, especially in industrial areas, although the general practitioner delivered the majority in market towns and some rural areas.[38] A report published in 1806 showed that Nottingham had eleven midwives and fifteen surgeon-apothecaries all practising midwifery, while the county of Nottinghamshire (excluding Nottingham) had twenty-five surgeon-apothecaries all practising midwifery

[35] Northampton CRO, 'Letters of Lady Drayton', D(CA) 988.

[36] Sarah Stone, *A Complete Practice of Midwifery* (London, 1737).

[37] John Blunt (pseud. of S. W. Fores bookseller of Piccadilly, London), *Man-Midwifery Dissected* (London, 1793).

[38] 'Report of the Infant Mortality Committee of the Obstetrical Society of London', *Transactions of the Obstetrical Society of London*, 12 (1870), 132–49, and 13 (1871), 388–403. Also *Report of the Select Committee on Midwives Registration*, PP 1892, p. 144 and Q. 931.

and 123 midwives.[39] The ratios are less important than the clear statement that all the surgeon-apothecaries in the county included man-midwifery in their practice. Before the fourth decade of the eighteenth century, therefore, surgeons willing and able to undertake man-midwifery were few, and when they were involved it was only in complicated cases. After the 1730s an increasing number of medical practitioners attended normal labours as well as abnormal ones as part of the routine of their practice. That was the essence of the obstetric revolution.

The revolution in obstetrics took place at two levels. At the upper level, there were both the fashionable physician-accoucheurs and the pioneers of obstetrics as an academic discipline. The latter laid the foundations for understanding the mechanism of labour, the anatomy and physiology of the uterus, and the pathology of obstetrics. Amongst them the two outstanding figures were William Smellie (1697–1763) and William Hunter (1718–83). Works such as Smellie's *Treatise*, published in 1752 and Thomas Denman's *Essay on Natural Labours* (1786) are based on an obvious wide experience of normal as well as abnormal labours. They convey the authors' enthusiasm for the art of midwifery as an advancing and important activity for medical practitioners which required as much skill and knowledge as any other branch of medicine. They wrote, in other words, for medical men, where their predecessors wrote for the most part for the instruction of midwives. These works were both a stimulus, and a response to, the growing demand from students and young practitioners for obstetric instruction; for man-midwifery was clearly seen by them as a new and exciting discipline which was going to play a central part in their careers. Richard Kay's account of instruction under Smellie in London in 1744 is one of the earliest accounts of a systematic course of theoretical and practical instruction that was to become standard by the late nineteenth century, although the quality of teaching was probably better in 1744.[40] Likewise, Haighton, a well-known teacher at the 'Borough Hospitals', published a *Syllabus of Midwifery* (1806). It contained a summary of his remarkably full and comprehensive lectures with blank pages for the student's own notes. It also reveals the existence of a well-developed system of practical instruction, first in a lying-in institution, and then in the community.[41]

[39] Replies to Dr Edward Harrison published in the preface to *Medical and Chirurgical Review*, 13 (1804).

[40] W. Brockbank and F. Kenworthy, 'Diary of Richard Kay' (1968).

[41] Wellcome MS 2665–6, J. Haighton, 'Syllabus of Lectures on Midwifery', 1806–14. Haighton was the first lecturer in midwifery at the combined schools of Guy's and St

The lower level of the revolution in obstetrics was that of the rank-and-file practitioners. As we have seen, midwifery became a routine part of the practice of the large majority. The surgeon-apothecary became the surgeon-apothecary and man-midwife. The growing demand for obstetric training was evidence not only of the increasing involvement of medical men in midwifery, but of the importance they attached to this aspect of their practice. What was it, however, that determined the patient's choice of a midwife on the one hand or a medical practitioner on the other to attend her in labour? Price is the obvious answer, and probably it was the most important. Nevertheless, it must be remembered that in London, at least, there were fashionable midwives with thriving practices amongst the rich, the aristocracy, and even royalty. So, too had the fashionable practitioners, and it was, perhaps, at this level of rich private practice that the enmity between practitioner and midwife was greatest, although mutual hatred spread down to the lowest levels in provincial towns and in the country. In general, however, it is probably true that money was the most important deciding factor, although there were many records of men-midwives delivering the poor for very low fees or for no fees at all.

The most difficult of all questions is why the obstetric revolution occurred when it did; why man-midwifery became rapidly so popular amongst practitioners from about 1730. A frequent explanation is the introduction of the forceps which produced a sudden market for the surgeon man-midwife. Forceps, invented in the early seventeenth century by the Chamberlen family, were kept secret for three generations.[42] The design of forceps was published in the 1730s in works by Giffard and Chapman, although, as Wilson has pointed out, they were probably used and known by few practitioners other than the Chamberlens in the late seventeenth and early eighteenth century.[43] Moreover, in some

---

Thomas's Hospitals. He was by no means the first to publish a syllabus of lectures on midwifery. An equally detailed and comprehensive *Syllabus of the Lectures on the Theory and Practice of Midwifery* by John Leake was published in 1776 after his *Lecture Introductory to the Theory and Practice of Midwifery*, published in 1773. These syllabuses by Haighton and Leake are testaments to the new demand and the high standard of midwifery teaching in London by the late eighteenth century.

[42] See Glaister, *Dr. William Smellie* (Glasgow, 1894), H. R. Spencer, *The History of British Midwifery* (London, 1927), note 31, and J. Chassar Moir, *Munro Kerr's Operative Obstetrics*, 6th edn. (London, 1956), 501–8.

[43] Adrian Wilson (1984), note 32, instances John Drinkwater of Brentford in Middlesex who practised there between c.1697 and 1728 and who possessed, and presumably used, Chamberlen forceps.

parts of England man-midwifery developed long before the use of forceps became general.[44] Probably a more important factor than the use of forceps was the substantial rise in the status and prosperity of the surgeon-apothecary, who looked for ways of expanding his activities, increasing his income, and—through midwifery—acquiring a practice of regular and faithful patients. At the same time, the arrival in England of practitioners trained in Edinburgh and Glasgow was certainly influential. The establishment of the lying-in hospitals was a result rather than a cause of the revolution in obstetric care, in which the voluntary hospital principle was adapted to midwifery.[45] Some would suggest that the birth of man-midwifery was an offshoot of the rapid rise in surgery which was such a feature of the eighteenth century. Against this suggestion one can point out that midwifery was never the sole province of the surgeon. It was also practised by physicians and apothecaries. For example, at the Westminster General Dispensary in London the rules required that the accoucheurs should be physicians; across the river at the Surrey General Dispensary the accoucheurs were recruited from surgeons. The difference points to the indeterminate position of midwifery in the eighteenth century.

Perhaps one has to appeal to a number of reasons in the search for explanations for the rise of man-midwifery. Once the rise had started, however, it was rapid and substantial, and it occurred in spite of the indifference of the medical corporations and in spite of quite formidable opposition; for midwifery differed from physic and surgery in one important respect. The need for medical men at normal labours was hotly disputed—not only by midwives but also by some influential and vociferous laymen and medical men. It was, for instance, often argued that there was nothing 'more unnecessary or unmanly than for a surgeon

[44] Jonathan Toogood, MD, 'On the Practice of Midwifery, with Remarks', *PMSJ* 7 (1844), 103–8. When Toogood arrived in Bridgewater in *c.*1800 he was surprised to find that delivery with the aid of the forceps or vectis was unknown.

[45] The first of these institutions was established by Sir Richard Manningham in 1739 and became the General Lying-In Hospital in 1752 and then Queen Charlotte's Hospital. The British Lying-In Hospital (later the British Hospital for Mothers and Babies) was established in 1749, the City of London Lying-In Hospital in 1750, and the New Westminster Lying-In Hospital (later the General Lying-In Hospital, York Road) in 1765. The Middlesex Hospital was the first general hospital to open a maternity ward in 1747. In addition there were a number of lying-in charities for delivering the poor in their own homes and some dispensaries also included maternity departments for delivering the poor at their homes. Collectively the dispensaries and lying-in charities delivered far more women than the in-patient institutions and did so with much better results, as discussed in I. Loudon, 'Deaths in Childbed from the Eighteenth Century to 1935', *Medical History*, 30 (1986), 1–41. See also Spencer, *History of British Midwifery*.

or physician to neglect his patients, to sit by a lady's bedside for hours together in a natural labour which any female of prudence could manage'.[46] There are at least three arguments buried in this sentence which are important because they recur at regular intervals until the mid-nineteenth century in the publications of the opponents of man-midwifery. First, that the attendance of medical men at normal labours is robbing midwives of their 'right' to the practice of normal midwifery; second, that the absence of a medical practitioner at a midwifery case meant that he was unavailable for medical and surgical cases, especially emergencies; and third there was the imputation of something close to effeminacy in any man wishing to undertake what was properly 'women's work'. Midwifery was, as the writer put it, 'unmanly' as well as unnecessary. It was a slur that was emphasized by the well-known cartoon which represented the man-midwife as half a man and half a woman.

But the opponents to man-midwifery went further than that. It was even disputed that medical men would always be required to deal with the complications of labour, on the grounds that men created the very complications by which they justified their intervention. Midwifery should therefore be left to women. Childbirth, it was argued, was a natural process, and attitudes to midwifery were reinforced by the naturalistic philosophies of the eighteenth century associated, for example, with Rousseau. There is, indeed, a seemingly close affinity between recent pronouncements on natural childbirth and those which were current in the eighteenth century; but it is an affinity with a difference. In the eighteenth century the poor were believed to be healthily prolific in their breeding because they were closer to the savage and natural state. In contrast, the rich with their luxurious and indolent lives, deprived of pure fresh air, were most at risk from barrenness and complications of pregnancy and labour.[47] There was a certain logic in employing men-midwives for the rich rather than for the poor. However, tradition and questions of delicacy ensured a market, albeit a declining one, for the educated and literate midwife. It is a nice question whether the early eighteenth century (when the midwife was supreme) bred a larger number of educated midwives than the nineteenth when the midwife was suffering from the intense competition of medical prac-

---

[46] T. Champney, *Medical and Chirurgical Reform* (London, 1797).

[47] J. S. Lewis, 'Maternal Health and the English Aristocracy: Myths and Realities', *Journal of Social History*, 17 (1) (1983), 97–114.

titioners.[48] Unfortunately questions of this sort are hard to answer, partly because our picture of the nineteenth-century midwife is dominated by the stereotype of Sarah Gamp, and partly because the evidence on the quality of female midwifery in the nineteenth century comes largely from the heavily biased pens of medical practitioners. But it does seem likely that the fashionable society midwife known to most of the rich families in London in the mid-eighteenth century had largely, if not completely, disappeared by the mid-nineteenth century.

The opposition to man-midwifery from those who regarded it as unnecessary, unmanly, or immoral was not in the end of great importance. The accusations that were bandied about in books and pamphlets were too unbalanced and strident to have much appeal.[49] The opposition of the medical corporations—an opposition all the worse for being characterized by a mixture of indifference and disdain—was much more important. As we saw in the first chapter, none of the corporations believed that midwifery came within their province. The situation in Scotland was quite different. The first professor of midwifery in the world was appointed in Edinburgh (by the city, not the university, however) in 1726, while the first professor of midwifery in England, Dr David D. Davies, was only appointed in 1828, at University College in London, followed by Robert Ferguson at King's College in 1831. Both were physicians. Obstetrics was therefore a respectable medical subject north of the border long before it was in England, and the difference had a profound effect on obstetric practice. The London College of Physicians had always regarded intra-partum care as somebody else's job, although they agreed that disorders of pregnancy and the lying-in period were part of the practice of physic. In 1783 they instituted a licence in the 'ars obstetrica'.[50] One must not be deceived into believing

[48] See William Farr, *5th Annual Report of the Registrar General for 1841* (London, 1843), 186–96; 'Deaths in Childbed', *LMG*, NS 1 (1843–4), 747–9; and D. N. Harley, 'Ignorant Midwives: A Persistent Stereotype', *Bulletin of the Society for the Social History of Medicine*, 28 (1981), 6–9. This paper is discussed by Adrian Wilson in ibid. 32 (1983), 46–9, and by B. Boss and J. Boss, ibid. 33 (1983), 71.

[49] Some of the most notable contributions to the attacks on men-midwives were: John Blunt, *Man-Midwifery Dissected* (London, 1793); 'Proprietas', *Address to the Public on the Propriety of Midwives instead of Surgeons Practising Midwifery* (London, 1826); N. Adams, *Man-Midwifery Exposed* (London, 1830); John Stevens, *Man-Midwifery Exposed* (London, 1849); W. Talley, *He, or Man-Midwifery*, (London, 1863); Anon., *The Accoucheur and the Accoucheuse* (London, 1864). See also 'Sir Anthony Carlisle and Man-Midwifery', *Lancet* (1826–7), ii. 177–9 and 456–61. There is also a prolonged correspondence by Dr Kinglake and others on the supposed evils of man-midwifery in *MPJ* 34, 35 and 36 (1815–16).

[50] Sir George Clark, *A History of the Royal College of Physicians of London*, (2 vols. Oxford, 1964, 1966), ii 588–9.

that that indicated a change of heart however. This licence was no more than a recognition that a few distinguished physicians not only practised midwifery, but did so with such success that it seemed expedient to recognize the fact. The licence implied no responsibility on the part of the College for the teaching, examination, or organization of obstetric care, and it was in fact discontinued in 1800, probably because 'it occurred to the learned body, that since they were prohibited by their own laws, from exercising the Act of Midwifery, they are not the proper persons to decide upon the pretensions of obstetrical candidates'.[51]

In the view of the physicians the messy and indelicate business of deliveries belonged to surgery since it was essentially a manual operation.[52] But the Company of Surgeons, and its successor in 1800, the Royal College of Surgeons of London, was intent on creating a small, tight élite of London hospital surgeons who devoted, in theory, all their time to surgery and nothing else.[53] In fact, all surgeons in the early nineteenth century practised physic as well because there was not enough 'pure' surgery to keep them fully employed. But they singled out the practice of pharmacy and midwifery as the two activities in which they would take no part. They were considered the hallmarks of the rank-and-file practitioner, and any surgeon who combined either of these activities with surgery was barred from election to office within the College. Both the medical colleges rationalized their position on midwifery, the physicians by saying that delivering babies was a surgical operation, and the surgeons by saying that surgery had now become so vast that no man with the pretence of being a proper surgeon could afford to dissipate his energies in the practice of midwifery. But the attitudes of the medical corporations towards midwifery was merely one of thinly veiled contempt for such an unmanly occupation.[54] Although some physicians and surgeons, especially in the provinces, continued to practice as man-midwives or 'accoucheurs' in the nineteenth century as well as in the eighteenth, midwifery became increasingly regarded as the province of the lower ranks of the profession, and thus, almost by default, it became associated with the general practitioner. Midwifery became the central point of general practice in the nineteenth century. What was its importance to the surgeon-

---

[51] Edward Harrison, *Remarks on the Ineffective State of the Practice of Physic* (London, 1806), 13.
[52] Sir Henry Halford, PRCP, in *SCME*, Part I, 223–33.
[53] *SCME*, Part II, Q. 4725, and, indeed, the whole of the evidence of G. J. Guthrie for its illuminating account of surgical attitudes.
[54] J. Donnison, *Midwives and Medical Men* (London, 1977).

apothecary in the eighteenth century? Was it just an important source of income and no more?

The advantages and disadvantages of obstetric practice

In the eighteenth and early nineteenth century, although it was undertaken by nearly all of them, the rank-and-file practitioners had mixed feelings about the practice of midwifery. It was a hard way to earn a living. Richard Smith of Bristol maintained that 'the man-midwife, as he was termed, cannot be compensated at all by the mere lying-in fee, unless it leads to other business. I know of no surgeon who would not willingly have given up attending midwifery cases provided he could retain the family in other respects—but that is unprofitable as every accoucheur knows—I do not speak of the metropolis.'[55] Robert Hull expressed a similar view that all general practitioners are forced to practice obstetrics: 'to some it is so odious they officiate in the Army, they suffer the Navy, rather than act as midwives . . . yet it is essential, unavoidable, in civil practice.'[56]

In country areas the practitioner had little choice but to attend when called, whether it was to sit through a normal labour or answer the summons of a midwife in a difficult case. The nature of ordinary provincial obstetric practice is shown by the records of a Lincolnshire practitioner, Matthew Flinders (1750–1802) who, in 1775, recorded in his diary, forty-three deliveries. He stayed in continuous attendance in the patient's house for over twenty-four hours in two cases, from twelve to twenty-four hours in four cases, and from four to twelve hours in eleven cases. In March 1775 he attended two cases in succession and noted that he 'had not been in bed or my boots off for 40 hours'. All but a few were 'easy', 'normal', or 'excellent' labours, or at worst 'lingering ones'. It is not clear who all the patients were, but the suggestion is farmer's wives, tradesmen's wives, and probably some labourers. His usual charge was 10s. 6d. a case, sometimes 15s. or 1 guinea. His total income for 1775 was £222 of which only £32 came from his obstetric cases. As a young practitioner with a growing family, struggling to make a living, he could not afford to refuse a case; indeed, once when called to a village where he had not previously been employed, although at a distance, he 'hoped it would lead to further midwifery employment'. As he got older he complained of the weariness of midwifery as an

[55] BIBM 2, 157.
[56] Robert Hull, 'On the Divisions of Medical Labour', *LMG*, NS 2 (1841–2), 473–5.

occupation, especially when he was suffering from one of his recurrent bouts of malaria in the summer.[57]

Richard Paxton of Maldon in Essex, who practised at almost exactly the same time as Flinders, also left an account of his work in the country which he compiled at the end of his life. It was the difficulties of obstetric practice that stood out. Often he or his partner was booked to attend by the patient, but on several occasions he was fetched by the midwife to attend a dreadful late complication of a labour with which the midwife had struggled without effect. One was a woman 'who had formerly borne children, was now and had been three days in labour under the hands of a midwife'. She had been ill with diarrhoea, was in 'a dying condition with a high breech presentation and an os only the size of a half-a-crown'. Paxton dilated the os, brought down one leg and then with great difficulty the other. He delivered a dead and putre-fying baby and placenta, and his description of the smell is graphic. The patient 'revived beyond expectations but she died within twenty four hours'. While much of his obstetric practice consisted of normal, if prolonged, labours, the cases he recalled when he sat down to write 'the hysteries … being only the result of memoranda or loose papers compiled and put in some kind of form' were those which stretched his skills to the very limits. Many involved intensely difficult intra-uterine manoeuvres carried out in distant houses and cottages with no possi-bility of outside assistance. Often he remained in attendance for many hours and occasionally for two or three days, always with the dread, after a successful delivery, of losing his patient from puerperal fever.[58]

It is not surprising that some eighteenth-century practitioners in towns and cities who were able to make a good living from physic and surgery avoided obstetrics, but some adopted it for the enjoyment of exercising a skill so manifestly in demand. Danvers Ward, a Bristol surgeon, was one who practised between about 1780 and 1823. In 1822 he boasted that 'in one twelvemonth he "put to bed" 246 women of which number 20 were confined in one week.'[59] His failure to obtain a post as surgeon to the Bristol Infirmary may have robbed him of the opportunity of practising as a 'pure' surgeon. But his extensive obstetric practice was at least partly due to his enjoyment of the practice of midwifery. He 'went for low fees' according to Richard Smith, and the

[57] Lincolnshire Archives Office, Lincoln. The diaries of Matthew Flinders.
[58] Wellcome MS 3820, the case-book of Richard Paxton of Maldon in Essex.
[59] BIBM 3, 203, and 4, 48–50.

chance discovery of his accounts for 1787 show that he then delivered 121 women, the payments received being as follows:

Payment	Number of cases
None recorded	15
Half a guinea	77
One guinea	15
Two guineas	12
Three guineas	2
TOTAL	121

In the same year he noted 161 non-obstetric cases. Although the nature of these is not known in detail, they included the usual minor conditions that formed the content of surgical practice—dental extractions, opening abscesses, venesection, and the treatment of fractures and dislocation. When a midwifery case would often take up the greater part of a day or night, surgical treatments were usually simple and brief. Yet it can be calculated that Ward's average fee for midwifery cases was 14.4 shillings while that for a non-obstetric case was 14.3 shillings.[60]

Dr John McCulloch (1757–1853) practised obstetrics in Liverpool, working chiefly amongst those of modest means and the poor. His register of cases from 1798 to 1806 shows a range of fees closely similar to those of his Bristol contemporary Danvers West.

Dr McCulloch of Liverpool: Midwifery Cases 1798–1806

Fee	Number of cases
No fee listed	969
Less than one guinea	26
One guinea	1,694
One to two guineas	31
Two guineas	167
More than two guineas	10

His annual income from these fees was £248 for an average of six deliveries a week. The number of patients delivered free of charge rose sharply in 1800 (a year of great poverty) and his income from obstetrics fell from £402 in 1799 to £261 in 1800 and £128 in 1803.[61]

Practice in London, as Smith had hinted, was a different matter. Thomas Denman, when he was becoming established and only three years after his appointment as physician man-midwife to the Middlesex

    [60] Gloucestershire CRO, cash-book of Danvers Ward of Bristol, surgeon, 1786–7, ref. D. 1928. A3.
    [61] I am deeply grateful to Dr Paul Laxton of the Department of Geography, Liverpool University, for supplying me with data on the practice of Dr McCulloch.

Hospital, earned £400 from practice, £100 from lectures, and £70 from his appointment as surgeon to the royal yacht.[62] This was in 1772, and later when he became a fashionable accoucheur he earned much more. The position as far as surgeons were concerned was explained by G. J. Guthrie in 1834 in his usual style:

A practitioner in midwifery is a gentleman who makes his election at a particular period of time. He says, when he commences the profession, 'If I practise surgery alone, I shall be 30 years of age before I get £30 a year.' Then seeing the prospect in that branch of the profession is so bad, he says, 'What else am I to do? I cannot starve; I will be a practitioner in midwifery.' He knows that the public demand for practitioners in midwifery is very considerably greater than for practitioners in surgery; that the same circumstances are not required to enable him to get into practice in midwifery, as in surgery; because Mrs. Such-a-one will send for anybody as a man-midwife, who is known to be of respectable character. But persons do not go to a surgeon upon such an understanding. They usually come to him only in consequence of his great public reputation, or extensive private recommendation, or by the recommendation of the general practitioner in attendance upon the family. Consequently, a gentleman can get himself into an excellent practice as a midwife at a very early period of life.[63]

The ambitious London surgeon with his sights on a place on the College Council would renounce midwifery as soon as possible. The provincial surgeon would often continue a lifetime as an accoucheur, even when he was senior surgeon to a provincial hospital. John Greene Crosse of Norwich (1790–1850) was an example who, through extensive private and consulting practice, became exceptionally skilled in complicated labours.[64] Crosse arrived in Norwich in 1815. It was sheer bad luck that his second midwifery case died of puerperal fever in 1815, and the circumstances injured his reputation for several years.

Whilst I was detained with her during a tedious labour, a woman in the city whom I had engaged to attend gratuitously, was attended by an old woman in the absence of all other assistance and did well—such a co-incidence placed the value of my abilities in a very unfavourable light and contributed to retard my progress in the acquiring of midwifery practice even to the present [1819].[65]

---

[62] H. R. Spencer, *History of British Midwifery* (1927).

[63] *SCME*, Part II, Q. 4801.

[64] This account is based on the two remarkably full and valuable midwifery notebooks of John Greene Crosse, the first dated 1816 and the second 1833, Wellcome MS 1916–17. See Also V. Mary Crosse, *A Surgeon in the Early Nineteenth-Century* (London, 1968).

[65] Wellcome MS 1916, 'Introduction'.

By 1819, however, he was engaged to attend 65 cases and delivered 63; in 1820 he delivered 93; in 1821, 125; and in 1822, 124. In 1823 he was appointed assistant surgeon to the Norfolk and Norwich Hospital (and subsequently full surgeon) and he reduced his private midwifery practice. Between 1833 and 1843 he only attended some twenty to thirty cases a year, but his consulting practice (which he recorded separately) increased greatly. Sometimes these were cases where the patient engaged a midwife who, after hours or even days of an unproductive labour, called in a young general practitioner who would attempt a delivery, fail, and call in one or even two senior practitioners; and when they, too, had failed Crosse would be called in. Often the patient was moribund from blood loss due to placenta praevia, or a labour obstructed by a transverse lie in which, on one occasion, a previous attendant had opened the foetal thorax with a perforator, mistaking it for a head; or, most often of all, a retained placenta with an hour-glass contraction of the uterus and a snapped-off cord. These were the problems with which he dealt, always, of course, in the patient's home without anaesthetic or antisepsis.[66]

There is no record of Crosse's midwifery fees, but his total earnings in full career are thought to have been £3,500 a year. By 1843–4 his own private midwifery cases (separate from the consultation cases) had amounted to a total of 1377; of these, 5 per cent were stillbirths, and about nine of every one thousand deliveries resulted in maternal death. The forceps or 'vectis' (essentially a single blade of the forceps) was employed in 6 per cent of cases. As if the latter was considered on the high side, he explained, interestingly, the difference between institutional and private practice.

In public institutions, instruments may be used late owing to the negligence or absence or indolence of the accoucheur, but never more early than is deemed necessary because her solicitations will not be attended to; whereas in private practice the impatience of the patient or the interference of her friends may so teaze the Practitioner as to bias his judgement sooner than he deems to be absolutely necessary.[67]

In the 1840s, when Crosse listed his many activities, the list, and the order of the list, is revealing. 'A large general practice in medicine, surgery and midwifery; a consulting practice from 80–100 doctors a year; senior

66 Wellcome, MS 1917; see e.g. p. 68.
67 Ibid., MS 1916.

surgeon to the [Norfolk and Norwich] Hospital; surgeon to the Magdalen Hospital and much vaccination—30–40 weekly at my home.'

A survey of obstetrics in the eighteenth century inevitably leaves a sense of confusion and a large number of unanswered questions. Published works on obstetrics tend to tell us what was known and what was taught; generally, however, they tell us very little about day-to-day practice at the ordinary level. Thus our knowledge tends to be based on midwives and medical practitioners who, by the very fact that they wrote and published, were atypical. Questions concerning the generality of midwives—what was their background? what was their status? how much instruction did they obtain? how much did they earn? what persuaded them to take up midwifery?—these are largely unanswered. Wilson, however, has produced important evidence that suggests the workload of midwives in East Anglia and London during the seventeenth and eighteenth century was often surprisingly low; perhaps twenty to, at most, 50 cases a year each. This suggests to him that midwifery may have been only one of their occupations and their involvement in deliveries so slight that they may not have seen midwifery as the basis of their sense of identity.[68] Probably they spent as much, or more time, in treating sick neighbours, especially children, and in doing such duties as laying out the dead, than they spent in the practice of midwifery. But this is speculation.

If our knowledge of the work of the surgeon-apothecary and man-midwife is rather more complete it is almost entirely due to the preservation of a few scattered case-books and diaries of the kind quoted in this chapter. From these, at least, we obtain a consistent picture of man-midwifery as an increasingly important, time-consuming, and often exhausting branch of practice, poorly paid in terms of time and energy expended, but undertaken largely because of its central importance in building up and keeping a practice of patients. In a period when practice was becoming steadily more competitive, the importance of midwifery grew until it formed the central feature of the general practitioner and family doctor of the mid- to late nineteenth century; but the foundations of midwifery in general practice were, as we have seen, laid firmly in the eighteenth century.

[68] Adrian Wilson (1984).

5

The Eighteenth-century Practitioner: His Income and Practice

Medicine—a profitable occupation

IN the last three chapters the background, education, and clinical practice of the surgeon-apothecary and man-midwife have been the subjects. Here, we return to some of the queries raised at the beginning of chapter I and attempt to answer the general question, what sort of men were the rank-and-file practitioners of eighteenth-century England? In chapter I two contrasting views were offered: the traditional view of the semi-illiterate, shop-keeping apothecary, and the more recent view of Holmes that, by 1730, the 'doctor' in the form of the surgeon-apothecary had 'arrived in English Society'.

It is fair to say that standard histories of medical practitioners in the eighteenth century usually suggest a race consisting of a few giants and a multitude of pygmies, but with no one in between. The giants of the century—the Hunters, Heberden, Lind, Smellie, Percival, and Jenner, being the obvious examples—have received the attention due to them. But remarkably little is known of the ordinary practitioners who, if considered at all, seem to be overshadowed by the nineteenth-century general practitioner. Belief in the inevitability of progress in medical knowledge and medical education suggests the transition from the surgeon-apothecary and man-midwife of the mid-eighteenth century to the general practitioner of the mid-nineteenth was a major advance in the status and competence of the rank and file of the medical profession. It is sometimes argued that the Apothecaries Act of 1815 was not only the generator of medical education as known today, but that it also led towards a united medical profession by transforming the general practitioner into a scientifically trained professional man.

Waddington,[1] in a recent account of the medical profession in the

---

[1] I. Waddington, *The Medical Profession in the Industrial Revolution* (Dublin, 1984). The author's views on medicine in the eighteenth century and the question of professionalization were included in I. Loudon, 'The Nature of Provincial Medical Practice in

industrial revolution, describes the transition from the eighteenth century to the nineteenth using the concepts of professionalization, especially those of Freidson. Certainly there is a stark contrast, even at the simplest level, between the two centuries in terms of the medical corporations, medical associations, and state intervention in the form of statutory licensing and registration. The College of Physicians, the Company and College of Surgeons, and the Society of Apothecaries were largely irrelevant to the realities of everyday practice in the eighteenth century. The numerous associations of practitioners whose purpose was partly or wholly medico-political were a feature of the first half of the nineteenth century. Waddington argues cogently that there was no single united profession in the eighteenth century by standard criteria of professionalization, and also that it is not just the external features of professionalization that are important, but also the market for medical care. Then, however, he makes a number of assumptions about medical practice in the eighteenth century—assumptions of central importance to understanding the transition of medicine from 1750 to 1850—which must be questioned.

He believes that eighteenth-century regular or 'qualified' medical care was available only to a minority of wealthy people.[2] The market for 'qualified' medical care was limited not only for financial reasons, but also because of the persistence of attitudes which led the majority of people to prefer domestic remedies and irregular practitioners. For reasons of poverty, tradition, and a preference for irregular sources of medical care, people in general 'were not in the habit of calling in a doctor in times of illness'.[3] As a consequence, the market of regular practitioners was so slight they were forced to follow a second occupation to make ends meet. The nature of the medical consultation is described in terms of Jewson's theory that 'eighteenth-century medical men were dependent upon the favours of a small group of upper-class patients . . . who held ultimate control in the consultative relationship.'[4] This, it is suggested, led to a client-dominated rather than a practitioner-dominated form of medicine as typical of medical practice as a whole in the eighteenth century, and this concept is extended to account for some of the ideology of medicine in that century. Medical practice, in

Eighteenth-century England', *Medical History*, 29 (1985), 1–32. See also E. Freidson, *Profession of Medicine* (New York, 1972).
  [2] I. Waddington (1984), chapter 9, p. 181.
  [3] Ibid., 182.
  [4] Ibid., 191. N. Jewson, 'Medical Knowledge and the Patronage System in Eighteenth-century England', *Sociology*, 8 (1974), 369–85.

other words, consisted in the eighteenth century of an upper level of subservient practitioners dictated to by aristocratic and wealthy patients and, at the lower level, a sparse degree of regular medical care because of the poverty of the general population below the aristocracy and the thriving condition of domestic, self-administered and irregular medical care.

All of these assumptions are contradicted, however, by the direct evidence from eighteenth-century sources considered either in this or in previous chapters. The diaries, case-books, and ledgers of Richard Kay of Baldingstone, the Pulsfords of Wells, Flinders of Lincolnshire, Lee of Hampshire, Misters of Worcestershire, Harrison of Chester, Paxton of Essex, and the accounts of numerous practitioners in the Bristol Infirmary Biographical Memoirs suggest, on the contrary, that the provincial surgeon-apothecary and man-midwife of the second half of the eighteenth century was generally active, busy, and prosperous within the consumer society of that period. He was also very much an entrepreneur. If he followed a second occupation it was usually a means of investing his money to increase his wealth. Often country practitioners owned land and farmed it. One would not want to exaggerate the picture of relative wealth. Beneath the respectable carpet of medical prosperity one can speculate that there may have been an underfelt of poor and struggling apothecaries about whom few records survive. But the picture of non-élite medical practice provided by Waddington is incompatible not only with the manuscript evidence, but also with the comments in 1747 on the profitability of the trade of the apothecary,[5] that many in the country were 'eminent in their way',[6] and that surgeons were always assured of a steady living.[7]

It is also incompatible with the expansion of the activities of the rank-and-file practitioners in the second half of the eighteenth century shown by the phenomenal growth of man-midwifery and medical education, and with the ability of ordinary practitioners after 1740 to raise their fees substantially. Evidence in this and previous chapters, moreover, shows that the market for regular medical care came from a wide range of social classes and that people did indeed frequently consult the regular practitioner not only for serious disorders but also for minor self-limiting ones.

While it is reasonable to suppose that some medical practitioners were overawed by their aristocratic patients, to suggest that this was the

---

[5] R. Campbell, *The London Tradesman* (London, 1747).
[6] Anon., *A General Description of All Trades* (London, 1747).
[7] R. Campbell (1747).

dominant mode of the practitioner/patient relationship in the eighteenth century is at the very least highly misleading. The wide variety of patients treated by the regular practitioners (the aristocracy and the wealthy forming only a small minority) led to a range of subtly different attitudes of medical men to their patients ranging, as the sources show, from subservience through feelings of social equality to downright authoritarianism. The attempt to impose an all-embracing model of a client-dominated type of medical practice amongst the wealthy to medicine as a whole in the eighteenth century finds no justification in the historical evidence. While it is true that the labouring classes could rarely afford a regular practitioner, the importance of poor law medical care (both for patient and practitioner) which was touched on in the last chapter and is considered in more detail in chapter 11, is left out of the account in Waddington's portrayal of eighteenth-century practice. Finally, there is no evidence that the market for irregular practice was larger in the second half of the eighteenth century than in the first half of the nineteenth. Quantification is very difficult. Such evidence as there is suggests the contrary (see chapter 10).

To illustrate some of these points, the specific example of an ordinary and undistinguished surgeon-apothecary and man-midwife is considered in the next section of this chapter. Matthew Flinders has been chosen because of the richness of his diaries, part family history and part business ledger. Probably there were thousands like him who lived and worked all their lives in one area and, in the end, received the accolade of a memorial tablet on the wall of the local church. In this instance, the tablet can be found close to the altar: 'Matthew Flinders, Surgeon to this Parish. A Man of exemplary Manners and superior Abilities. Died May the 1st, 1802 aged 52 years.' If the name seems familiar it is because his oldest son of the same name achieved fame as a naval officer, hydrographer, and explorer of Australia where certain geographical features and a university bear his name.

Portrait of an eighteenth-century practitioner

Matthew Flinders (1750–1802) of Donington in Lincolnshire was the grandson of a farmer and grazier who moved from Nottinghamshire to Lincolnshire, and the son of John Flinders, surgeon, of Donington.[8] In 1770, at the age of twenty or twenty-one, he took over his father's

---

[8] Lincolnshire archives office, Lincoln, the diaries of Matthew Flinders (2 vols.); plus additional material from wall tablets, etc. in the church at Donington, Lincs.

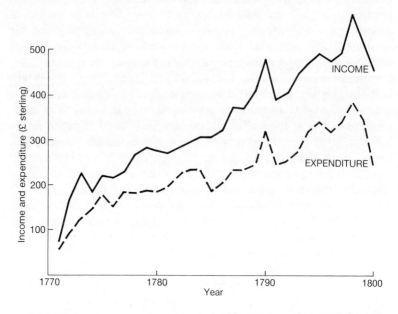

Fig. 1   Annual income and expenditure of Matthew Flinders, surgeon in Lincolnshire, 1771–1800
Source: The diaries of Matthew Flinders, Lincoln archives office, Lincoln.

practice in the market town and the surrounding flat, malarial fenland. It was neither a rich nor a particularly attractive area. Donington probably had a population of between one and a half and two thousand and a busy market, later replaced to a large extent by the market at Boston. There were few if any rich patients.

   In the meticulous financial records which Flinders kept throughout his life one finds numerous patient's bills, but small ones, seldom reaching as much as twenty pounds and usually much less. His income rose from £72 in his first year to a level of between £200 and £300 p.a. reaching a peak of £582 in 1798 (see Figure 1). Parsimonious to a fault, he kept his expenditure so firmly in hand that after twenty-seven years in 'business' he had saved and invested £2,786. He tended to agonize over small expenditures. In 1778 he closed two windows in his house 'reducing the number I pay for to 12, an annual saving of 3/4d.— now pay 17/-.'[9] But only three years later he embarked on extensive

[9]   Flinders's diaries, i, f. 30.

improvements to his property.[10] Likewise, deciding that a mangle would provide 'a very considerable saving of coals, time and trouble as regards to ironing the clothes', he paid a Mr Parker to make one for £3, but only when 'my wife and Mrs Goodwin agree to join in its use.'[11] His only servants were a maid and a lad, or rather a succession of both, one of the maids being his wife's niece. Neither servant was paid handsomely: 'Our maid Mary Goodyer is to have the same wages as before, viz. £3 [p.a.] and 3s. earnest money—my servant boy John Harmiston, I have been obliged to raise his wages to 50s. [a year] and 2/6d. earnest money . . . the lad is ingenious and can do many things which other boys cannot; as jobs in carpentry, masoning, painting, lettering bottles, etc. by which he has, and will, save me the additional wages, nor are we fond of new faces if we are any way near well.'[12] This lad's successor, less ingenious in his ways, was dropped to 30s.[13]

In 1779 Flinders toyed with the idea of an apprentice for a premium of not less than 80 guineas, and 'If I take him I intend to have some form of writing to prevent him fixing over near me'. It came to nothing, however, possibly because Flinders was terrified of opponents.[14] This showed when a young practitioner from Boston, a Mr Wrangle, settled in Donington in September 1789 and, failing to make a living, departed in less than two years.[15] Just when Flinders was complaining of the incessant work and how much he would like some help, a second opponent arrived in 1795, fresh from an apprenticeship in Spalding. Flinders promptly tried to buy him out because 'the business is very limited for two', but the young man, Ayliff, refused to go.[16]

One of the major expenses, accepted because of its importance, was the horse on which Flinders, like all country surgeons, depended. On the bad roads of the eighteenth century a chaise or carriage was impractical and a horse could cut across fields and bridle paths. At regular intervals Flinders bought a new horse paying between twelve and eighteen guineas and insisting it must be a 'good fast walker'.[17] In the early days, when Flinders and his wife went visiting, they 'went

[10] Ibid. i, (1781), f. 52.
[11] Ibid. ii, (1785), f. 8.
[12] Ibid. i, (1777), f. 21.
[13] Ibid. i, (1775), f. 13.
[14] Samuel Foart Simmons' *Medical Register* (1783) records Flinders as the only practitioner in Donington. His nearest colleagues were in Boston (2 physicians, 1 surgeon, and 8 surgeon-apothecaries) and Spalding (2 physicians and 3 surgeon-apothecaries).
[15] Flinders's diaries, ii, ff. 40 and 52.
[16] Ibid. ii, f. 77.
[17] Ibid. i, f. 52, and ii, f. 8.

double on the mare'.[18] Later he borrowed or occasionally hired a chaise for social occasions but never owned one.

Flinders resented the expense of his children, much more than his horses. He was not by nature cold or incapable of affection for his family, but he showed few signs of affection for his children when they were small and worried continually how much they cost him.[19] He delivered all his own children at home and thanked God for saving him an unwelcome addition to his family when his wife was delivered of premature, stillborn twins. This apparent lack of affection may well have been due to the habit of sending them all 'out to nurse', often for a very long time, so that they eventually returned as strangers to their family.

John, the second son, was 'put to nurse' when less than a fortnight old 'at Bett Wells's (the Lab[r]. wife) at 2/6d. a week and 1d. milk a day of Jno. Kendall ... I hope this woman will prove a good nurse'.[20] There John stayed until he was three, returning in April 1784 and recorded in the diary by the sole comment: 'this has been a very expensive child'.[21] Samuel, the third son born in November 1782, was sent 'out to nurse' until June 1784 and

Came from nurse ... [when] ... he has just begun to go alone. I have now all my five children with me, which causes a considerable additional trouble but is not so much as expected and saves me 5/6 per week in my Pockett.[22]

As they grew older there was the worry of their education. He managed this as long as he could, teaching them Latin at home. Matthew (jnr.) was sent at the age of eleven 'only half days to Mr Whitehead ... my present intentions is not to send him [to a grammar school] until twelve years old.'[23] In fact he was sent to a private school at the cost of eighteen guineas p.a.,[24] while the cost of the other boys' schooling was sixteen guineas p.a., 'but I expect every expense included with it will be not less than £20'.[25]

It was not as if he could claim to be poor. From his early days of

---

[18] Flinders's diaries, i, (1775), f. 5.

[19] Flinders's account of his wife and of her premature death are sufficient to remove any suspicion that he might have been a man incapable of love or affection. See entries for March 1783. in vol. i.

[20] Flinders's diaries, i, f. 51.

[21] Ibid. i, f. 52.

[22] Ibid. i, f. 72.

[23] Ibid. i, f. 75.

[24] Ibid. ii, f. 16.

[25] Ibid. ii, f. 57. John and Samuel were sent to school aged 11 because they had fallen in with some 'rough companions' and had developed 'very unpolished manners'.

practice, Flinders assiduously bought cottages, houses, and land, a few acres here, a few there, but always increasing in quantity. By 1792 about a quarter of his income (viz. £120) came from rents and invest-ments,[26] the largest being an estate of thirty acres with house, farm, and outbuildings which he bought for £915 in 1788, which produced a rent of £45 p.a., and which sold for £1,500 six years later.[27] In the 1790s he sold most of his land and invested extensively in '5% Stock'. His final wealth is unknown, but it is unlikely to have been less than £5,000 and may have been more. He inherited nothing from his father. His father's second wife, no friend of her stepson, made sure of that. Such wealth as Flinders acquired came from his practice and his ability to save and invest wisely. From the financial point of view he was successful and, towards the later part of his life when his children had grown up and his own financial anxiety had tempered, he was a contented man.

In this respect, Flinders was in no way exceptional. But in spite of his ample income and investments he appears to have been careful to make no show or display. His neighbours may well have mistaken his tight-fistedness for relative poverty; it often happens. And there is nothing to suggest that Flinders was socially ambitious, not even as far as his children were concerned.

Matthew, the oldest, was intended for a surgeon, but rebelled and took himself off with Capt. Bligh as midshipman to 'circumnavigate the Globe'.[28] Bligh liked him, helped him in his career, and he rose to the rank of captain and to fame. Samuel imitated his brother, joined the Navy, but never rose above the rank of lieutenant. John was always a trouble. He was apprenticed first to a printer, then to a chemist and druggist (for seven years at a premium of £50)[29] but failed at both, returned home 'deranged', and was sent to York asylum.[30] One daughter was apprenticed to a milliner in Boston for a premium of £30 because

I think it best as my young ones grow up to put them in some creditable way to obtain an honest living ... I pray God gives us his blessing in this affair, may she be a good girl and industrious, which will repay us this trouble and expence, to save the expence of an attorney I filled up a printed form of Indenture and proper stamps which I suppose will answer every necessary purpose.[31]

[26] Ibid. i, f. 70.
[27] Ibid. i, f. 31.
[28] Ibid. ii, f. 49.
[29] Ibid. ii, f. 78.
[30] Ibid. ii, ff. 106 and 110.
[31] Ibid. ii, f. 72.

His other daughter by his first marriage married, to her father's delight 'Mr Harvey, our worthy draper—he is a worthy man and as to property far beyond what we ought to expect.'[32]

Flinders seldom left home for long, fearing the loss of a midwifery fee. Social visits were rare and the only journey of note was a holiday in London with his wife in October 1796 when he stayed in private lodgings, visited 'The Abbey and theatre', and with money sent ahead and £500 he carried with him, bought £1,000 of stock. 'We both agreed', he wrote, 'this was the most agreeable jaunt we ever had.'[33]

His main recreation was reading. Although he sometimes reproached himself for the extravagance, he bought books regularly and subscribed to a succession of periodicals. His choice was eclectic. Amongst the general periodicals to which he subscribed were the *Annual Register*, the *Universal Magazine*, and the *Gentleman's Magazine*. He bought 'Dean Swift's Miscellany (3 vols.); the Laws of England; Burn's Justice (2 vols.); Hervey's Geography for £3.8.0; the entire works of the late good Bishop Newton in 9 vols. for £3.3.0 and The Beauties of England.' Purchases of medical works included 'Garth's Dispensary, a poem; the Medical Magazine, Medical Commentaries and Medical Transactions; Hamilton's Midwifery and Dr Mead's Medical Works in 3 vols.'[34]

As a staunch but critical Anglican, Flinders often travelled some distance to hear a sermon, but was usually unimpressed. Social occasions seem to have been rare, but in 1796 he helped establish a local medical society.

Drs Wilcox, Lane and six of us surgeons and apothecarys have established a monthly meeting at the Red Cow at Donington during the summer to discuss Medical Subjects and raise a small Fund for the purchase of New Medical Books. We have had two meetings—I hope it may prove a useful institution.[35]

Flinders's house stood solid, plain, and four-square, like a farmhouse; adequate rather than big. Today it might very well be the home of a doctor or local solicitor. The records of this practitioner suggest a thriving market for orthodox medical care from the local practitioner in a locality that was poor rather than prosperous. Ordinary people, it seems, came to him for major and minor illnesses and paid his fees. There is no evidence of competition from less expensive, irregular practitioners.

---

[32] Flinders's diaries, ii, f. 78. This daughter died, probably of phthisis, a few years later.
[33] Ibid. ii, f. 83.
[34] Ibid. (1775–88), i, ff. 1, 27, 45, 73; ii, ff. 3, 11, 12, 97.
[35] Ibid. (Oct. 1796), ii, f. 82.

Comparison with the records of other surgeon-apothecaries suggest that Flinders was a typical country practitioner of his time.

The income of medical practitioners in the eighteenth century

Most of the research on the income of medical practitioners in the eighteenth century has suffered from the emphasis on celebrated practitioners, nearly all practising in London. Some of these, of course, were very wealthy indeed. In the provinces, incomes were generally lower, but the financial importance of an honorary appointment to a hospital applied to both London and the provinces. The first of the provincial voluntary hospitals to be established were at Winchester and Bristol (1736–7), York (1740), Exeter (1741), Bath (1742), Northampton (1746), Shrewsbury (1747), and Liverpool (1749). The effect of hospitals on medical incomes was confined to physicians and surgeons and occurred almost entirely in the second half of the century. Likewise, the income of the rank-and-file practitioners increased, as we have seen, between about 1740 and 1750. There is no reason to see any connection between the latter and the voluntary hospitals except in so far as the hospitals enhanced the image of medicine and, directly or indirectly, medical practitioners as a whole profited.

James Ford, born in 1719, the son of a minor canon and prebendary of Wells in Somerset, practised in Bristol and in his first year, aged twenty-one, earned £42. At the age of twenty-four he was appointed surgeon to the Infirmary and his income leapt to £495. Twelve years later, in 1758, he earned £1,763 and in 1760 he left Bristol to become a London physician-accoucheur with an appointment at the Westminster lying-in hospital.[36]

John Townsend, elected surgeon to the Bristol Infirmary in 1754, worked endlessly and 'was greedy for money but often generous'. His annual income was said for many years to be between £1,200 and £1,500 but 'he spent nothing like it and left, when he died, £62,000'.[37]

William Moncrieffe, physician to the Bristol Infirmary from 1775 to 1816 earned for about twenty years an average of £2,000 a year.[38] Joseph Metford was appointed surgeon to the Bristol Infirmary at the age of twenty-eight in 1783. He earned £115 in the first year and this

---

[36] BIBM 1, 54.
[37] BIBM 1, 95.
[38] BIBM 3, 154.

was considered a good start. He died wealthy, although there are no data on his income when he was well established.[39]

The physician Andrew Carrick (1767–1838) was slow in becoming established. It was said he only earned £5 in 1789 at the age of twenty-two. In 1795 his income was £423 and in 1805 £1,287. But after his election to the Bristol Infirmary his income rose to £2,000 a year.[40]

It would be wrong to assume, however, that incomes of £1,000 or over were only available to physicians and surgeons with hospital appointments, or that the rich employed these practitioners exclusively. The example of William Broderip was mentioned in chapter 3. Broderip's income 'in full career' reached the unusual level of £4,000–£5,000 p.a.[41] Joseph Shapland, Broderip's mentor and one-time senior partner, was another highly successful apothecary who attended many of the 'best families' in Bristol.[42] From about 1740 to the end of the century a number of city apothecaries became very popular with fashionable society, but, for reasons which appear in the next chapter, the rich apothecary was rare after 1800. It was Richard Smith's opinion that, by 1808, few if any apothecaries in Bristol earned as much as £1,000, with the possible exception of 'Mr Thos. Griffiths—but then he had his diploma and also practised as a physician.'[43]

In country areas it was rare in the eighteenth century to achieve an income anywhere near £1,000 a year. Records of incomes for the first four decades are sadly very few. An apothecary who practised near Leeds at the beginning of the century, however, left a detailed record of his income from 1703 to 1710. He was busy, but visited few patients at home. Most of his practice was conducted over the counter of his shop. His income varied from £69 to £106 p.a., and was not all collected from medical practice. Thus, in the year 1 January 1703/4 to 31 December he earned £56 from medical practice and £14 from farming.[44] The records of a Dorset practitioner, probably from Wareham, show a rising income from £140 p.a. in 1697 to £260 in 1716.[45]

The records of Claver Morris of Wells are exceptionally interesting. The son of a clergyman, Claver Morris became a physician, graduating from Oxford University and acquiring the extra-licence of the Royal College of Physicians of London. He practised briefly in Salisbury before

[39] BIBM 3, 98.   [40] BIBM 8, 645.   [41] BIBM 1, 46.   [42] BIBM 1, 43–5.
[43] BIBM 1, 64.
[44] Anon. day-book of a medical practitioner near Leeds, Yorkshire, 1703–10, library of the Royal College of General Practitioners, London.
[45] John Chaplin? (provenance uncertain) of Wareham, Dorset. Medical notebook, 1667–1715, Dorset CRO, Dorchester, 15, PHI.

moving to Wells where he stayed through the first quarter of the eighteenth century. He treated the poor and the rich, but he had a high proportion of patients amongst the gentry and local aristocracy not just in Somerset but over the whole of south-west England. His reputation was as high as anyone in that part of the country, but this was the early part of the century. By comparison with the end of the century his fees were low and his income was only £100–£150 up to 1710 and between £200 and £300 thereafter.[46]

It is interesting from several points of view to compare Claver Morris, working between the start of the century and 1725, with another physician a hundred years later, Dr Lubbock of Norwich. Lubbock, in the first decade of the nineteenth century was reputed to earn £4,000 a year.[47] While Claver Morris was the son of a rector and a graduate of Oxford University, Dr Lubbock was the son of a Norwich baker, initially apprenticed to Mr Rigby, a well-known surgeon in Norwich, and afterwards a graduate of Edinburgh University. It is a striking contrast in social background and level of income, and it is not too far from the truth to say that in both respects Claver Morris and Lubbock were typical provincial physicians of their time.

But there is another and even sharper contrast, and that is between Claver Morris and the Pulsfords. The Pulsfords were surgeons in the same Somerset town (Wells) practising only some twenty-five to thirty years later than Claver Morris but practising on a much more limited and parochial basis. We know much more about the social structure of their practice, and it was certainly amongst people of a lower socio-economic level than those treated by Claver Morris. Yet, although mere country surgeons with no degrees or diploma, they earned about twice as much—probably about £400 a year each and this is not allowing for the often forgotten method of payment which was probably common in the country—payment in kind, where a farmer would pay by giving a load of hay, or when, as in the case of the Pulsfords, the surgeon and the blacksmith would sit down with a bottle of wine, calculate how much they owed each other and settle the difference.[48]

This level of income—£400 p.a.—is the level of income suggested by

---

[46] E. Hobhouse, *Diary of a West-Country Physician* (London, 1934).

[47] James Greig (ed.), *The Farington Diaries, 1793–1821*, 8 vols. (London, 1922–8), iii, 115.

[48] For details of the calculation of incomes of the Pulsfords of Wells, see I. Loudon, 'Medical Practice in Provincial England', *Medical History* (1985). Richard Smith of Bristol recorded how, in the 1790s, he was similarly paid in goods by a patient who was a woollen draper: BIBM 2, 152–3.

the records of the surgeon Mr Thomas Misters of Shipton-on-Stour, and calculated by the size of the fees he charged and the amount of business he did.[49] A similar method of calculation suggests that Thomas Roots, an apothecary of Kingston-upon-Thames, in 1752 achieved an income of between £250 and £300 from medical practice.[50] It is unlikely that Mr Lee of Odiham in Hants earned less than £250 a year of which at least £25 came from parish work, and judging by his fees it may well have been much more in the years before his presumed death in 1779; but the sparsity of the records makes accurate computation impossible.[51] Adam Smith's calculation in the *Wealth of Nations* suggests that the country apothecary in the second half of the eighteenth century would earn between £400 and £500 a year.[52]

Job Harrison is another example. He was an apothecary in Chester, whose education was apprenticeship and a spell of one year in Edinburgh where he attended lectures but took no examination and obtained no formal qualification. On his return he went into partnership with his former master in a well-established practice. Harrison died prematurely, aged thirty-six, in 1789. Outstanding bills amounted to between £200 and £300. It would be unusual for such bills to exceed annual income and it seems likely that Harrison was earning at least £300 a year.[53] For comparison, Thomas Denman illustrates the greater wealth of London practice. As we saw in the previous chapter he was earning £650 a year in 1772.[54] Danvers Ward, also mentioned in the previous chapter, who worked as a busy surgeon-accoucheur but in Bristol, not in London, achieved an income of £300 a year in full career.[55]

Scotland, in passing, was notorious for the poverty of medical practice. Glaister, in his life of Smellie, reproduces a bill from a practitioner to a writer (lawyer) in Lanark, covering a period of seventeen years from 1759–76. It includes one 'attendance', two 'cutting a child's tongue' and twenty-one items of medicine. The grand total was £1. 4s. 3d.[56] Likewise, the records of the surgeon James Steedmean of Kinross in the second half of the eighteenth century show medicines

[49] Wellcome MS 3548.
[50] Wellcome MS 4254.
[51] Wellcome MS 3974.
[52] Adam Smith, *Wealth of Nations* (London, 1776).
[53] Chester CRO, the Harrison papers, G/HS/72–106.
[54] H. R. Spencer, *The History of British Midwifery from 1650 to 1800* (London, 1927), 133–4.
[55] Cash-book of Danvers Ward, surgeon of Bristol, Gloucester CRO, D, 1928, A3.
[56] J. Glaister, *Dr. William Smellie and his Contemporaries* (Glasgow, 1894), 16–17.

dispensed for only a few pence, a quarter or less than the equivalent charges in the south of England.[57] Gideon Grey, the surgeon and hero of Sir Walter Scott's *The Surgeon's Daughter*, a novel set in the late eighteenth and early nineteenth century, travelled five thousand miles a year in his practice for an income of less than £200 p.a.—fictional, but probably accurate as Gideon Grey was modelled on an actual practitioner practising in the borders. Dr Allison's revelations of the operation of the poor laws in Scotland should be contrasted with the relatively generous payments to parish surgeons in England. In Scotland the poor-law practitioners were frequently not paid at all, and when they were, to quote one instance, it was three shillings for twelve years' attendance on seventy constant and thirteen occasional paupers.[58] Medicine, and often food, was paid out of the practitioners' own pockets. From Scotland it was also reported in the 1850s that:

In an important and populous country [area] adjoining that of Edinburgh, where the tax upon incomes of £150 was, some time ago, first established, only one medical practitioner was found to possess an income large enough to bring him under the operation of the law.[59]

Here is one very good reason why so many Scottish-born and Scottish-trained practitioners flocked to the south to settle in England, join the armed forces, or go abroad.

There is, therefore, evidence that the country surgeon-apothecary in mid- to late-eighteenth-century England could expect to earn on average £400 a year once he was well established. In provincial cities, hospital physicians and surgeons and a few fashionable apothecaries could earn an income in the thousands rather than hundreds of pounds. These were considerable incomes.

Joseph Massie's estimates of income for 1759–60 were £100 p.a. for the superior clergy and £50 for the inferior; £100 for persons professing the law and £150 for the richest farmers.[60] Possibly these are underestimates. The legal profession in particular grew richer from the growth of non-litigious business about the same time as medical practitioners.

[57] Wellcome MS 4702.

[58] W. P. Allison, *Remarks on the Poor Laws of Scotland* (1844).

[59] John Brown, *Medical Reform: Our Gideon Greys*, pamphlet reprinted from *Edinburgh Medical Journal*, Dec. 1857, in Royal Society of Medicine Tract A7. Reprinted as 'Our Gideon Greys' in *Rab and his Friends* (1858).

[60] P. Mathias, 'The Social Structure in the Eighteenth Century: A Calculation by Joseph Massie', *Economic History Review*, second series, 10 (1), (1957–8),30–45.

Holmes suggests £100–£200 as the income of the minor clergy, c.1740, and at least £250 for the middle ranks.[61]

Thus, in the early years of the eighteenth century the 'trade, business or profession' of the surgeon-apothecary may have been poorly paid; from the mid-eighteenth until the end of the century it was not. It was probably the rule that rank-and-file practitioners were men of property and substance in the country. In the cities, while it was probably true that the poor practitioners were sometimes very poor, the richest could be very rich indeed. Their grandsons and great-grandsons may well have looked back at them with envy.

The patients of the surgeon-apothecary

To have achieved such incomes required a substantial number of patients able to pay high fees. The popular belief that there was, somewhere on the social scale, a divide above which all employed a physician and below which all employed the rank-and-file practitioner, is not supported by the evidence. There may have been a tendency for such a divide in large towns and cities where physicians were plentiful, but it was not the normal state of doctor/patient consultations. The surgeon-apothecary especially in country areas was the regular medical attendant to a wide range of social classes. Two sources from the second half of the eighteenth century provide a profile of patients: one from a surgeon-apothecary in Hampshire,[62] and the other from the Pulsfords of Wells in Somerset, where there was at least one physician in the town.[63] The occupational status of these practitioners can be seen in tables 15 and 16. Job Harrison of Chester (c.1754–89) was an apothecary whose family, originally yeoman farmers, rose to become mill-owners, iron-founders and mayors of Chester. Harrison was a close friend of Drs John Haygarth and William Currie, and his regular patients included a peer, an 'esquire', clergy, lawyers, army officers, a surgeon, an alderman, tradesmen, and innkeepers.[64]

These were the patients of the rank-and-file practitioners; but who were their social equals? It is difficult to answer that question. A grocer,

[61] G. Holmes, *Augustan England: Professions, State and Society 1680–1730* (London, 1982).

[62] Wellcome MS 3974.

[63] The physician in Wells from c.1750 to 1771 was Henry Harington (1727–1816), a noted composer of music who later moved to Bath. He is mentioned twice in the ledger of William Pulsford (*DNB*).

[64] Chester RO, the Harrison papers, G/H/72–106.

Table 15 *William Pulsford's cases*[a]—*occupation or status of patients*

'The Hon. Esq.'	1	'Serjeant' (Army)	1
Esq.	1	Clerk	1
Attorney	3	Silversmith	1
Captain (Army)	1	Carpenter	1
Clergy	1	Millwright	1
Farmer	12	Tanner	1
Innkeeper	7	Peruke maker	1
Servant	6	Glover	1
Servant boy	3	Hatmaker	1
Gardener	1	Organ builder	1
'Gardener at the Pallace'	1	Glazier	1
'Porter at the Pallace'	1	Brazier	1
Shoemaker	5	Thatcher	1
Shopkeeper	4	Wheelwright	1
Apprentice	3	Staymaker	1
Stocking maker	2	Pine maker	1
Mason	2	Chandler	1
Blacksmith	2		
TOTAL			73

[a] A record of occupation or social status was only made in about a quarter of the cases; the list, therefore, may not be representative of William Pulsford's practice as a whole.
Source: as for table 11.

Table 16 *Occupation or status of patients treated by a Hampshire practitioner,*
1777

Baronet	1	Carpenter	1
Right Hon	1	Sawyer	1
'Gentleman of the Hunt'	2	Potter	1
The Revd	1	Glazier	1
Farmer	9	Gardiner [sic]	1
Shepherd	1	Collar maker	1
Wagoner	1	Baker	1
Wheelwright	1	Servant	1
Blacksmith	2	Mason	2
Miller	1	Paper maker	1
Malster	1	[Game] keeper	1
	Widow	3	
	Plain Mr or Mrs	14	

Source: Prescription book of an unidentified practitioner in Hampshire (probably Mr Lee of Odiham), Wellcome MS 3974.

after all, might boast of regular customers from the same social profile as the surgeon-apothecary, but neither he nor his customers would assume a social relationship on that basis. As long as the rank-and-file practitioner kept to his 'surgery' or 'shop' the counter was a physical and social barrier between him and his patient. Visiting patients at home, however, and becoming the confidant of family affairs, put the practitioner more on a par with the solicitor than the grocer, and tended to break down, if only to a limited extent, the social barriers. It is known that home-visiting played a steadily increasing part in the practice of the eighteenth-century surgeon-apothecary, but little is known of the extent to which he saw patients in his own house or set aside a room specifically for that purpose. Possibly it was so usual, so commonplace, that it was rarely recorded. Richard Kay referred on a number of occasions in his diary to 'home patients' and the context suggests they were local patients who came to Kay's house to consult him or his father. Richard Kay's diary is valuable not only in this respect, but even more because, unusually, he recorded the details of daily routine practice and his attitudes to his work and to his patients.[65]

He makes several references to dividing the day with his father, one staying for the 'home patients' while the other 'rode abroad' visiting. Thus, on 18 May 1742, 'This Day in the morning, I assisted Father in a Throng of Patients, in the afternoon Father waiting on some Patients abroad, I served them at Home.' Likewise, on 11 April 1747, 'This day after attending a while upon Patients at Home, I visited several sick Patients Abroad which is my general Method of spending every Day.' The Kays, father and son, were busy and had little free time. On 13 August 1746 when he was thirty years old and his father sixty-two ('and at the best age for doing business'), he wrote: 'we have daily Business, God be thanked for our daily success.' That day he had travelled twelve to fourteen miles and visited a young woman 'bad in her belly with a dangerous fever', a young man with a fever whom he bled, a girl with a 'strumous disorder' under her chin, 'an Antient woman with a bad pain in her hip', a young woman anxious about her first pregnancy, 'A Brother and Sister both consumptive', a woman with a sore leg and another with a 'very sore stinking leg', and 'A Man under a Strumous Disorder in his arm. These particulars have been the occurrences of the Day.'

Frequently Kay returned late from such a round, only to be called out again, as on 24 April 1746 when, having 'returned home this Evening betwixt 10 and 11 o' th' clock and not many Minutes afterwards [I] was sent for to visit a Person who was seized very bad this

---

[65] W. Brockbank and F. Kenworthy, 'Diary of Richard Kay', *Chetham Society*, 16 (1968).

Evening in his Belly, waited upon him till three o' th' clock this morning.' On frequent occasions Richard Kay travelled many miles on horseback, perhaps to visit a patient in the night and stay for hours or even until the morning, not leaving until he was sure the patient was improving or that there was nothing more he could do. He was a man of great compassion.

in the course of my business [I] have frequently to deal with Persons where their disorders are attended with favourable and many Times with unhappy Circumstances; I am not an idle Spectator, an unconcerned Visitor, when I see the Afflictions and Distresses of my Neighbours and fellow Creatures; yet the Lord hath hitherto in some good Measure helped me; by his Grace I am what I am.[66]

So busy was Richard Kay that his only concern was the neglect of his religious devotions.

I do not spend near that Time in my Closet I formerly did, neither have I leisure time so much for Closet Duties, yet I beg I may never be a Stranger to my Closet; my employment at present is of a much more Publick Nature, it is my duty to be about my Father's Business; I am sent for, I am called upon in Haste, I must go; we seldom have a leisure Hour.[67]

Other sources are seldom as informative on when and where practitioners saw their patients. John Townsend, however, who lived in Broad Street, Bristol and practised as a surgeon, had a surgery to which the patient could admit himself discreetly at night by a door in a side-alley. The reason was Townsend's many syphilitic patients.[68] But this was a special case. Generally the successful practitioner of the mid- to late eighteenth century owed his success to visiting patients at home, especially in the country. As William Carr remarked in the 1780s: 'The Business of a Country Surgeon will greatly depend on his riding about much; if he does that he will be fully employed; if he stays i' th' house he'll not get employed in the country.'[69] Two things above all were essential for success as a country practitioner: a good reputation and a good horse.

Medical men and their transport

It was, therefore, no more than stating the obvious when a *Lancet* editorial asserted in 1841 that 'the country doctor's horse is as indis-

---

[66] Ibid., 28 Mar. 1748/9.
[67] Ibid., 11 Apr. 1747.
[68] BIBM 1, 95–7.
[69] Diaries of William Carr, Wellcome Institute, London.

pensably necessary as himself to the pursuit of his practice.'[70] The practitioner's most valuable piece of equipment, his horse, was neither highly bred, elegant, nor (within the wide range of prices) expensive. But it had to be reliable, possessed of unusual stamina and, as Flinders emphasizes, 'a good fast walker'.[71] If the country doctor today is sometimes apt to talk at length on the choice of his car, his predecessor in the eighteenth and nineteenth century was even more concerned with the care and choice of his transport. Flinders in Lincolnshire preferred mares. Richard Kay in Lancashire rode a temperamental bay stallion.[72] William Carr junior in Yorkshire bought a chestnut pony.[73] If the three of them had been able to meet they would have found common ground in the talk of horses and argued at length, as experts will, on the merits of various breeds. But they would have agreed on the cardinal qualities—stamina, strength, and safety. John Simpson, MD, as a young physician in Bradford in 1825, took the greatest trouble over the choice of a horse, going everywhere on horseback and rarely by carriage. Having parted with one which had 'bad feet', he was shown another with a stiff way of going and an ugly, long back. But he bought it in the end because it was strong and safe, and called it 'Weasel' from its general appearance. His uncle had a beautiful animal that he would have given his nephew but it was known to be unpredictable and unsafe—not a horse for a doctor. Weasel cost Dr Simpson £20.[74]

Throughout the eighteenth and nineteenth centuries the rank-and-file practitioners bought or hired horses chosen for their ability to withstand an arduous life. In fact the introduction of the railway system in the nineteenth century, while abolishing the need for long-distance coach horses, stimulated the breeding of just such small tough horses, suitable for short distances. The increase in such horses in city, town, and country throughout the nineteenth century has been documented recently by a number of historians.[75] By the end of the nineteenth century an author and expert on horse-hiring knew exactly what was required for medical practitioners.

[70] *Lancet* (1841–2), ii. 95.
[71] Flinders's diaries, Lincolnshire archives office, i, f. 30 (1779).
[72] Brockbank and Kenworthy (1968).
[73] The diaries of William Carr, Wellcome MSS 5203–07.
[74] E. Willmott (ed.), *The Journal of Dr John Simpson of Bradford* (Bradford, 1981).
[75] See F. M. L. Thompson, *Victorian England: The Horse-Drawn Society* (Bedford, College, University of London, 1970) and chapters in F. M. L. Thompson (ed.), *Horses in European Economic Society: A Preliminary Canter* (British Agricultural History Society, 1983).

The man with a consulting practice wants a different sort of horse to the humbler general practitioner. The consulting man must have a pair that go fast and well, and cover long distances, and draw up at the door in a style that will inspire the patient ... and move the general practitioner to envy. The said general practitioner must have a horse that is ready for work at all hours, and looks none the worse for standing about in the rain; in other words one wants a coach-horse, the other a good hackney, which some would consider the better horse of the two. There is no doubt that the typical doctor's horse, the horse of a hard-working general practitioner, has a trying life. Like the maid-of-all-work, his work is never done, and he must be exceptionally sound and robust to stand the wear and tear of day and night ... He may not look so well as the animal driven by the country medico, who generally takes a pride in his horseflesh, but he costs quite as much and does not last as long. Six years work is as much as can be expected of him ...[76]

Thirsk tells us that riding on horseback, relatively uncommon before 1500, became increasingly the common man's way of getting about by the end of the seventeenth century.[77] By the eighteenth and nineteenth century the importance of the horse was such that it had become the most privileged of all species of animals, treated with care and credited with semi-human attributes.[78] Few amongst the professional classes were so utterly dependent on their horse as the country practitioner, and their devotion to their horses is often striking. Matthew Flinders, not usually given to the display of emotion, recorded in 1798 that 'My old Pony, poor Taffy, died—he shrunk to a skeleton, having for above two months refused Hay and Corn and would eat only a little grass—he has carried me I think more than 5 years, and I feel concerned for his loss.'[79] Mr Wells, the elderly, kindly surgeon of Bourton-on-the-Water in the early nineteenth century, would forgive his apprentice almost anything except over-riding his favourite mare who knew the practice so well that when the apprentice got lost in the hills and valleys of the Cotswolds he dropped the reins and the mare took him safely home.[80] There have been countless stories commending the wisdom of the horses; how they have been known to trundle home late at night with their exhausted master fast asleep in the saddle;[81] but the horse,

[76] W. J. Gordon, *The Horse World of London* (London, 1893), 121–2.

[77] J. Thirsk, *Horses in Early Modern England: For Service, for Pleasure and for Power* (University of Reading, 1978).

[78] K. Thomas, *Man and the Natural World: Changing Attitudes in England, 1500–1800* (London, 1983) esp. pp. 101–2.

[79] Flinders's diaries, ii, f. 90 (5 Mar. 1798).

[80] J. L. Mann, *Recollections of my Early and Professional Life* (London, 1887).

[81] John Brown, 'Our Gideon Greys' (1858).

too, could suffer exhaustion, and William Carr made careful notes in his diary on the need to carry a 'pocket-full of corn' or 'an oatcake' to prevent his horse from stumbling after four or five hours. A colleague told Carr he must build a shed for his horse in the winter and keep 'a tub filled with hay or corn' twice daily 'to renovate' its 'strength and agility'.[82] 'Many a one-horse doctor', wrote W. J. Gordon, 'walks his round on Sunday to give his weary steed a rest.'[83]

The horse deserved such care. He was a faithful servant, a constant companion, and an expensive item in the practitioner's budget. Thirsk has shown the wide variety of prices paid for horses at the end of the seventeenth century, from colts costing £2. 10s. to £3, to coach horses at £15 each, and fine-bred horses up to and beyond £200; and she has likened the breadth of the market to that of today in new and second-hand cars.[84] The country practitioner's horses were mostly in the lower middle range. Prices recorded in medical diaries and ledgers were never less than £10 and rarely more than £30.[85] Sometimes two horses were kept, one for the day and one for the night.[86]

It would be a mistake, however, to picture the country practitioner going his rounds on horseback as the personification of peaceful rural bliss. It was, especially in the winter, a hard slog, and often dangerous. Richard Kay fell heavily from his horse on a number of occasions, once breaking a favourite cupping-glass in his pocket.[87] Another time he had a narrow escape when, returning from visiting a patient 'under a fever' in the pitch dark, he and his horse fell over the parapet of a bridge into a river. Both were submerged. Kay's foot was caught in a stirrup and he thought his horse was dead; but, freeing himself, he pulled his horse

[82] William Carr diaries, 25 May 1803 and 16 Dec. 1807.

[83] W. J. Gordon (1893), p. 122.

[84] J. Thirsk (1978).

[85] Dr John Simpson of Bradford, however, complained of the price of horses in 1825. He spent £37. 10s. on a mare and complained: 'A decent hack cannot be got under £25 or £30 and a good hack not much under £40. Anything in the hunting way cannot be got under £50 and real good hunters not under £100. Carriage horses will be about the same as hunters. Some hunters fetch as high as £200 or £300, or even £500. I believe Sir Harry Goodricke refused last year £1000 for a hunter, but that price was enormous.' E. Willmott, *Journal of Dr John Simpson of Bradford, 1825* (Bradford, 1981), 15 Feb. 1825, p. 12.

[86] In Sir Walter Scott's *The Surgeon's Daughter*, the hero Gideon Grey had two horses— Pestle and Mortar. 'Dr Camomile', a caricature of the country general practitioner of the 1850s, had 'a stable with two stalls whose inmates are never destined to enjoy each other's society, as Dr Camomile drives one about all day and rides the other round the country all night.' 'The Income Tax and its Oppressive Effects on General Practitioners', *PMSJ* (1851), 111–12.

[87] Brockbank and Kenworthy (1968), Apr. 1738, June 1749, Mar. 1749/50.

to its feet and found they were both, miraculously, uninjured. Next day he measured the height of his fall and it was six yards.[88]

In 1709 James Clegg was 'riding double' with his wife when his 'headstrong horse boggled, ran away with us and cast us off in a very dangerous place'. They were unhurt, but in 1732 Clegg's young mare fell and Clegg was 'so stunned by the Fall as to be taken up for dead'.[89]

But in spite of the dangers and fatigue, riding on horseback was out of necessity the preferred method of the majority of country practitioners in the eighteenth and nineteenth centuries. Nor was it confined to the rank and file. Richard Smith senior in the late eighteenth century, even when he was the senior surgeon to the Bristol Infirmary, invariably rode on horseback.[90] Returning home in the early summer of 1791, unusually exhausted from visiting patients, he finally conceded that 'he would indulge himself in keeping a carriage'; but the fatigue was the first sign of his final illness and he died a short time later.[91] Mr Wells of Bourton-on-the-Water was forced through lameness to travel in a 'donkey-chaise', but it was 'dreadfully slow' in the hilly country.[92] Broderip was a rare example of an apothecary who employed a coach and a coachman; but Broderip was rich and excessively fond of displaying his wealth.[93]

Two advances in road transport led to increased use of carriages. The first was in carriage design, especially between 1750 and 1770;[94] and the second was the improvement in the roads, associated especially with Thomas Telford (1757–1834) and John Loudon MacAdam (1750–1836), during the early nineteenth century.[95] To an increasing extent from about 1820 medical men used carriages. But they were apt to be expensive and were taxed. In the 1790s the average four-wheeler cost, depending on size, between £16 and £24. A 'Whiskey' could be bought for as little as £9, a gig for £11, and a curricle (mainly for the quality trade as it needed two horses) for £15.[96] Country gigs of the kind used

[88] Ibid., Dec. 1748.

[89] Vanessa Doe, 'Diary of James Clegg', *Derbyshire Record Society*, 3 vols. (1978, 1979, 1981), i. 2, 151.

[90] The father of the Richard Smith whose memoirs are used so extensively in this study.

[91] BIBM 2, 558–66.

[92] J. L. Mann, *Recollections* (1887).

[93] BIBM 2, 156–64.

[94] See especially William Felton, *A Treatise on Carriages* (London, 1794); Anon., *The Book of Carriages* (printed for the SPCK, London, 1853); H. McCausland, *The English Carriage* (London, 1948); and M. Watney, *The Elegant Carriage* (London, 1961).

[95] Sir Walter Gilbey, *Early Carriages and Roads* (London, 1903).

[96] W. Felton (1794).

by farmers were often roughly built. In 1790, if they cost less than twelve pounds and had 'taxed cart' painted on the side, tax was only twelve shillings. Above that, tax was £3.17s. for two-wheelers and £8 16s. a year for four-wheelers.[97]

To the initial costs of horse and carriage one had to add tax, feeding, and maintenance. It could be an expensive affair, but it was essential for the young physician setting up in practice to demonstrate his status and worth by his horses and carriage. The author of *A General Description of all Trades* in 1747 remarked that when a physician set up in business 'the first object of his Care is a Chariot, the next an Apothecary, both with the same view, that of introducing him to Business.'[98] Claver Morris of Wells at the beginning of the eighteenth century rode in a calash (a light low-wheeled carriage) while the surgeons, Benjamin and William Pulsford, some twenty years later went everywhere on horseback.[99] The first physician in Bristol to own a carriage was Dr Middleton in the 1730s. His carriage 'was a great lumbering thing without springs ... the horses never went beyond foot-pace ... it was in fact a sort of genteel waggon.'[100] Thomas Shute, a surgeon, ran 'a small sulky, just large enough to hold him and no more' and looked very odd in it in his eccentric clothes.[101] But it was the surgeon John Townsend who was the most eccentric. He was an endless worker who would 'often eat standing up, a slice off the spit in a patient's house'. In the 1770s he employed a day and night coachman at a cost of £100 a year to drive a carriage of his own design with special pockets to hold tins of ointment, spatulas, tooth instruments, forceps and splints—'ready for any emergency'.[102]

Surgeons and physicians, practising in cities and earning high incomes, could afford the hire of coach and coachman, but it was expensive. Dr Ludlow of Bristol, who had raised himself from surgeon to the Infirmary to physician by purchasing the MD St Andrew's in 1771, hired a coach on a long-term basis in 1775 from Weekes and Ross of the Bush Tavern, Corn St, Bristol, with a pair of horses. The

[97] M. Watney (1961), G. A. Thrupp, *The History of Coaches* (London, 1877), and W. B. Adams, *English Pleasure Carriages* (London, 1837).

[98] Anon., *A General Description of all Trades* (London, 1747).

[99] E. Hobhouse, *Diary of a West-Country Physician* (1934), and ledger of William Pulsford, Somerset RO, Taunton, DD/FS Box 48.

[100] BIBM 1, 38–9.

[101] Hence the name 'sulky' as opposed to the 'sociable' with room for two. BIBM 2, 860.

[102] BIBM 1, 95.

cost was £50 for a half-year. A Dr Lean hired 'a coach for the day and two drivers' from the same firm for a charge of 1 guinea.[103] From various sources it seems that practitioners in the nineteenth century who owned a carriage used it in the daytime for the ordinary round of visits but went out at night on horseback.[104] The time and energy required for harnessing a horse in the carriage at night would be an obvious explanation.

Physicians were often mocked for their ostentatious choice of horses, coaches, and coachmen. An army officer in *Pendennis* grumbled at the outrageous arrogance of Dr Goodenough for presuming to possess 'as foin a pair of high-steppin' horses as ever a gentleman need sit behind, let alone a Dochter'.[105] In one of a series of 'intercepted letters' published in the *Lancet* in 1833, the young physician was advised to keep a carriage and liveries in rich colours, driven in an appearance of perpetual hurry and filled with loose papers and notes. The carriage should be out all day, the horses sweating and mud-spattered, to give the impression of a busy and popular physician. 'The late Mr Heaviside always contended that his cream-coloured carriage picked out in skyblue, and a pair of grey horses, hooked many a patient for him.'[106] When, in Worcester in 1825, a vacancy occurred at the Infirmary, the young physicians 'Hastings, Malden and Lewis ... made a grand exhibition of gigs and highly decorated horses and footmen, driven with such rapidity through the streets that "merciless death was never before so closely pursued".'[107] Even the quacks, or at least the most prosperous, took a leaf from the physicians' book. Dr Day in 1775, a well-known empiric, 'kept an elegant carriage with two footmen in green livery'. It was considered to be the height of impertinence.[108]

There is a social history of medical practitioners and their transport which has yet to be written. Until this century a large and finely graded variety of horses, carriages, fitments, and footmen's livery, provided

[103] PRO, chaise-books, Messrs Weekes and Ross, C/104/139–40. The driver of 'Dr Townsend' was paid 11s. a day and two other drivers only 9s. a day. Driving a doctor may have been more prestigious, or more arduous, or both, than the ordinary run of hirings. My gratitude to Dr Jonathan Barry for this reference.

[104] 'Dr Camomile', for example; see note 86.

[105] W. M. Thackeray, *Pendennis* (London, 1850).

[106] 'Intercepted Letter: Advice to a Young Physician', Letter IV, *Lancet* (1833–4, no. 1), 797–8. The author of the series of 'Intercepted Letters' was the surgeon James Wardrop, J. F. Clarke, *Autobiographical Recollections* (London, 1874).

[107] An interesting sidelight on Dr Chas Hastings, the founder of the British Medical Association, in his youth, in *Gazette of Health*, 10 (1825), 338.

[108] 'Quacks and Empiricism', Letter II, *MPJ* 12, (1804), 137.

evidence of relative wealth or poverty, of sound conservative taste, or uncalled-for flamboyance. The discerning eye of patients and fellow-practitioners would have noted these finer points and judged accordingly that 'Mr' or 'Dr So-and so' was doing well, doing badly, was thoroughly respectable, or given to vulgar display. The infinite variety of horse-flesh and equipment by which the medical man could be judged makes the mere choice of a car today seem pale and mundane by comparison. But sources on the socially significant details of personal transport in the eighteenth and nineteenth centuries are rarer than might be supposed. Here we have only touched on the subject in order to make a few broad generalizations which can be summarized as follows.

In the eighteenth century the rank-and-file practitioner travelled, with few exceptions, on foot or on horseback.[109] Most physicians and some surgeons travelled in a carriage, at least in towns and cities. In the nineteenth century the enormous improvement in the roads made light, cheap, one-horse vehicles a practical proposition.[110] To an increasing extent the town general practitioner owned, or more often hired, a one-horse carriage; while any physician worth his salt ran a carriage and pair. In the country much depended on the roads within the practice area. Riding was often the most practical, if not the only method of visiting patients. Nevertheless, the country doctor in his horse and trap became increasingly familiar in the late nineteenth and early twentieth century. The richest general practitioners would rival the physicians in the grandness of their 'turn-out'. There is a touching and revealing item in the 'medical news' of the *Lancet* for 1853:

An act indicative of the kindest sympathy and highest respect has recently been shown by the patients of Mr Jackson, Surgeon of High Wycombe, Bucks, in the presentation to him of a handsome brougham, built by Hoadley, of Kensington, upon his recovery from an illness, as a mark of regard, and their anxiety for the maintenance of his health.[111]

---

[109] At Birmingham Dispensary the visiting apothecary who visited the sick poor in their homes complained that he walked the length and breadth of Birmingham visiting up to 79 patients a day. In 1825 the Committee of the Dispensary agreed to provide him with a horse. Records of the Birmingham General Dispensary, committee minute books, Birmingham Dispensary, Birmingham.

[110] Edward Taylor, a practitioner in Wakefield who had many patients outside the town, was the first in his area to 'set up a gig'. H. Clarkson, *Memoirs of Merry Wakefield* (Wakefield, 1887).

[111] *Lancet* (1853), ii. 615

Mr Jackson (MRCS 1842, LSA 1832) was a general practitioner. Patients and fellow practitioners would no doubt have appreciated the implied significance of 'Hoadley of Kensington'. On such details was the scale of worth and respect constructed. It was, at all events, a handsome present.

PART 2

Medical Reform and the Creation of the General Practitioner, 1794–1850

6

The Rise of the Druggist and Medical Reform

The acrimony of the period of medical reform

THE period from 1794 to 1858—that is, from the foundation of the General Pharmaceutical Society of Great Britain to the Medical Act—is known as the period of medical reform. In many ways the remarkable feature of this period was not so much the reforms accomplished as the extraordinary degree of hostility and bitterness generated within the profession. Intra-professional conflict was one of the outstanding features of the transition from the disparate group of mid-eighteenth-century practitioners based on a more or less tripartite structure, to a structured and unitary profession in the mid-nineteenth in which the ranks and divisions within the profession were clearly demarcated and are recognizable still as the main divisions in the medical profession of Britain. The bitterness and hostility of this period arose largely from the struggle for position, status, and power between the new majority, the general practitioners, and the old-established minority of established physicians and surgeons and their representative corporations. The questions that need to be answered are why the transition took place, and why it took place at that particular period.

There is, at first sight, no obvious reason why the period of medical reform should have begun at the end of the eighteenth century. As we have seen, for the majority of practitioners the second half of the century appears to have been one of increasing prosperity and status, when medicine was one of the commodities in growing demand through the 'birth of the consumer society'. Of course, there were exceptions. There were impoverished practitioners as well as prosperous ones, and there was rivalry and competition and at least a certain degree of antagonism between the physicians and the rank and file. Yet, in the end, we are left with the paradox that the period of medical reform appears to have followed a period of general contentment and prosperity when the established practitioners increased their incomes and investments and the younger generation enthusiastically improved their medical education.

Periods of reform, perhaps, require two sorts of preceding events. A preliminary period of growing discontent and awareness of the need for change, and a trigger factor, often of apparent triviality, which initiates the reform movement. For the period of medical reform, the trigger factor seems to be clear. It was the rise of the dispensing druggist; the difficulty is to identify reasons for discontent of a more solid and convincing nature.

One could, of course, argue that medical reform was forced on medical practitioners by the nature and the rapidity of change that was occurring in the country at the time. There is no need to spell out the extensive changes which characterized the late eighteenth and early nineteenth century, except to say that industry and rapid urban growth produced a crisis in health for which the structure of medical institutions and the organization of medical men were ill-prepared. Was this the generator of medical reform? To say 'yes' might be to suggest that medical men saw what was going on around them and made a conscious decision to reform themselves in response to these changes; in other words, reform was instituted for the improvement of the public health. There is, however, little evidence of any such public-spirited motivation although lip-service was paid to such ideas on frequent occasions.

Alternatively, it could be argued in more general terms that the impetus for progress and change in a world which seemed to be going faster and faster was so powerful that it picked up the small world of medicine and swept it along on the tide of electoral and other reforms that were so conspicuous during this period. It is tempting to follow this idea and to cast the general practitioner as the radical reformer demanding change, and to set him against a reactionary élite of physicians and surgeons committed to the status quo. A detailed examination of the political and religious beliefs of all who were active in medical reform might, for instance, reveal a loose association between medical reformers on the one hand and political radicals and religious dissenters on the other. On the whole, however, this does not stand up to close examination. There was little evidence of a close correspondence between the world of general politics and that of medicine, although a glance at some of the major figures might suggest that there was. Thomas Wakley, the irascible editor of the *Lancet*, is the outstanding example of a raucous medical reformer who was also a political radical.[1] James Parkinson was, in general politics, a radical of impeccable cre-

---

[1] S. Squire Sprigge, *The Life and Times of Thomas Wakley* (London, 1897).

dentials and a member of a secret society who narrowly escaped prosecution for his involvement in the 'pop-gun' plot.[2] In the field of medical reform, however, his reforming zeal was much less radical. Both have achieved a place in the history of the period—Wakley for his journal, Parkinson for the description of the disease which carries his name. Other practitioners, radical to a greater or lesser degree, could be cited, but they are hard to find amongst the majority. Most, it seems, were of the same mind as the medical man who wrote to the *Lancet* and introduced himself by saying, 'although I am Tory to the backbone in General Politics, I am Radical to the heart's core in Medical Politics.'[3]

Medical reform was remarkably inward-looking, and medical men who took a political stance kept their politics in watertight compartments as far as medicine and general affairs were concerned. Of course the reformers were children of their time and can not have been immune to the prevailing atmosphere of their age, but there were few connections between the state and medicine and little reason for the politics of the one to reflect the mood of the other. It is notable that the general public heard little and understood less of the politics of medicine, and would probably have been startled to learn that in the opinion of an unusually perceptive physician, Dr Barlow, 1813 was a time when

so strangely perverted and unharmonised has the whole medical profession become in this country that it is impossible to conceive any change that could be as productive of equal recriminations. The surgeon exclaims against the apothecary, the physician answers both, the apothecary retorts and thus they go on mutually exasperating each other by every vilifying epithet and opprobrious insinuation until they have rendered life such a scene of heart-burning animosity and contention, that the strongest feeling of every liberal mind must be a desire to escape for ever from the profession and its bickerings ...[4]

Dr Barlow makes it sound remarkably like a family quarrel, and so, in a sense, it was. The key to understanding medical reform may be that medicine as a whole had grown up so rapidly in the eighteenth century that it was outgrowing its institutions. It was doing so mainly because

[2] L. G. Rowntree, 'James Parkinson', *Bulletin of the Johns Hopkins Hospital*, 23 (1912), 33–45. While Parkinson's radicalism was more evident in general than in medical politics, Wakley was the opposite, noted for his violence in the cause of medical reform, but quieter in Parliament.

[3] 'Castigator', 'Insults offered to Surgeons in General Practice', *Lancet* (1836–7), i. 560 (first published in *The Medico–Chirurgical Review*).

[4] 'A Disinterested Physician' (Edward Barlow—see below), *MPJ* 30 (1813), 265–96, esp. p. 286.

of advances in the training and status of the surgeon-apothecary and man-midwife, the rank-and-file practitioner. The pressure was coming up from below. In the late eighteenth and early nineteenth century, well before the Apothecaries Act of 1815, the talented and enthusiastic student could find for himself a medical education which was reasonably comprehensive, and better than anything available at the beginning of the eighteenth century. With this behind him he could enter practice with some confidence and pride. But many others with the same title and rank, so to speak, went into medical practice with nothing but a brief apprenticeship behind them, and sometimes not even that. There was no uniformity, no control, no clear public distinction between the educated regular practitioner and other practitioners, and no guarantee to the public that their local doctor had any sort of proper preparation for his career.

For those who sought a formal qualification, no less than sixteen separate medical bodies in Britain provided licenses, degrees, or diplomas which varied immensely in difficulty and merit.[5] Some were granted after a formal course of instruction, as in Edinburgh, Glasgow, and Dublin. Some could be bought, as in Aberdeen and St Andrew's, and in certain continental universities. In the two English universities of Oxford and Cambridge, the teaching of medicine was virtually moribund, and the medical corporations of England accepted no responsibility for teaching, believing that if they conducted examinations and granted licences and diplomas, teaching could be left to look after itself.

In the mid-eighteenth century, when only a minority of students attended hospitals, a private system of lectures and demonstrations based largely on the London teaching hospitals may have seemed adequate. By the early nineteenth century, however, with increasing numbers of students, medical education, although a thriving industry as far as the teachers were concerned, was beginning to be seen for the chaotic system it was. To an increasing extent it was recognized that in the absence of an organized system of training and qualification the public could never distinguish between the regular and irregular

[5] In England the universities of Oxford and Cambridge, the Royal College of Physicians of London, the Company of Surgeons, and the Society of Apothecaries. In Scotland, the universities of Edinburgh, Glasgow, St Andrews, and the two universities of Aberdeen; the Royal College of Surgeons of Edinburgh and the Faculty of Physicians and Surgeons of Glasgow. In Ireland, the University of Dublin, the College of Physicians of Ireland, the Royal College of Surgeons of Ireland, and Apothecaries Hall of Ireland. If the Lying-In Hospital of Dublin is included (since it offered a diploma in obstetrics) the total (counting the two universities of Aberdeen separately) is seventeen.

practitioner, between the trained and honest doctor and the untrained fraudulent quack. Improved medical education led to rising aspirations to professional status; it also increased greatly the cost of entering on a medical career. Up to a point, expectations of a prosperous career were an adequate compensation for initial costs. But when practitioners saw, or thought they saw, an increase in irregular practitioners to such an extent as to threaten their livelihood, demand for reform was inevitable. And the worst of the irregular practitioners, as far as the surgeon-apothecary was concerned, was the dispensing druggist. He was the trigger which set off the period of medical reform.

The rise of the druggist

There is no obvious explanation for the rise of the druggist in the 1780s and the 1790s. One can speculate that the druggist as wholesaler had, in the second half of the century, observed the profits to be made from pharmacy and decided to imitate the apothecary. It is also possible that druggists as wholesalers had increased to a sufficient extent that they were forced to find a new outlet as retailers, but such evidence as there is about the trade of the chemist and druggist before 1780 provides no support for such a theory.[6] But it does seem certain that the dispensing druggist appeared and multiplied in the last two decades of the eighteenth century.

Richard Smith recorded the rise of the dispensing druggists in Bristol in the 1790s and the sudden appearance of their shops all over the city.[7] Jackson was the most successful in 1795 and 'made a fortune'. He was the first to open 'a *splendid* shop—he had immensely large and elegantly painted jars in the windows'.[8] Profits were large in comparison with initial costs. Apprentices and shopmen were employed and soon followed their masters' example and set up on their own. ' "Dispensing Establishments" soon began to multiply everywhere ... in a word, the apothecary became more and more eclipsed.'[9] The physicians of Bristol, no friends of the apothecaries, colluded with the druggists to dispense their prescriptions. Some even attended at stated hours in the druggists' shops to give advice 'gratis', splitting the fees with the druggists for

---

[6] Druggists were also colourmen and suppliers to the building trade. Jonathan Barry has suggested that the decline in the building trade in the 1780s and 1790s may have forced the druggists to find other outlets. (Personal communication).

[7] BIBM 1, 94, and 6, 350.

[8] Ibid. 6, 350.

[9] Ibid. 1, 167, and 2, 163.

the medicines dispensed. In addition, the physicians, freed from their dependency on the apothecary, 'began to inform their patients that there was no need of their paying eighteen pence to an apothecary when the draught might be had for sixpence elsewhere—and that if a physician were alone employed he would have no inducement to order such a load of "apothecary's stuff" '. The apothecaries soon found that 'families where they had been in for a good thing for many years ... slipped from their fingers altogether'. In a short time the apothecaries were forced to lower their prices and sold 'pennyworths of drugs'.[10]

William Broderip, it will be recalled, earned an exceptionally large income as an apothecary in Bristol, and lived with every outward appearance of a gentleman of means. His fall, when it came, was as dramatic as his previous success. Notorious for his high charges and the multitude of patients who demanded his attention, he was suddenly able to see 'a storm gathering upon the horizon and he flew for shelter to the bottle'. By the beginning of the nineteenth century he was forced to lower his fees more and more until he, too, was selling pennyworths of drugs. His country house, his town house, his carriage, furniture, and pictures had all been sold by 1815. 'If you chanced to pass him in the street he hurried by you under a confused salute and it was painful in the extreme to all those who had partaken of his hospitality when fortune smiled upon him.'[11] What had happened in Bristol, happened elsewhere as dispensing druggists sprang up all over England providing a new and cheaper form of medical care in competition with the rank-and-file practitioners who began to suffer for their often exorbitant prices. In 1818 'C.H.' from Ipswich wrote, 'I have a family of four children and until I grew wiser by experience I annually paid 20 to 30 pounds for their little ailings, for which I now get medicine for about as many shillings at a neighbouring druggist.'[12] One druggist moreover could, by staying in his shop, supply a much larger population than the surgeon-apothecary going his rounds on foot or on horseback. The ready market for the dispensing druggist was shown by the rapid increase in their numbers.

In Bristol, for example, the population rose from an estimated 50,000 in 1775 to 124,000 in 1845. The ratio of physicians to population (1:6250 in 1775; 1:5000 in 1845) remained about the same. Surgeons and apothecaries decreased from 1:900 in 1775 to 1:1200 in 1845.

---

[10] BIBM 2, 161.
[11] Ibid. 2, 164.
[12] 'Increase of Medical Fees', *Monthly Magazine*, 44 (1817), 498–9.

Table 17 *The rise in numbers of the dispensing druggist during the late eighteenth and early nineteenth century, in selected towns*

Town	Date	Physicians	Surgeons and apothecaries	Chemists and druggists
Bristol	1755	8	56	3
	1793–4	18	52	12
	1819	21	89	29
	1826	25	94	44
	1835	22	104	56
	1845	25	108	61
Wiltshire				
Chippenham	1783	0	4	0
	1793–8	0	5	0
	1822	1	3	2
	1839	2	5	3
	1842	1	7	5
Devizes	1783	0	3	1
	1793–8	2	4	1
	1822	0	6	2
	1839	1	7	5
	1842	4	5	6
Salisbury	1783	3	6	1
	1793–8	2	8	1
	1822	3	10	3
	1839	3	13	8
	1842	4	10	8
Dorset				
Dorchester	1793	1	5	0
	1823–4	0	3	3
	1855	1	9	5
Blandford	1793	1	5	0
	1823–4	1	2	2
	1855	1	9	6
Northamptonshire				
Daventry	1784	0	4	0
	1823	0	5	1
	1830	0	8	3
	1841	2	8	8

Sources: BRISTOL: Sketchley's Bristol Directory (1775); Matthew's Annual Bristol Directory (1793–1845); WILTSHIRE: Bailey's Western and Midland Directory (1783); P. Barfoot's and J. Wilkes's Universal British Directory (1793–8); Pigot's Commercial Directory (1822 and 1842); Robson's Commercial Directory (1839); DORSET: Universal British Directory (c.1793); Pigot's Directory (1823–4); Slater's Directory; NORTHAMPTONSHIRE: Bailey's British Directory (1784); Pigot's Directory (1823, 1830, 1841).

Dispensing druggists however increased enormously. In 1775 there was one to every 17,000 inhabitants, in 1793–4 one to every 4,000, and by 1845 one to every 2,000. It is not surprising if the rank-and-file practitioners saw this as an invasion of ordinary medical care (see table 17).

The parallel between the rise of the apothecary in the late seventeenth century and the rise of the dispensing druggist in the late eighteenth was noted with wry amusement.

The apothecary, who was formerly only a druggist, had become a physician; and, as the apothecary was still more than ever required, the druggist took possession of his vacant stool and thus excited the same jealousy in the new physician as the encroachments of the apothecary had done in the mind of the old physician. ... The apothecaries were certainly wrong for becoming grand, and shutting-up their own shops, because they hastened the sad catastrophe; but we believe that nothing would have prevented it.[13]

Who were these dispensing druggists and where did they come from? Dr J. Power of Bosworth wrote in 1806:

The Druggists are generally persons who have served an apprenticeship to Grocers and Tea dealers, who had acquired their own knowledge of drugs in the same kind of service, and are generally incompetent to judge betwixt good and bad drugs. ... These persons make up physicians' prescriptions, occasionally prescribe and visit patients; many serious accidents have arisen from their selling one medicine for another, or giving them in improper doses.[14]

Another correspondent at the same time complained that some of these druggists were 'making their fortunes by pills which they compound and advertise, but they are not the only persons who do so, for there are booksellers and schoolmasters who have their pills and embrocations'.[15] Faced with this serious threat to their livelihood the reaction of the apothecaries and surgeon-apothecaries was to form an association, the General Pharmaceutical Association of Great Britain, established in 1794. It was the first of the many medico-political associations formed in the following fifty years, and it ushered in the period of medical reform. But it was short-lived and almost totally ineffective. The name of the association is confusing, suggesting an association of chemists and druggists. It was, of course, exactly the opposite, being an association formed by medical men to protect their monopoly of dispensing medicines.

The idea of an association originated in spring 1793 when 'several respectable apothecaries formed themselves into a society for the inves-

[13] 'Letters to the President of the Associated Apothecaries' *MPJ* 43 (1820), 496–510, esp. p. 501.
[14] J. Power, letter lvi, *Medical and Chirurgical Review*, 13 (1806), pp. clxxi–clxxii.
[15] Anon. letter xi, ibid. p. xxxvi.

tigation of the source of existing evils'.[16] In June 1794 a meeting of two hundred apothecaries took place at the Crown and Anchor tavern in the Strand and the Association was formally established. It was calculated that in London the druggist had already deprived each apothecary of £200 a year, and it was noted that although the increase in druggists began in London it spread rapidly to all the large towns and cities; 'nor stopped the contagion here ... so general was the disease there was scarcely a village or hamlet without a village or hamlet druggist.'[17]

It was undoubtedly a serious threat to medical practice, as the history of William Broderip has shown. But it was difficult to arouse the support of the public on this alone in an age of *laisser faire* and free competition. Therefore the Association concentrated on attempting to show that the dispensing druggists were ignorant, uneducated, and a public menace, dispensing medicines improperly composed from adulterated drugs and even encroaching on other departments of the medical art by setting fractures. In short, the druggist was denounced as a quack or irregular all the more dangerous because the public could be deluded into believing he was just another, but cheaper, form of medical practitioner possessed of skill in the practice of pharmacy.

This became the recurrent and most important theme in the prolonged war between the general practitioners and the druggists. In spite of the superficial similarity between the dispute of the physician *v.* the old apothecary and that of the new style apothecary *v.* the druggist there was this essential difference which it is important to understand. The rise of the apothecary at the time of the Rose case was seen as the rise of a medical man who was expanding his activities. The apothecary was sometimes condemned for stepping outside the confines of his shop, but he was never stigmatized as a quack; the druggist was. The

---

[16] John Mason Good, *The History of Medicine so far as it relates to the Profession of the Apothecary* (London, 1796); and Jacob Bell, *Historical Sketch of the Progress of Pharmacy* (London, 1843).

[17] J. Bell, *Historical Sketch*. In Suffolk in 1806 a practitioner wrote: 'The Chemists and Druggists are of late become numerous. In the principal town in this county there are five and in every market town one or more.' *Medical and Chirurgical Review*, 13, (1806), pp. clxxi–clxxii. 'The truth is that the chemists and druggists were becoming an important body in the City of London and suburbs, and were, as compounders, pressing hard upon the interests of the apothecaries; as the latter had, at a former period, been encroaching upon the privileges of the physicians.' John Davies, MD, *An Exposition of the Laws which relate to the Medical Profession* (London, 1844). See also R. M. Kerrison, *An Inquiry into the Present State of the Medical Profession* (1814), 40–1, and 'On Medical Education: A Critical Analysis', *LMPJ* 43 (1820), 500.

Pharmaceutical Association, having collected its evidence, presented addresses to the three London medical corporations and, in 1795, petitioned Parliament.[18] Nothing seems to have come from this form of protest, and shortly afterwards the Pharmaceutical Association faded away, leaving the druggists unscathed.

The most that can be said of this Association is that it attracted attention to a new threat to the livelihood of medical practitioners and stimulated interest in the extent of unorthodox practice. But it also began the association of the various predecessors of the general practitioners, bringing them together to make plans to protect their living and to improve their position in the world of medicine. There had been no large-scale meetings of this kind before 1794, and no previous attempts to collect evidence on the state of medicine in England. It was, from this point of view, an important step forward, for all its feebleness.

Dr John Latham and Dr Edward Harrison (1804–9)

Following the failure of the General Pharmaceutical Association in 1795, there were no further attempts to institute reforms by the surgeon-apothecaries for seventeen years. Instead, three physicians took up the subject of the state of medical practice in Britain and suggested measures for reform. Two of them, Dr Latham and Dr Harrison are well known; the third, Dr Edward Barlow is not.

John Latham was the first to propose a plan and he differed from the other two in being a Royal College of Physicians' man to his backbone. Born in 1761 the son of a Cheshire clergyman, he entered Brasenose College, Oxford, in 1778, and proceeded MB in 1786 and MD in 1788. He practised briefly in Manchester and Oxford before settling in London where he was elected a fellow of the College of Physicians at the age of twenty-seven. By the age of thirty-five he had been appointed physician successively at Manchester Infirmary, the Radcliffe Infirmary, Oxford, the Middlesex Hospital and St Bartholomew's Hospital in London; he had also become influential in College affairs, reorganizing the College library (for which he was voted £100) and became censor, Goulstonian lecturer, and Croonian lecturer. He was elected President of the College in 1813 and re-elected each year up to and including 1819.[19]

Clearly he was an unusually active man with a flair for organization.

---

[18] John Mason Good (1795); Jacob Bell (1843).

[19] W. Munk, *The Roll of the Royal College of Physicians of London* (London, 1878) ii. 393–5; and Sir George Clark, *A History of the Royal College of Physicians of London*, (Oxford, 1966) ii. 624.

His plan for medical reform was produced in 1804 and presented to the College for consideration. It was a classic example of armchair strategy, breath-taking in the Napoleonic sweep of the measures he proposed. The main proposal was the division of England into sixteen districts and Ireland into eight. The number for Scotland was undecided and Wales was overlooked or assumed to be part of England. In each district, according to his plan, a district physician would

> have authority to call upon all physicians practising with in his district, to exhibit their Diplomas and Licenses to practise; and that he shall, either by himself or his assessors, examine every surgeon, apothecary, chemist, druggist or vender of medicine touching upon their qualifications and abilities ... and that he shall report to the Quarter Sessions, or to the Judge of the Summer Assize, the results of his visitation.[20]

Such a grandiose and authoritarian scheme might have attracted some support if the post of district physician had been open to free election by medical men who lived in the district. Instead, Latham proposed that the various posts should be offered to the most senior fellows in each of the three colleges of physicians in England, Scotland, and Ireland. If they refused, it should be offered to the next most senior, and so on down the line. At the very time that Latham was producing his plan, the London College of Physicians was asking Counsel to examine the extent of its jurisdiction in the provinces and the validity of their extra-licence.[21] They knew that in fact, if not in law, they possessed no influence over the provincial physician. Latham must have known this, and been aware of the complex legal arguments over such matters as the interpretation of the original College statutes of Henry VIII in the light of the Act of Union with Scotland of 1707 and whether this Act conferred the same status on the Scottish universities as it did on Oxford and Cambridge. Latham's plan, it it had been accepted, would have made the problem of the extra-licence redundant. The London College of Physicians would have obtained complete power over all forms of practice, orthodox and unorthodox, throughout England. In this respect, Latham's plans were unique. No other plan was ever as sweeping, as autocratic, or as blindly insensitive towards provincial medical men or the realities of provincial practice. The College of Physicians considered it and buried it firmly out of sight.

[20] Sir George Clark (1966), note 19 above, appendix VII, pp. 772–5 gives in full the plan of Dr John Latham. The plan was printed in Feb. 1806 and published with the authority of the College, in the *Medical and Chirurgical Review* of 1806.

[21] Ibid. 629.

Here it may be remarked that throughout the period of medical reform the College of Physicians was remarkably consistent in its resistance to change. Inertia may have played a part because it was not a vigorous institution. It also sees to have believed that the tripartite division of medical men was the best that could be devised. But the rise of the rank-and-file practitioner was, as we see in later chapters, a threat to the future of the physician. Resistance to change was partly, if not largely, inspired by the fear of losing power, privileges, and position. Hard on the heels of Latham's plan came another one; and this one could not be dismissed so lightly. It was all the more threatening because it was reasonable, it was practical, and it came from an outsider who consistently refused to recognize the authority of the College and was tactless enough to say so openly and publicly on more than one occasion. This was the plan of Dr Edward Harrison of Lincolnshire, backed by a number of influential men. The effect of Dr Harrison was to alert the College to the formidable and growing power of the movement for medical reform. No longer were the reformers to be taken lightly or dismissed with contempt as mere trouble-makers.

There are several detailed accounts of Harrison's plans for reform and of his ultimate defeat by the College of Physicians.[22] Here a summary of that story is all that is needed, except for one aspect which has been largely neglected. The basis of Harrison's proposals was the scandal of the extent of unorthodox practice in the provinces, and he spent a considerable time collecting evidence on this from various parts of Britain. Not all the evidence has survived, but a substantial part was published. It was the first time, as far as we know, that anyone had attempted to discover the extent of unorthodox practice in more than anecdotal terms; and for this reason it is uniquely valuable. First, however, the plan proposed by Harrison and its origins.

The physicians in Lincolnshire were unusual in establishing a benevolent society by which they took it in turn to provide a medical service for the poor. It was this society, the Lincolnshire Benevolent Medical Society, which initiated an enquiry that grew from a county affair to a national one. In 1806 Harrison published his first report, *Remarks on the Ineffective State of the Practice of Physic in Great Britain with Proposals*

---

[22] For an excellent modern account of Harrison and his plans for reform see Sir George Clark's *History* (note 19). The main primary sources are Edward Harrison, *Remarks on the Ineffective State of the Practice of Physic* (London, 1806) and *An Address to the Lincolnshire Medical Benevolent Society* (London, 1810). See also the evidence of Edward Harrison in *SCME*, Part I, Q. 4401–30.

for its Future Regulation and Improvement. The title was chosen with care, because Harrison had two purposes in mind. The first was to expose the problem of the quacks, empirics, or irregulars, and to emphasize that virtually all the chemists and druggists, as well as the midwives, belonged to this category because they had served no apprenticeship and received no training. His second purpose was to outline a plan of reform for regular practitioners, to be introduced into Parliament as a Bill.

It was clear that improvement of the regular practitioners depended on the provision of a better and more uniform medical education for all classes of medical men. There was nothing controversial here except for his insistence that the authority of the College of Physicians ceased at the seven-mile border from the centre of London.[23] This may have been obvious, but it was provocative; yet it was necessary, perhaps, to justify the intervention on the national scene of a provincial physician and provincial medical society; and Harrison took care to state that none of his proposals would interfere with the existing rights of the medical corporations.

In his proposals, published in the medical press in 1806,[24] it was suggested that physicians must have reached the age of twenty-four, surgeons twenty-three, and apothecaries twenty-one. Physicians, who would be graduates, would be required to study physic for five years at least at a university and a respectable medical school, not less than two of those years being spent at the university where they took their degree. Surgeons would be required to spend five years in apprenticeship with a surgeon and two studying anatomy and surgery at a reputable school. Apothecaries would serve five years' apprenticeship and at least a year in some reputable school of physic. No medical man should practise midwifery unless he had attended anatomical lectures for a year and received practical instruction from an experienced accoucheur, including assistance at 'real labours'. All chemists and druggists would be required to serve a five-year apprenticeship.

Before these proposals were produced, Harrison had obtained some powerful support. First he had gone to the President of the Royal Society, Sir Joseph Banks, who lived near Horncastle, was a patron and trustee of the Lincolnshire Benevolent Medical Society, and may even have

---

[23] E. Harrison (1806).
[24] They appeared in, among other places, the *EMSJ*, 2 (1806), 252–3, 437–40, 487–91.

been a patient of Harrison's.[25] Sir Joseph Banks was generous in his support, suggested that Harrison went to London, and lent him his town house in Soho Square. Initially Harrison spent five months in London, and altogether between 1805 and 1809 made three more visits each of several weeks.[26] He must have lost a certain number of patients by his devotion to the cause of reform.[27] Harrison wrote for support to a number of people including Samuel Whitbread, MP for Bedford, who had more than a passing interest in medical affairs;[28] and he obtained the support of a number of physicians including the rich and influential Sir Walter Farquhar, as well as Sir John Hayes, and Drs Blackburn, Garthshore, Pearson, Stranger, Robert Willan (junior), and Henry Clutterbuck; Sir Gilbert Blane also attended meetings once or twice.[29] Some of these men were critical of the College of Physicians and most were senior, respected, and well-known figures in the medical world.[30] These physicians formed, with Harrison, a committee 'to confer and correspond with the different public bodies in the United Kingdom, upon the subject of the proposed regulations.'

By this time Harrison had sent out a questionnaire to various parts of Britain for which the Treasury allowed the privilege of free post. Harrison asked his correspondents to answer certain questions.[31] The first concerned the number of 'regular' practitioners and how many of these were incompetent compared to those 'whose education and talents rendered them deserving of the confidence of patients'. He also asked for the number of chemists and druggists, the number of midwives, and the number of quacks and empirics, and invited suggestions on how things could be improved. An initial survey in Lincolnshire had been carried out in two districts—Horncastle and Market Razon. The results of this initial survey, and of those from other areas which provided the necessary figures, are shown in table 18. The evidence came back partly in quantitative terms and partly in anecdotes. Harrison himself described the druggists in Lincolnshire who undercut the apothecaries and sold very large quantities of opium (which was perfectly legal) for

[25] Harrison had corresponded with Sir Joseph Banks many years before in 1795. See Warren R. Dawson (ed.), *The Banks Letters* (London, 1958).

[26] Evidence of Dr E. Harrison, *SCME*, part I, Q. 4401–4430.

[27] Was this a contributory reason for his moving to London in 1820?

[28] See 'The Whitbread Correspondence' in Bedfordshire CRO for this period.

[29] *SCME*, part I, Q. 4410.

[30] Sir George Clark's dismissal of Harrison's associates as a 'gathering of the discontented critical' does not stand up to examination. Clark, *History of the College of Physicians* (1966), ii. 631.

[31] The list of queries can be found in full in the *EMSJ*, 2 (1806), 253.

Table 18 *The numbers of regular medical practitioners and irregulars reported to Edward Harrison in his investigation of the state of the practice of physic in England, 1804–6*

	Lincolnshire		Nottinghamshire		Durham	Total of all five areas (%)
	Horncastle District	Market Razon District	Nottingham District	Nottingham-shire District		
Physicians	5	0	4	0	2	0.2
Surgeons and apothecaries	11	7	15	35	5	12.0
Druggists	25	9	13	13	3	11.0
Irregulars of both sexes over and above the druggists	40	17	35	114	7	36.0
Midwives	63	32	11	123	2	39.0

Sources: E. Harrison, *Ineffective State of Physic* (1806), and *Medical and Chirurgical Review*, 13 (1806).

the pacification of small children whose mothers went out to work; and he described a farrier who practised medicine and midwifery, 'hurrying many persons of all ages to an untimely grave'.[32]

From Suffolk came the complaint that apothecaries were in the habit, after a few years in their shops, of buying an Aberdeen or St Andrew's MD and setting themselves up as physicians. In addition there were two empirics in the leather line and 'a cobbler and cutter who do much business'. The latter worked 'by imagination', muttering and moving fingers, and steadfastly gazing into the face of his female patients who felt much better for this primitive form of hypnotism. There was also an irregular who specialized in curing ulcerated legs.[33]

In another part of Suffolk a clergyman was reputed to give a prescription in return for a pound note 'whilst his wife goes daily to administer her nostrums to her neighbours'.[34] Cambridgeshire reported a 'failed grocer' turned bone-setter and man-midwife, and complained that the country was invaded by itinerant quacks in the summer. Previously, in the county, there were many 'smallpox doctors' but 'Jenner has nearly ruined this class of beings'.[35] In Northumberland it was estimated that there were five empirics to every regular practitioner, while Yorkshire had its 'Greenland doctors ... These ... are a set of mechanics of various descriptions who, failing in their respective vocations, too often from profligacy, learn to bleed and are then qualified for the place of surgeon on board a Greenland ship. On their return ... they go into the country and are doctors until the next Greenland season.'[36]

Liverpool reported a multitude of irregulars, a surprisingly large number of them, apart from the midwives, being women.[37] From all areas the midwives were reported as consisting largely or entirely of 'un-instructed irregulars'. In the Horncastle district of Lincolnshire, 'not one of the sixty-three had received any instruction'.[38]

Middlesex had the double complaint of 'the impudence of quacks' and 'an inundation of medical men': the penalty, no doubt of being so near

[32] E. Harrison (1806), 15–16. For a modern account of the use of opium in the Fens, see V. Berridge and G. Edwards, *Opium and the People* (London, 1981).

[33] *Medical and Chirurgical Review*, 13 (1806), pp. xxiv–xxviii.

[34] Ibid., pp. xxxviii–xxxix.

[35] Ibid., p. xlii. Smallpox doctors were lay inoculators, some of whom, like the Suttons, inoculated thousands of people and made a large income by doing so.

[36] Ibid., pp. lxxiii–lxxiv.

[37] Ibid., p. lxix.

[38] E. Harrison (1806).

the Metropolis where 'many foolish and fond parents who cannot give their son a decent, much [less] a classic education, are induced partly from pride and partly from a great demand for young men in the army and navy, to place them as apprentices to apothecaries ... to learn the art of blacking shoes and making up medicines'.[39]

In Manchester it was Ferriar who replied that 'the number of quacks and irregular practitioners is very great in this town and neighbourhood ... even the chirurgical practice in the town suffers from such interlopers' and the income of country practitioners was seriously affected.[40] A letter from St Neots signed by ten medical men stated that 'irregulars' outnumbered the 'regulars' and half the latter (physicians, surgeons, and apothecaries) were judged incompetent.[41]

From Ripon in Yorkshire, on the instigation of George Cayley, MD, nine medical men and forty-two other gentlemen signed a petition of support for the reform of medicine and the outlawing of quackery.[42] Amongst these reports, sent in response to Harrison's circular, there were many florid anecdotes of the more extreme forms of quackery. For example, one of the correspondents from Suffolk (unnamed because Harrison usually suppressed the names of his correspondents in the published letters) wrote about 'A man within four miles of this town, formerly a collector of geese for public sale, now a practitioner in physic, boasts that he expends £200 a year with his druggist, keeps his chaise, and is sent for through a district of thirty miles diameter.'[43] Another practitioner from Lancashire wrote:

Persons not engaged in the practice of medicine &c. could scarcely credit the extent of the injury done to society by unqualified practitioners. Many instances might be furnished, from this town, of joints being reduced that never had been dislocated, and bones treated as fractured which had never been broken. In some of these cases, there is every reason to believe that mortification of the limbs had been induced by the improper treatment, whilst the subsequent amputation and examination of the limbs has proved the bones to be entire.[44]

From Dorset a correspondent complained bitterly of the damage he had suffered from the unfair competition of the multitude of quacks: 'the surgeons without diplomas, instruments or knowledge' and 'apoth-

---

[39] *Medical and Chirurgical Review*, 13 (1806), pp. lxxiii-lxxvi.
[40] Ibid., p. cxxxvi.
[41] *Medical and Chirurgical Review*, 13 (1806), pp. cv-cvi.
[42] Ibid., pp. cv-cvi.
[43] Ibid., p. xxxix.
[44] Ibid., p. lxxxi.

ecaries who had never been beyond the precincts of their parish ...
accoucheurs ignorant of the shape and formation of the female pelvis
... grocers and stationers turned chemist and druggist ... quacks and
empirics, both stationary and itinerant'. This correspondent, on the
other hand, had served his apprenticeship with two respectable
surgeons, studied two winters in London (under Fordyce, Hunter, Pott,
etc.) and one winter in Paris (at *La Charité* under M. Sabatier, etc.), and
obtained his diploma at Surgeon's Hall. He had 'now attained the
summit of my profession in this town and district around' yet he had
difficulty in providing for his family and his old age and was forced to
continue working to a late age because of the competition of ignorant
quacks.[45] There is no doubt that in most areas the 'regular' members
of the medical faculty believed that quacks were outrageously dangerous
to the public and that they stole business which properly belonged to
the regulars.

But the pattern was not consistent throughout Britain. In Scotland
part-time empirics were few and full-time ones unknown—with reason.
'They can hardly be expected to thrive in so poor a country as Scotland,
and we have none of them here.'[46] Over-production of medical men in
Scotland, poverty, and the very low fees charged by the medical faculty,
combined to scare off the unorthodox. It is more surprising, however,
to find that replies from Devon, Berkshire, and Essex indicated only a
small number of irregular practitioners and, in the case of Essex, their
number was decreasing when other areas reported an increase.[47] Likewise a physician from Sherborne (Dorset) told of twenty competent and
regular practitioners in his neighbourhood but only six druggists and
one or two irregulars who acted as bone-setters and used toads in bags
as charms, with one regularly educated surgeon-apothecary who acted
in the manner of an empiric to whome 'the ignorant flock in multit-
udes'.[48] But the revelations were scandalous enough. Sir Walter Farquhar
had a word with the Prime Minister about it. Pitt said he was 'convinced
that something is wanting' and some measure of reform necessary. He
even said 'I will carry it into effect', but he died in February 1806 and
nothing was done.[49]

Between 1806 and 1809 Harrison struggled to win over the medical

---

[45] *Medical and Chirurgical Review*, pp. lxxix–lxxx.
[46] Ibid., pp. cxliii–cxliv.
[47] Ibid., p. lxxvii.
[48] Ibid., p. lxxvii.
[49] *SCME*, part I, Q. 4414.

corporations. His approach to the Society of Apothecaries received 'a short very cold answer'. The College of Surgeons was 'ardent at first but cooled afterwards'.[50] But the defeat of Harrison was due most of all to the obduracy of the College of Physicians. Repeatedly, Harrison was asked to leave his proposals with the College who would consider what reforms were needed. Harrison refused, saying he 'could not commit the provincial faculty' to the College.[51] It was a trying time for him as he continued his single-handed campaign and learnt from sore experience of 'the feuds, jealousies and the discontent, which have unfortunately set the Metropolitan faculty against each other'.[52] In 1809, however, when he felt success might be in sight, he was told (on 22 December) suddenly and brutally by Sir Lucas Pepys, PRCP, that the College considered the Bill for reform to be 'highly objectionable ... and that it will be incumbent on the College to oppose its enactment'.[53] No reasons were given, and when Harrison offered to alter the Bill, Pepys gave it as his private opinion that the College would still remain hostile, regardless of any alterations. At this, Harrison gave up and remained implacably and understandably bitter at the behaviour of the College. An account of Harrison's failure was included in the 'Sketch of the Progress of Medicine' in the *Medical and Physical Journal* of 1811.

Those who held privileges, and those who held none; those who believed themselves deprived of their rights, and those who feared a change on the grounds that all change was dangerous, united into a phalanx compact, formidable and impenetrable. Against this host, drawn together by various motives and feelings, but all looking to particular interests, fearing the loss of some good already possessed, or apprehending the demolition of some expectancy, it would have been unwise to contend; and Dr Harrison, judiciously perhaps, suspended his projected plan of reform.[54]

Dr Barlow and the agenda for medical reform

In the meantime, Dr Edward Barlow, MD of Bath, became increasingly interested in medical reform. Like Harrison he was an Edinburgh graduate and a stern critic of the London College of Physicians. His first publication on medical reform was in 1807 before Harrison had been forced to admit defeat. No copy of this has been found, and his sub-

---

[50] Ibid., Q. 4408 and 4414.
[51] E. Harrison (1806).
[52] Ibid.
[53] E. Harrison (1810).
[54] Leading article, *MPJ* 26 (1811), 2–5.

sequent essays on medical reform show that he differed from John Latham and Edward Harrison in one important respect. He foresaw, correctly, the central position of the general practitioner in the movement of medical reform, and he wrote extensively between 1813 and 1834 on the importance of supporting the principle of a corpus of educated and able general practitioners as the central feature of the medical profession. Latham and Harrison, although their proposals differed, based their plans on the continuation of the tripartite division of the medical profession, and accepted as their starting point the perpetuation of the rigid differentiation of medical men that was already outmoded by the end of the eighteenth century. Within the limited field of medical politics, Barlow, who saw further than his predecessors, began as a radical and ended as an orthodox reformer; and the fact that he did so without a significant shift in his views is a measure of the change that occurred, and possibly a tribute to his influence.

His first essay was published under the pen-name 'A Disinterested Physician' in the *Medical and Physical Journal* of October 1813.[55] The second and third were published anonymously in the *Edinburgh Medical and Surgical Journal* in 1818 and 1820.[56] Anonymity was a sensible precaution for a young physician who was fiercely critical of the Royal College of Physicians and a strong supporter of the general practitioner. His fourth essay in 1827 was published under his own name and disclosed the authorship of the previous two articles.[57] By this time his views were shared by many of his colleagues. A fifth essay was published in 1833–34.[58] Barlow's style, like so many physicians of his time, was apt to be ponderous, verbose, and repetitive, and his excursions into the history of the profession in the later essays were almost always unfortunate. But in spite of this he was a perceptive and outspoken observer.

In contrast to Harrison he was remarkably unconcerned with the problem of quackery, not because he approved of unorthodox practice, but only because he felt it was unimportant and would disappear when

---

[55] 'A Disinterested Physician' (Ed. Barlow), leading article in *MPJ* 30 (1813), 265–97. Confirmation of Barlow's authorship can be found in a letter from Barlow to Samuel Whitbread, MP for Bedford, written at the end of 1813, and preserved in the Whitbread correspondence in the Bedfordshire CRO.

[56] Anon. (E. Barlow), 'An Attempt to develop the Fundamental Principles which should guide the Legislature in Regulating the Profession of Physic', *EMSJ* 14 (1818), 1–26, and anon. (E. Barlow), 'Exposition of the Present State of the Profession of Physic in England, and of the Laws enacted for its Government', *EMSJ* 16 (1820), 479–509.

[57] Edward Barlow, 'An Essay on the Medical Profession', *EMSJ* 28 (1827), 332–56.

[58] E. Barlow, 'An Essay on Medical Reform', *LMG* 13 (1833–4), 899–905, 936–43.

with better education and licensing of medical practitioners, the public would make the obvious choice of the orthodox man. Barlow's main concern was the chaotic state of medical education, and the lack of uniformity amongst the medical corporations. Many changes were needed, but much the most important was one already beginning in 1813—the transformation of 'that excellent species of practitioner, the surgeon-apothecary' into the general practitioner. He welcomed this innovation because he believed the public needed and demanded a well-educated generalist: 'on the competency of this class must the great mass of the population rely for the preservation of health and removal of disease. To by far the largest portion of society they are the sole physicians, and even the highest ranks are known to depend with the fullest confidence on their skill and ability.'[59] The young men entering the profession would see this and 'naturally qualify themselves for that line which is most likely to prove both most lucrative and most respectable'.[60] Physicians, he wrote, could not take the place of general practitioners for they lacked all knowledge of surgery and pharmacy. Fewer physicians would be needed in the future and 'they must be satisfied to exist in the greater towns and more populous districts, where, only, the separate departments can be specially maintained'.[61]

This was certainly an unorthodox view for a physician to hold and one which was based on an optimistic future for the general practitioner: 'As one body of practitioners increase [the general practitioners] the other will sensibly decline.'[62] But who would undertake the training and examination of the future general practitioners? Significantly, the Royal College of Physicians was never considered. Barlow had no doubt that it should be the Royal Colleges of Surgeons in England, Scotland, and Ireland. The Edinburgh College was already carrying out this function. The course and examination for the LRCS (Edin.) was not purely surgical but included physic, pharmacy, amd midwifery. It was deservedly popular as a complete training for the generalist. Barlow went to great lengths to praise the London College of Surgeons as a far-sighted and liberal institution and hoped the College would model itself on its sister in Edinburgh.[63] But there was never the slightest chance of the London College doing anything of the sort. Instead, the London

[59] E. Barlow (1813), 277.
[60] Ibid. 293.
[61] E. Barlow (1818). See also evidence of Benjamin Brodie, *SCME*, part II, Q. 5752–6.
[62] E. Barlow (1813), 273.
[63] Ibid. 275–6.

College was preoccupied with the creation of an élite of 'pure' surgeons based largely on the London teaching hospitals. As Wakley was to show later, nepotism was rife amongst the small close-knit group of surgeons at the London teaching hospitals who dominated their college and retained for themselves all positions of privilege and power. Barlow was curiously obtuse in his failure to recognize this state of affairs. Perhaps he was unduly influenced by his experience of Dublin and Edinburgh; perhaps he hoped to win over the London College of Surgeons by flattery and persuade them to support the new general practitioners, but if he did, he underestimated them.

If the Colleges of Physicians and Surgeons rejected responsibility for the education of the general practitioner, what about the Society of Apothecaries? In Barlow's view to link the general practitioner with the Apothecaries would be a disaster. They were a City company, not a medical college. It was true that pharmacy was important for general practice, and it was also true that medical cases predominated over surgical. Nevertheless, it was well known that all surgeons treated medical cases as well as surgical, and that the growing tendency towards conservatism in surgery meant that many cases previously treated by operation were now treated medically. The College of Surgeons was the appropriate institution to take the general practitioners under their wing.

Following this discussion of the training and licensing of the future general practitioner, Barlow commented on the state of the medical corporations. Edinburgh, Glasgow, and, to a lesser extent, Dublin were singled out for praise. For Aberdeen and St Andrews, who granted medical degrees on the basis of a fee and two letters of recommendation, he had nothing but scorn: 'These universities possess no competent schools of physic. Their degree is obtained without resident study or examination, and on the sole grounds of private certificates'; they were characterized by 'gross venality and shameless corruption'. Oxford and Cambridge were scarcely better, for although they required 'a certain observance of acts and terms' they did not require any proper qualifications in 'the art of curing diseases; yet these graduates possess privileges such as no other men enjoy, and are entitled to demand admission as fellows of the London College of Physicians.' There were some scathing observations on the College of Physicians. Why, for example, should candidates for the licence of the College be subjected to examination when they were already medical graduates? And why did anyone bother to take the extra-licence of the College (by which the

College maintained the pretence of power over the practice of physic in the provinces) when the extra-licence was known to have no legal force? The College of Physicians should confine itself to confirming the validity of the medical degrees of those who applied for its licence; if they were valid, there was no reason for withholding the licence. This was revolutionary stuff, but he added for good measure a condemnation of the College for its method of granting fellowhips. In Barlow's opinion, fellows should be elected by the vote of all members of the College, including the licentiates. In fact, Barlow had written the agenda for the subsequent and increasingly acrimonious debate on medical reform. Features stressed in the 1813 essay, and repeated in his subsequent ones, reappear again and again over the whole of the first half of the century. They include:

1. The need for a medical practitioner trained and competent in physic, surgery, midwifery, and pharmacy who would undertake the large majority of medical care of all sections of the population, including the higher ranks.
2. The fulfilling of that role by the general practitioner who had evolved directly from the surgeon-apothecary.
3. The consequent decline of the physician except in the centres with large populations, where a limited number of 'pure surgeons' would also be found.
4. The need for a new comprehensive process of education, examination, and licensing for the general practitioner and the belief that this ought to be the responsibility of the College of Surgeons.
5. The justification of this belief on the theoretical grounds that surgery was expanding to incorporate much of physic; and on the practical grounds that the College of Physicians would not contemplate taking on the task, and the Society of Apothecaries was unfit to do so being a City trading company and not in any way an academic body.
6. The need for greater uniformity amongst the medical corporations, and the urgent need for the reformation of some, in particular Aberdeen and St Andrews and the London College of Physicians.

Other themes were debated too, but these were the central ones. And, as Barlow was writing his essay in 1813, they were already being debated by the first and the most important of the many general practitioner associations founded in the first half of the nineteenth century: the Association of Apothecaries and Surgeon-Apothecaries, founded in 1812.

7

The Association of Apothecaries and Surgeon-Apothecaries, and the Apothecaries Act of 1815

The Association of Apothecaries and its proposals

THE Apothecaries Act of 1815 was the product of the fourth attempt to introduce a plan for the reform of the medical profession. The plans of the General Pharmaceutical Association, John Latham, and Edward Harrison had failed in the sense of producing no material or legislative changes, but they had succeeded in bringing the need for reform to the attention of medical men so that some enactments were inevitable; the first of these was the Apothecaries Act.

In spite of its name this Act had nothing to do in the first instance with the Society of Apothecaries. The Society was brought in, somewhat reluctantly, at the insistence of the Royal College of Physicians during the half-way stage of a long, bitter and controversial attempt to improve the education and status of the rank-and-file practitioners.[1] The initiative came at a meeting of practitioners held at the Crown and Anchor tavern in the Strand in London, on 3 July 1812. The meeting had been called to protest against the new heavy tax on glass, only one of a

---

[1] The main sources for this chapter are: *The Transactions of the Associated Apothecaries and Surgeon-Apothecaries*, 1 (1823), pp. 1–cxxviii; The *Medical and Physical Journal* and the *London Medical and Physical Journal* (*MPJ* and *LMPJ*), especially vols. 29, 30, and 31 (1813–14); *The London Medical, Surgical and Pharmaceutical Repository*, especially vol. 1 (Jan.–June 1814); G. M. Burrows, *A Statement of Circumstances connected with the Apothecaries Act and its Administration* (London, 1817); R. M. Kerrison, *An Inquiry into the Present State of the Medical Profession in England* (London, 1814); and, from the Guildhall Library, London, the records of the Society of Apothecaries, especially the minute book of the committee relating to the Apothecaries Act, MS 8211/1, and papers relating to the Association of Apothecaries, MS 8299, referred to here respectively as Guildhall MS 8211/1 and 8299. For secondary sources see especially C. Wall, H. C. Cameron, and W. A. Underwood, *A History of the Worshipful Society of Apothecaries of London* (London, 1963), and S. W. F. Holloway, 'The Apothecaries Act 1815: A Reinterpretation,' part I, 'The Origins of the Act', *Medical History*, 10(2) (1966), 107–29; part II, 'The Consequences of the Act,' *Medical History*, 10(3) (1966), 221–36.

number of tax increases introduced to pay for the war. Since the trade of the apothecary was heavily dependent on glass bottles, this increase— 'from eight to forty-five shillings'—was 'almost equivalent to another income tax' as far as medical practitioners were concerned. It was 'deeply felt by all apothecaries and roused them to endeavour to remove or modify it. Accordingly, meetings for that purpose took place; and, as is common when persons having similar sentiments and pursuits assemble, other subjects of complaint were discussed and various means of relief were proposed. And, with this intention an association ... was formed.'[2]

George Man Burrows, who, more than any other individual, played the central part in the reform of the medical profession and the establishment of the general practitioner, was appointed chairman of the association. Writing about this meeting some years later, he stressed the fact that those who attended the meeting were 'the first in rank, ability and character amongst the London Practitioners'.[3] Robert Masters Kerrison was also at pains to emphasize that the meeting 'was not the conflux of a few discontented men, without practice, or public estimation, but the assemblage of nearly all the reputable practitioners in London, and many from Distant Counties'. Over two hundred attended the meeting. Those from 'Distant Counties' consisted of two each from Surrey, Colchester, and Kent, and one each from Hendon, Hadham in Hertfordshire, Swaffham in Norfolk, Sheffield, and Liverpool.[4] By 1813 the published list of subscribers showed that although the association was initially dominated by London practitioners it rapidly became representative of England and Wales as a whole.[5]

At the meeting on 3 July it was Anthony Todd Thomson, then a prosperous practitioner in Sloane Street and later Professor of Materia Medica and Medical Jurisprudence in the University of London, who opposed one of the resolutions on the price of glass. He did so on the grounds that it was 'an object too trifling for the attention of such a meeting, when there were evils of much more importance, that required their most serious reflections, and proportionate energy to correct'.[6] His suggestion, that medical reform should be their subject, struck a

---

[2] G. M. Burrows, *A Statement* (1817), 3.
[3] Ibid.
[4] R. M. Kerrison (1814), Introduction.
[5] See list of subscribers in *MPJ* 29 (1813), 168–72, 258–8, 340–7.
[6] *The London Medical, Surgical and Pharmaceutical Repository*, 1 (1814), 512.

sympathetic chord. As soon as it was agreed by all that an association should be formed a committee was elected consisting of twenty-four members from London and seven from the provinces.[7]

Initially the association was known as the London Association of Apothecaries and then changed to the London Association of Apothecaries and Surgeon-Apothecaries. With the rapid increase in provincial membership it became the Associated Apothecaries and Surgeon-Apothecaries. Some believed the title archaic. A correspondent wrote to the chairman of the association in 1813 to say: 'The Bill might with a great deal of propriety be termed that of the general practitioner in medicine, surgery and midwifery ... the character of the general practitioner was always respectable, whilst the regular apothecary of the present day retains little else than the name of his predecessor.'[8] For legistlative purposes, however, the term 'general practitioner' had no status or agreed definition, and it was not until 1826 that the Associated Apothecaries and Surgeon-Apothecaries became the Associated General Medical and Surgical Practitioners. Here, the term 'Association' will be used to cover all the changes of title.

When the Association was established, George Man Burrows accepted the chair reluctantly and later wrote that he would have declined had he known what would be involved. Between 1812 and 1815 he attended 130 committee meetings each of several hours, and answered personally more than 1,500 letters sent to him as the membership rose from the intitial 200 to over 3,000 in three years.[9]

The rapid growth of the Association showed the magnitude of change in attitudes and expectations of the rank-and-file practitioners. The apothecaries and surgeon-apothecaries of the eighteenth century, individual entrepreneurs who owed no allegiance to corporations or associations, had now become the nineteenth-century general practitioners who saw themselves increasingly as professional men with a growing sense of collective identity, a determination to reform, and a new pride in their position in medicine and in society as a whole. The impulse behind reform was not solely due to anger at the encroachments of the druggists and irregulars. 'Public advantage had a higher place in their deliberations', and the Association was 'actuated by far more philosophical views' than mere 'calls of private interest'.[10] The reason why

[7] R. M. Kerrison (1814), pp. v and vi.
[8] *MPJ* 30 (1813), 478–81.
[9] G. M. Burrows (1817).
[10] *Transactions of the Association*, 1 (1823), pp. vi–vii.

change was essential was spelt out as clearly as possible in 'An address, explanatory of the Motives of the present Application to Parliament by the Apothecaries and Surgeon-Apothecaries'. The sentiments expressed in the address may seem obvious, even banal, to us today, but in 1812 they were new. Nothing similar appears in the eighteenth century in connection with the surgeon-apothecary.

> The duties [of the apothecaries and surgeon-apothecaries] are of very serious and individual interest, the lives and health of by far the greater part of the community being entirely confided to their care, without in many instances the possibility of obtaining other advice; yet there are allowed to practise without any examination or test of competency whatever; so that, any person, however destitute of medical or even common education, may assume with impunity the character and functions of the apothecary.[11]

From July to November 1812, the committee of the Association drew up an outline plan for reform and presented it to the second meeting of the Association on 6 November which 'enumerated the grievances and difficulties with which the apothecary has to contend ... within the last thirty years [and which had caused] the condition of the apothecary gradually to decline'.[12]

With a poor appreciation of their own history, the Association complained that the apothecary had become degraded from a gentleman to a tradesman 'by the mode in which he is remunerated', and it was believed that their income had remained level for a century although costs had doubled. But the main concern was the usual one of the encroachment of druggists and 'improper persons' and the absence of a system which placed the 'apothecary, surgeon-apothecary and the practitioner in midwifery under the direction of a proper controlling body'.[13] It was decided to send the outline plan to Sir Joseph Banks and the executives of the Colleges of Physicians and Surgeons and the Society of Apothecaries, who were asked to 'concur and unite in an Application for an Act of improvement and better regulation of the Apothecary throughout England and Wales.'[14] This outline formed the basis of a parliamentary Bill which was drawn up by the Association's solicitor in January 1813. Whatever the feelings of the members of the Association towards the medical corporations they saw they would need, and believed they would get, their blessing.

---

[11] *MPJ* 29 (1813), 347.
[12] *Transactions of the Association*, p. vii.
[13] Ibid., p. vii.
[14] Ibid., p. viii.

Meanwhile, a deputation consisting of four senior members of the Association, Mr Brande, apothecary to the King, Mr Upton, and two surgeon-apothecaries, A. T. Thomson and G. M. Burrows, waited upon the Chancellor of the Exchequer, Mr Vansittart. The latter expressed his wholehearted approval for the plans of the Association and arranged with the Postmaster General that the Association could circulate letters to practitioners throughout England and Wales free of postal charges.[15] By the end of the year 1812, the Association had reason for guarded optimism. The rank-and-file practitioners in London and the provinces and even the Government had expressed warm approval. Opposition must surely have been anticipated from the medical corporations, but so far the corporations were sitting, side by side, on the fence. The Society of Apothecaries would express no opinion until it had heard the opinion of the College of Physicians. The College of Physicians said it was not their business, it was the concern of the Surgeons and Apothecaries and their opinion must come first. The College of Surgeons, however, merely said that it did not intend to interfere with the plans of the Association, but it was certainly not going to give its approval.[16]

The outline proposals were eleven in number.[17] The first stated that the Bill should not be retrospective; that is, its measures would not apply to anyone in practice when the Act was finally introduced. The second required all new entrants to have served an apprenticeship or 'to produce testimonials of a suitable medical education'. The third, fourth, and fifth were concerned with the examination and licensing of candidates and stamp duty. The sixth spoke of a superintending body and the seventh, which ended ambiguously, proposed that England and Wales should be divided into 'a certain number of medical districts, of which London shall be the superior, and where only certificates for qualifications can be obtained'. The eighth dealt with the examination of assistants and the ninth proposed that practitioners should be able to charge legally for advice 'as visits or journeys' and would reduce charges for medicine. The tenth proposed new regulations for attendance on the parish poor and the eleventh, foreshadowing the Act of 1858, proposed a register of licensed practitioners. During its passage from an outline plan to a Bill there were certain modifications, but the

---

[15] *Transactions of the Association*, p. x, and *MPJ* 30 (1813), 166.

[16] See 'Appendix' to the report of the London Committee of Apothecaries and Surgeon-Apothecaries, *MPJ* 30 (1813), 472–7 where the correspondence between the Association and the medical corporations was published.

[17] *MPJ* 29 (1813), 348–9.

majority of the above proposals were included in the Bill presented to parliament by William Wilberforce, John Calcraft, Samuel Whitbread, and George Rose. It received its first reading on 8 March 1813, only nine months after the Association was founded. If the Bill was remarkable for the number and scope of the changes it suggested, it was also in certain parts unintentionally provocative.[18]

It was entitled 'A bill for regulating the practice of Apothecaries, Surgeon-Apothecaries and Practitioners in Midwifery and Compounders and Dispensers of Medicine throughout England and Wales.'[19] The preamble explained the reasons for the Bill—the health of the community, the decline in the status of the apothecary and surgeon-apothecary, and the difficulty of getting apprentices. The first clause suggested that the Act should be administered by a committee consisting of the presidents and master of the Colleges of Physicians and Surgeons and the Society of Apothecaries, four censors of the College of Physicians, two governors of the College of Surgeons and four wardens of the Society of Apothecaries. These would be joined by twenty-four surgeon-apothecaries who had been in practice for more than ten years in London or within ten miles of the metropolis. This was sure to anger provincial members and, since the surgeon-apothecaries would outnumber the dignitaries of the medical corporation by more than two to one, the latter would be certain to object. The second to tenth clauses were concerned with committee procedures, and the eleventh with the foundation of a medical college in London under the direction of the committee which would form the nucleus of a 'fourth body'. The twelfth clause proposed that sixteen districts should be created for the licensing of practitioners, each governed by a committee containing a JP, a physician, and four apothecaries or surgeon-apothecaries, two of whom should be practitioners in midwifery.

Further clauses proposed that no one should practise as a surgeon-apothecary without the diploma of the College of Surgeons. This was an additional requirement to that which proposed that no one should practise as an apothecary, a surgeon-apothecary, or man-midwife without having been first examined and licensed by the body appointed for that purpose. But there were exceptions. First the Act would not be retrospective. Secondly, those serving as surgeons in the armed services

---

[18] R. M. Kerrison (1814), and *Transactions of the Association*, p. xiii.

[19] This account is based on Guildhall MS 8299, 'papers relating to the Association of Apothecaries'. The Bill was published in full in *Transactions of the Association*, pp. xiii–xxix with an abstract of the amended Bill on pp. xxix–xxxv.

at the time the Act was introduced should be able to enter civilian practice without the necessity of being examined, except in midwifery, and with the rights and privileges of existing English universities or the medical corporations.

There were other important clauses. Candidates for the certificate or licence would be required to provide evidence of apprenticeship *or* sufficient medical education, and the latter was defined in the amended Bill as six months at a London hospital or one year at a provincial hospital or dispensary. The possibility of qualifying for the proposed licence without serving an apprenticeship was later removed; apprenticeship was made compulsory. The clause which allowed practitioners to charge for journeys or advice was not as revolutionary as it seems since it merely asked for legal sanction for established practice. It was also proposed that there should be a register of qualified practitioners in each district which should be open to the public. Finally, there were the proposals closest to the hearts of most members of the Association: those which proposed that chemists and druggists and midwives should be required to submit to examination and be licensed. They would then come under the control of medical practitioners.

Almost at once the College of Physicians opposed the Bill, refusing to give any reasons,[20] and petitioned against it in Parliament on 15 March 1813.[21] A similar petition followed from the College of Surgeons and another from the chemists and druggists of the City of London and Westminster.[22] The Association was called to a general meeting on 23 March which lasted twelve hours. In a state of near desperation the Association attempted to withdraw the clauses on the proposed London College and the licensing of druggists. A message to that effect failed to arrive in time for the second reading on 26 March 1813. Mr Calcraft, one of the Bill's sponsors, gave it such lukewarm support that the Association was advised to withdraw it, and agreed.[23] Fearing that it would appear that the committee had given in too easily to the opposition from the medical corporations, A. T. Thomson explained that the 'Committee had tried their fullest strength to get that Bill passed into a law; but they were opposed in all quarters—by the Medical Bodies—by the Legislature—by the Public. It would have been madness to per-

---

[20] Letter from Mr Hervey, registrar of the College of Physicians, *Transactions of the Associated Apothecaries*, p. xxxvii.
[21] *Journal of the House of Commons*, 68 (24 Nov. 1812–1 Nov. 1813), 314.
[22] Ibid. 343.
[23] *Hansard Parliamentary Debates* (11 Mar.–10 May 1813), 350–1.

severe: they wisely withdrew the Bill.'[24] It was, after all, a very small affair at a time when the country was preoccupied by war and by fears of riots and revolutions. It is unlikely the public was either informed or interested in the affairs of the apothecaries and surgeon-apothecaries, and it was true that the Association was in no position to challenge the joint opposition of the medical corporations and Parliament. Moreover, as critics were quick to point out, in many ways the Bill was a careless and ill-thought-out document.

The imperfections of the Association's proposals

Samuel Fothergill, the editor of the *Medical and Physical Journal*, referred to the Association's Bill in his 'report on the progress of medicine' in 1813.

It is evident that in framing this Bill the Committee must have had many jarring interests to reconcile ... much external opposition to conciliate or to conquer, arising out of public opinion, or out of private apprehension. Some thought it too extended, others deemed it too limited. Some asserted it did nothing if it did not humiliate the druggist. Some contended for the apothecary's right to demand fees. One district had this, another that local interest to satisfy ... Embarassed, probably, by intricacy of interests ... the Committee suffered clauses very loosely connected with this great principle [education] to be inserted in the Bill.[25]

The Bill, like the outline proposals before it, had the marks of amateurs in a hurry. Some proposals were trivial or unnecessary. For example, the suggestion that an oath should be taken by candidates, and the plan for an unnecessary annual licence. Others were clumsily provocative, such as the suggested composition of the body to examine candidates and administer the Act. The proposals for administrative districts, which appeared to hark back to the plans of Dr John Latham, had no basis in need, and the proposal that all candidates who intended to practise as surgeon-apothecaries should be required to hold the MRCS seems to have been made without prior consultation with the College of Surgeons. The decision to retain apprenticeship as the main form of medical education was much criticized, coming as it did at a time when apprenticeships in general were falling into disrepute; and the sole reason appears to be that the apothecaries and surgeon-apoth-

---

[24] 'General Meeting of the Apothecaries of England and Wales', *The London Medical Surgical and Pharmaceutical Repository*, 1 (1814), 513.
[25] *MPJ* 30 (1813), 3–6.

ecaries had grown dependent on an apprentice to mind the shop (literally) and carry out menial tasks. It was the Association itself, and not the medical corporations, which suggested the retention of the apprenticeship system, and the Association was later to regret it.[26] The defects of the Bill, which laid it open to scorn, deflected attention from the genuine need for reform and the kernel of worthwhile measures buried within the proposals. What was the real significance of these?

The Association was motivated by two main principles. First, the need for an improved medical education based on a broad curriculum and tested by examination, and secondly, for a process of licensing by which the irregular practitioners could be clearly distinguished by the public from the genuine educated medical man; only thus, it was believed, could quackery be defeated. But in another respect the Association hinted that it intended to go much further than these proposals. One of its aims was complete autonomy. The proposed London College was—and one has to add 'presumably' as this was never quite stated explicitly—the first step towards founding a Society or College of General Practitioners. Certainly it seems to have been interpreted as such by the Colleges of Physicians and Surgeons who saw the proposal as a serious threat to their dominance of medicine, and instantly opposed it. That the proposal was never close to the hearts of the Association is suggested by the alacrity with which this proposal was dropped at the first whiff of opposition. It might or might not have been regarded by members of the Association as either sensible or practical, but it was certainly radical, and it lay dormant for another thirty years.

Autonomy implied complete separation from the other medical bodies, and one notes the proposal to include the MRCS as part of the licensing of general practitioners. Why was this included in the original proposals if autonomy was an aim? The probable answer was the rapidly increasing number of students who, in the early years of the nineteenth century had sat for the diploma of the College. George Man Burrows estimated that nine-tenths of the membership of the Association held the MRCS and many referred to themselves as surgeons.[27] There was, and remained for the next thirty years, a strong feeling amongst many general practitioners that their future lay in cultivating a link with the

---

[26] 'If there were not apprentices, general practitioners in the country would find it difficult, I believe, to procure persons to give them the help which they require ... and if apprenticeship is not enjoined, I do not know where the masters are to procure persons to compound the medicine. That was the difficulty felt by general practitioners at the time of the Association.' G. M. Burrows, *SCME*, part III, Q. 322.

[27] *SCME*, part III, Q. 262.

College of Surgeons. Some who held this view preferred the title of 'surgeon in general practice' to 'general practitioner', seeing it as a means of denying their link with the apothecaries and the taint of trade. Some, when young, may have seen themselves as the future Abernethys or Astley Coopers of provincial towns and villages, holding a position of prominence in the local infirmary or, at worst, a dispensary. Others, more far-sighted, realized that surgery was only a small part of general practice and saw that subservience to the College of Surgeons (which had no intention of ever becoming a College of General Practitioners) would reduce the general practitioner to the status of a second-class surgeon. The indecision of the Association was shown by its first proposing that the diploma should be compulsory, then dropping the proposal and then, when the Royal College of Surgeons itself at a later date proposed it should be compulsory, opposing this proposal as well.[28] The Association was forced to accept that it had to make a choice. Either it should insist on autonomy and face the opposition, or it must court the physicians and surgeons with placatory proposals and hope for the best. It chose the latter course and saw the independence it had hoped for slip from its fingers. The future of the general practitioner thus lay in the hands of the existing medical corporations.

Opposition to the proposed reforms

The opposition of the medical colleges is not in the least surprising. The physicians had more to fear than the surgeons from a new generation trained, examined, and licensed in the practice of physic and pharmacy.[29] Dr Edward Barlow, as we have seen, had forecast, and even apparently welcomed, the probability that as the numbers of general practitioners rose, so the physicians would diminish in number and importance.

The surgeons, although less threatened, saw the danger of being swamped by run-of-the-mill, general practitioner surgeons just at the time when they were gaining a position of equality with the physicians at the top of the medical tree. Meanwhile, the Society of Apothecaries, disturbed from a comfortable life of profitable trade, 'professed to act according to the instructions they might receive from the College of Physicians'.[30] Indeed, the Society was in the awkward circumstance that some of the committee of the Association were also members of

---

[28] *Transactions of the Association*, pp. lxvi–lxvii.
[29] 'A Disinterested Physician', *MPJ* 30 (1813), 265–96.
[30] *SCME*, Part III, Q. 252, 253, 259.

the Court of Assistants of the Apothecaries. When instructed by the College of Physicians to oppose the draft Bill of the Association, they found themselves petitioning with one hand and rejecting the petition with the other. Hence the statement of the Society that it rejected the petition *as a body*.[31] What hurt the members of the Association of Apothecaries and Surgeon-Apothecaries was not the opposition of the medical bodies, which they must have expected, but the curtness of it. They

> saw with regret that they were treated with a coldness bordering on contempt, and they were afterwards opposed in Parliament, and *previously* to the introduction of the Bill, by letters written to individual Members, requesting their opposition to the measure when in the House, without assigning any reason, but resting merely upon their assertions that the Bill *ought to be opposed*.[32]

Finding the opposition to be implacable, they nevertheless pressed forward with plans to present another Bill, and work on this began in September 1813.[33]

The original clauses on founding a medical school, on the licensing of druggists, and on a committee to administer the Act which included all the heads of the medical bodies, were abandoned. With these modifications they applied once more to the College of Physicians for a meeting. The College only consented through the intercession of George Rose who, as the Member of Parliament for Southampton (he was first elected in 1794), was one of the four members who had introduced the first Bill. Rose's experience as a diplomat may have been useful and allowed him to act as 'the organ of communication between the parties'.[34] It was especially unfortunate for the Association that George Rose resigned his seat in December 1813 (he reentered Parliament in 1818 as Member for Christchurch), and, soon after, went to Munich as British Minister.

The Association soon discovered, however, that the College of Physicians had consented to reopen negotiations on one condition: that any Act would be administered by the Society of Apothecaries. There is no

[31] *MPJ* 30 (1813), 476.

[32] R. M. Kerrison (1814), p. x.

[33] *Transactions of the Association*, p. xl.

[34] *SCME*, part III, Q. 259. This George Rose is not to be confused with his father, also George Rose, who was elected member for Christchurch in 1790 and who corresponded with Sir Lucas Pepys, PRCP, on the subject of Edward Jenner and the Vaccine Institution. The Revd L. V. Harcourt, *The Diaries and Correspondence of the Right Hon. George Rose*, 2 vols. (1876), ii. 338–9.

evidence that the Society solicited such a task; indeed, it seems it was thrust on them by the College of Physicians. This ultimatum—for, in effect, that is what it was—was presented to the committee of the Association in January 1814[35] and the Society found itself rather unwillingly at the centre of the stage in a stormy play. It has to be emphasized that there was nothing about the Society of Apothecaries which made it the natural body to take over the training, examination, and licensing of the future general practitioners. It was not an academic body. It was not a representative association. The rank-and-file practitioners had not regarded it as 'their' corporation which understood their problems and was capable of looking after their interests. It was a City company, a wholesaler of drugs on a large scale, and, like other City companies, it possessed certain privileges which it was able to bestow on its members. Admission to high office was based on seniority, and many of the Court of Assistants, who were with few exceptions elderly men, had long since ceased to practise physic and pharmacy.[36] It was from these that the Court of Examiners would be chosen, and the Court of Examiners would be in a position of great power and influence. There were further details in the plan for an Act, which served to debase the emerging general practitioners. Instead of a new Act designed for the purpose, the Act would be an amendment to the existing Charter of the Society of Apothecaries.[37] Thus the College of Physicians preserved the old tripartite division by trying to ensure that although the general practitioner had a new title, he was no more than the old apothecary in a new coat.

To drive the point home even further, the College of Physicians insisted on the insertion of a clause to compel the 'apothecary' to compound and dispense the prescriptions of a physician, whether he wished to or not,[38] as if in retaliation for the defeat of the College of Physicians in the Rose case, more than a hundred years before (see chapter 1). This clause, which in fact was a trivial matter, was not without reason. For all the talk of collusion between physicians and druggists, most physicians still depended on apothecaries and saw the possibility of a new Act leaving them with no one to dispense their prescriptions. But the way it was introduced and surrounded with penalties and threats if the apothecary refused, was inflammatory.

---

[35] *Transactions of the Association*, p. xli.
[36] G. M. Burrows (1817), 35.
[37] *Transactions of the Association*, pp. xlii–xliii.
[38] *The London Medical, Surgical and Pharmaceutical Repository*, 1 (1814), 387.

When these plans as a whole were presented to a general meeting of the Association held on 12 May 1814, they caused a furore. G. M. Burrows and A. T. Thomson believed that the conditions imposed by the College of Physicians would have to be accepted, and accepted gracefully.[39] A. T. Thomson pointed out that many members of the Association might object to one or more of the provisions in the proposals; as befitted an Edinburgh graduate, he objected to the inclusion of apprenticeship. But if every objection was taken into account 'by attempting too much the whole might be endangered. It was impossible to enact provisions in a general Bill which would embrace every evil ... it was wise and politic to regard only the advantage to be derived to the whole of the profession.' He moved that the meeting should approve the *'basis* and *spirit* of the Bill ... which is about to be introduced to Parliament by the Society of Apothecaries, with the approbation of the College of Physicians'.[40] John Mason Good rose to object 'in a vein of severe sarcasm'.[41] He and Burrows had both been members of the weak and abortive General Pharmaceutical Association of 1794. Both had been disillusioned by the experience, and Good was as much of an old hand at the business of medical reform as the two previous speakers. Indeed, like them, he was on the committee of the Association, but too often an absent one because 'his other avocations had prevented his attendance as often as he wished'.[42] Good fastened on to the provision compelling apothecaries to dispense the prescriptions of physicians as especially obnoxious and made too much of it. More to the point, he observed that the Bill made no provisions for an examination in anatomy, surgery, or midwifery. The Bill as a whole, in his opinion, was 'a measure made up of restrictions, penalties and imprisonments, founded in tyranny and oppression'.[43] He was in favour of throwing it out. In doing so he took the most extreme stand, but in objecting to the Bill as a whole, and especially the provision on dispensing for physicians, he was not alone. Others objected to a tame acceptance of the way the Bill had been foisted on them. Mr Burrows, the chairman, was hard put to it to calm the meeting and persuade them that the greatest good would be obtained by acceptance of the motions put forward by A. T.

[39] For a report of this stormy meeting, see *The London Medical, Surgical and Pharmaceutical Repository*, 508–30.
[40] Ibid. 513–14.
[41] Ibid. 514–15.
[42] Ibid. 514.
[43] Ibid. 516.

Thomson. The meeting was prolonged, but in the end the motion was accepted by 'a large majority'.[44]

At this time Burrows, himself a member of the Society of Apothecaries, was convinced the Society would administer the Act with generosity towards the Association and with intregrity.[45] To reject the Bill outright would be to delay indefinitely the introduction of any measures of reform. Burrows was neither weak nor overawed by the medical corporations. In a period of less than two years he had, as he said himself, become more knowledgeable than any man living of the opinion of practitioners all over England and Wales.[46] Almost single-handed he had covered a great deal of ground and gone a long way towards the introduction of a Bill. Although the Colleges of Physicians and Surgeons had treated him with a 'coldness bordering on contempt', he believed there were grounds for optimism.

The period between the acceptance of the plan for a new Bill and the introduction of the Act was peppered with proposals and counter-proposals and promises made and sometimes broken. It was a period of muddle and complexity. The body charged with drawing up the new Bill was the Act of Parliament Committee of the Society of Apothecaries.[47] The committee found itself involved in many contentious matters. One concerned the position of medical officers on their retirement from the armed services. The Association believed it was insulting and unnecessary to force them to submit to an examination, except in midwifery (for which, in fact, there were no arrangements for an examination anyhow), since they would already have had to pass a qualifying examination and would be experienced pratitioners. The College of Physicians was insistent that entry to civilian practice as a surgeon-apothecary on the sole basis of service in the army and navy should not be allowed. All such candidates would have to take the examination and (although this was not altogether clear) they might even have to serve a five-year apprenticeship.[48] From April to June 1814 the argument continued about the clause compelling apothecaries to dispense physicians' prescriptions. The Physicians remained adamant and threatened in June to withdraw their support for the Bill if the clause was not accepted. The committee of the Society gave way but

---

[44] Ibid. 524.
[45] G. M. Burrows (1817).
[46] Ibid.
[47] Guildhall MS 8211/1.
[48] Ibid., 7 Feb 1814.

was moved to remark in July 1815 that they 'could not help observing with pain that from the time the Society have received their Charter the jealousy on the part of the Physicians which has existed towards the Apothecaries and which appears from the Records, continues with unabated force.'[49] They admitted that the Bill which was finally passed was imperfect in many respects, but protested that 'The Committee do not flatter themselves that they can by one effort put an end to the abuses of two hundred years endurance.'[50] While a number of proposed amendments still hung in the air, the Society of Apothecaries petitioned Parliament to bring in the Bill on 22 November 1814.[51] The Bill was read for the first time on 27 February 1815.[52] The Royal College of Physicians, the chemists and druggists, and a few apothecaries separately petitioned against the Bill in March and April,[53] but the Bill received its second reading and was sent to the House of Lords on 11 May 1815.[54] On 28 June the Lords sent it back with a number of amendments. One expressed the Bishop of Peterborough's dissatisfaction with the English translation of the preamble to the original Charter of the Society of Apothecaries. He demanded a better one. However, when this was attempted it was found that 'the original [was] so untractable that it scarcely admitted of a translation more intelligible than that which his Lordship rejected.'[55] The Bill was finally passed by the House on 11 July 1815[56] and, next day, it received the Royal assent. It came into operation on 1 August 1815. 'Thus ended this most arduous and most unsatisfactory struggle ... that it was very unsatisfactory may be seen by comparing the Apothecaries Act as it is with the Bill at first projected by the Association. Shorn, indeed, is the latter of its fair proportions.'[57] No one was really happy. The Colleges of Physicians and Surgeons opposed the measure on principle; the Society of Apothecaries found itself saddled with a new job it did not relish; and the far-sighted members of the Association achieved only a part of their original aims, but took heart from the belief that, having got thus far, they would succeed in the following years in putting the necessary amendments to the Bill and achieving their original aims.

[49] Guildhall MS 8211/1, 14 July 1815.
[50] Ibid., 14 July 1815.
[51] *Journal of the House of Commons*, 70 (8 Nov. 1814–7 Jan. 1816), 28.
[52] Ibid. 109.
[53] Ibid. 147, 156, 240.
[54] Ibid. 293.
[55] Guildhall MS 8211/1, 14 July 1815.
[56] *Journal of the House of Commons*, 70 (1815–16), 473.
[57] *Transactions of the Association*, p. lviii.

The Apothecaries Act of 1815

The full title of the Apothecaries Act was 'An Act for better regulating the Practice of Apothecaries throughout England and Wales, 1815.' The main provisions of the Act were as follows. The Act, which was to be an amendment to the Charter of 1617, gave to the 'Master, Wardens and Assistants' of the Society the power to carry the Act into execution. A Court of Examiners, consisting of twelve persons, was to be chosen by the Society to examine the candidates for the Society's licence and for granting a certificate to those who satisfied the examiners. The fee was to be ten guineas for those intending to practise in London or within a ten-mile radius, and six guineas outside that area. All candidates would have to have reached the age of twenty, have served a minimum of five years as an apprentice to an apothecary, and would be required to produce testimonials of having received a 'sufficient medical education'.[58] The Act became effective on 1 August 1815, after which no one could legally enter on a career as an apothecary without the licence. All who were in full practice as apothecaries (assistantships were not included) on the appointed day were exempted from the provisions of the Act. (These became known as the 'pre-1815' medical men.) The penalty for practising without a licence was fixed at £20, half of the fine going to the Society and half to the informer or informers. Specific clauses ensured that nothing in the Act should be construed as seeking to interefere with the chemists and druggists, the Universities of Oxford and Cambridge, or with the Colleges of Physicians and Surgeons. There were two hated clauses. One was that compelling the apothecaries to compound and dispense the prescriptions of physicians; the penalty for refusal was £5. The other conferred the power on the Society to enter and search the premises of any apothecary and destroy any faulty or contaminated drugs. Originally this power had been given to the College of Physicians. There were also regulations concerning the examination and certification of apothecaries' assistants which were never put into effect. There was, moreover, nothing in the Act concerning the

---

[58] 'A sufficient medical education' was defined as two courses of lectures on anatomy and physiology; two courses of lectures on the theory and practice of medicine; one course of lectures on chemistry; one course of lectures on *materia medica* and six months' attendance at a hospital or a dispensary. Candidates were examined in the theory and practice of medicine, pharmaceutical chemistry, and materia medica. From 1815 to 1840 the examination was oral only. Z. Cope, 'Influence of the Society of Apothecaries upon Medical Education' in *Some famous General Practitioners and Other Essays* (London, 1961).

position of surgeons in the Army and Navy.[59] The main difference between the Act of 1815 and the original Bill of the Association was the attachment of the Act to the Society of Apothecaries, and consequent loss of independence. Originally the Association had visualized an independent Act administered by general practitioners in co-operation with the established corporations. Part of this independence was the proposal for a medical school. This, of course, had been defeated. So had the measures for controlling the chemists, druggists, and the midwives, and the proposal permitting charges for visits and journeys and for surgical procedures. Nor was the plan for administrative districts or for registration included in the Act. From the Association's point of view, the worst of these omissions was the absence of any control over druggists and midwives. However, the Act as it stood should, in theory, provide some protection against the irregular practitioner. There was one minor point which angered G. M. Burrows. He claimed to have persuaded the Society that membership of the important Court of Examiners should be open to general practitioners who were not members of the Society. He maintained that this clause was removed surreptitiously at the very last moment without his knowledge or consent.[60] This, however, was only one of his complaints. Until the Act was introduced, Burrows appears to have been a model of patience, tolerance, hard work, tact, and diplomacy, unruffled by the contrary opinions he had to resolve and the contempt of the Colleges of Physicians and Surgeons. He was a successful mature practitioner, aged forty-one when elected chairman of the Association, which he served 'with untiring zeal, much to the detriment of his private interest and to the injury of his health'.[61] In 1817 he published an extraordinary pamphlet entitled *A Statement of Circumstances connected with the Apothecaries Act and its Administration.* In it he wrote of his bitter disillusionment. Although a member of the Society, before 1812 he had taken no part in its affairs. He had never intended that the Act should be placed in the hands of the Society, but once it became inevitable, he believed that the Act, with all its faults, would be administered fairly. The first important procedure after the

[59] The state of the medical officers remained unsettled until the Act of 1825 (5 George IV) which qualified all medical officers holding a commission or warrant in the Navy, Army or East india Company as apothecaries. That Act lasted from 6 July 1825 until 1 Aug. 1826 and then lapsed after which 'the law returned to its former state, and has continued in the same state ever since.' J. Davies, *The Laws Relating to the Medical Profession* (London, 1844) 66.

[60] *SCME*, part III, Q. 265.

[61] Obituary notice in Churchill's *Medical Directory* (London, 1847), vol. i, and *DNB*.

Act was passed was the appointment of the Court of Examiners, of whom Burrows was one. When this took place, Burrows was astonished to find that some of those elected 'did not know such an Act was in existence'.[62] When summoned before the Court the ceremony was perfunctory in the extreme: 'the most important occurrence that ever happened within those walls, passed as a trivial and ordinary affair!'[63] Then a member of the Court of Assistants placed himself firmly in the chair, 'pretty plainly indicating that that was his destined place. He was accordingly immediately and unanimously elected.' This was followed by the new chairman announcing that Mr Watson, his son-in-law, had been elected Secretary.[64] There are several pages indicating that the Court of Examiners were badly informed on the provisions of the Act, and lazy and self-seeking in its administration. Rules were ignored when it suited the majority to do so. Matters came to a head when a candidate, who had been apprenticed to a chemist and druggist, not an apothecary presented himself for examination.[65] Burrows objected to his admission and was overruled by the Court of Examiners. Burrows then entered a formal protest but it was refused and not entered in the minutes.[66] He wrote a letter to the Court of Assistants stating his complaint in detail, and later wrote a similar letter to the Master of the Society.[67] One of these letters appeared in the *Medical and Physical Journal* and in the *Medico-Chirurgical Journal*.[68] Burrows was naturally suspected of having sent the letter himself, and the editors stated that it had been sent anonymously. It is clear from the lengthy account of this trivial affair that Burrows, previously the friend of all and the master of diplomacy, had made enemies of most of the Courts of Assistants and Examiners. When confronted and questioned he was furious and refused to answer, although his published statement makes it clear that he did not send the letter to the medical journals. When he was finally arraigned before the master of the Society of Apothecaries he again refused to answer, and, bitterly hurt at the way he had been treated, he resigned.[69]

Burrows, it seems, had changed under the strain of the previous years of negotiations and disappointment. The administration of the reforms

---

[62] G. M. Burrows (1817), 9.
[63] Ibid.
[64] Ibid.
[65] Ibid., see letter VII in Appendix, p. vii.
[66] Ibid. 22.
[67] Ibid., letter VII and IX in Appendix, pp. vii and xi.
[68] Ibid. 24.
[69] Ibid. 32.

on which he had set his heart fell into the hands of elderly men with little or no knowledge of clinical practice,[70] but considerable expertise in nepotism. The Court of Examiners could fairly claim that members of the Association of Apothecaries and Surgeon-Apothecaries were well represented,[71] but the Court remained subservient to the all-powerful Court of Assistants. The general practitioners of 1812 had started with a sense of high optimism and youthful energy. They deserved to be administered by a body which shared these characteristics. Instead they ended up with an Act designed by the medical colleges for their suppression, and administered by a Society not fit for the purpose. It was a depressing outcome from all points of view.

[70] G. M. Burrows (1817), 35.

[71] The members of the Court of Examiners of the Society of Apothecaries, appointed in 1815, were the following. Those who were or had been members of the Association of Apothecaries are indicated thus:[A] and those who were Members of the College of Surgeons as well as of the Society of Apothecaries are indicated thus:[S] William Simons (chairman)[A], John Watson (secretary), Thomas Wheeler, James Hill, James Upton[A], Edward Browne[S], Henry Field[A], John Ridout, John Hunter[A], Richard S. Wells[A], George Johnson[S], George Man Burrows[SA], Everard Brande[A].

8

The Consequences of the Apothecaries Act

Contrary opinions on the Act

THERE are contrary opinions on the merits of the Apothecaries Act. Walter Rivington in the second edition of his Carmichael Prize Essay was almost as critical of it as he was of the Medical Act of 1858, and he quoted Gray, who observed in the supplement to his *Pharmacopoeia* 'This Act has had the singular fortune of being violently opposed as insufficient by those who were its original promoters, of being esteemed a burden by many of those it was meant to benefit, and of being looked upon with indifference by those against whom it was intended to act'.[1] During the present century, however, when the Act was receding into history and the anger it aroused had faded, a chorus of praise elevated it almost into a national monument. Carr-Saunders and Wilson in 1933 described it as a 'remarkable Act. ... It would not be astonishing to find it amongst the accomplishments of the Reformed Parliament.'[2] Bishop called it the great landmark in the history of the general practitioner and others who praised it even more lavishly saw it as a turning-point when the general practitioner was first established and, through state intervention, modern medical education was founded to provide a corpus of scientifically educated practitioners for all the people.[3]

Most who praised it so highly assumed that the Society of Apothecaries was responsible, if not for the initiative, at least for the design and content of the Act. This warm glow of approval was finally extinguished by Holloway in 1966, and his arguments are wholly convincing.

---

[1] W. Rivington, *The Medical Profession* (2nd edn., Dublin, 1888).

[2] A. M. Carr-Saunders and P. A. Wilson, *The Professions* (new edn. London, 1964).

[3] See for example, Sir Zachary Cope, 'Influence of the Society of Apothecaries on Medical Education', *British Medical Journal* (1956), i. 1–6; C. Newman, *The Evolution of Medical Education in the Nineteenth Century* (London, 1957); W. J. Bishop, 'The Evolution of the General Practitioner' in E. Ashworth Underwood (ed.), *Science, Medicine and History, Essays ... Written in Honour of Charles Singer*, 2 vols. (London, 1953) ii. 354; D. U. Bloor, 'The Rise of the General Practitioner in the Nineteenth Century', *Journal of the Royal College of General Practitioners*, 28 (1978), 288–91.

Holloway[4] pointed out that the Act was a muddled piece of legislation providing no clear definition of the apothecary. It perpetuated the hierarchical tripartite system. It degraded the general practitioner through the apprenticeship clause and the attachment to a trading company rather than a medical college. Its restrictions failed in their intention of outlawing irregular practitioners, and looked ridiculous when they were used in an attempt to outlaw well-educated Scottish trained practitioners. The Act was unpopular with practitioners at the time, and in general tended to lower the status of the general practitioner when the original intention had been exactly the opposite. Most of all, the Act was a shameful compromise forced on the general practitioners by the medical colleges in a naked struggle for power and status. It is certainly true that the Act was flawed, and in general, unpopular; but what about the long-term consequences? Can it at least be argued that it created the basis of modern medical education? This is a common view, but one which ignores the facts about medical education in the years immediately preceding the Act.

It was shown in chapter 2 that medical education was rapidly growing in London (and to a lesser degree in the provinces) throughout the late eighteenth and early nineteenth century. Before the Act was introduced the basis of a comprehensive system of lectures, anatomical dissections, and bedside teaching already existed and was attended by hundreds of students every year. It was a voluntary system, but it provided a foundation without which the Act could never have been introduced by 1815. The Act did no more than add compulsion and examination to certain parts of a pre-existing educational framework. Compulsory attendance and the examination may have raised the general standard of medical education, but the emphasis of that education was backward-looking rather than a bold initiative. Neither surgery nor midwifery were required for the Licence. Even when midwifery lectures were introduced after the first twelve years, there was no examination in the subject.[5] Instead, greatest emphasis was on Latin, chemistry, *materia medica*, and pharmacy. It was in fact a syllabus appropriate for the old-style apothecary, but not for the general prac-

[4] S. W. F. Holloway, 'The Apothecaries Act', part I, *Medical History*, 10 (2) (1966), 107–29; part 2, *Medical History*, 10 (3) (1966), 221–36. Holloway's views have largely been accepted by historians. See, for example, Ivan Waddington, 'General Practitioners and Consultants' in J. Woodward and D. Richards (eds), *Health and Care and Popular Medicine in Nineteenth-Century England* (London, 1977), and N. Parry and J. Parry, *The Rise of the Medical Profession* (London, 1976).

[5] See chapter 5 for the difficulties of teaching midwifery.

titioner. At best the Act could be seen as a step in the process of the professionalization of the rank-and-file practitioners: but it can not be claimed that it laid the foundation of medical education, and even less that it 'created' the general practitioner who preceded, in name and manner of practice, the introduction of legislation. As a contemporary put it: 'the Act of 1815, which first recognised the apothecaries as legitimate practitioners, was not the cause, but the consequence, of the change which had taken place in their condition'.[6]

Nevertheless, the majority of general practitioners saw the advantage of a system which, for all its faults, confirmed their new status as respectable professional men by giving them the right to put letters after their name. The term 'medically qualified' now had a clear meaning and if it had to be acquired at the cost of extra effort as well as money, it was worth it. There is a revealing letter, written in 1834, and sent to George Charleton, house-surgeon to Gloucester Infirmary from 1833 to 1868[7] by one of his friends.

I should have replied to yours of 25 Sept, but that I was then polishing up for a slap at the *Hall*—which slap I had on Thursday last and luckily came off victorious so that I am now MRCS, Licentiate of the Worshipful Company etc. etc. at your service.

I had a very fair practical examination of rather less than an hour and a half. Fortunately I happened to be rather strong on Chemistry and Materia Medica (of which latter they showed me 55 specimens) and came off with flying colours ... I mean to take a clinical clerkship or two this winter at the Hospital and give all my attention to the practice of my profession.[8]

There is a strong Dickensian flavour about the opening paragraph of this letter, and indeed, Dickens, in Martin Chuzzlewit (published in 1843–4 and famous for the character of Sarah Gamp) created Dr Jobling who tells his audience: 'We know a few secrets in our profession, sir. Of course we do. We study for that; we pass the Hall and the College for that; and we take our station in society *by* that.'[9]

---

[6] *The Quarterly Review*, 67 (Dec. 1840), 59. Likewise another contemporary remarked that if the general practitioners were better informed it was due to the enlightened spirit of the age not to the introduction of a compulsory Act, 'Remarks on the Apothecaries Act', *London Medical Repository and Review*, 6 (1827), 375–8.

[7] A house-surgeoncy in this period was sometimes a permanent post rather than a position occupied for brief periods by a succession of young medical men.

[8] Gloucestershire RO. Letter from R. Gray to George Charleton, dated 11 Oct. 1834, D 4432/3.

[9] Charles Dickens, *The Life and Adventures of Martin Chuzzlewit* (London, Chapman and Hall, no date), 419.

What, in the meantime, had happened to the Association of Apothecaries and Surgeon-Apothecaries? From 1812 to 1815 it was at the centre of the movement of medical reform. It might have been disbanded after the Act of 1815 was introduced, but instead it continued in the confident expectation of being able to improve the Act by the introduction of amendments. Although it was wholly unsuccessful in this, it actually increased its membership and was still in existence in 1833.[10] After that it disappears from sight.

G. M. Burrows continued as chairman until 1817. On his resignation he received the handsome present of five hundred guineas. He was succeeded by James Parkinson (of Parkinson's disease) and either in 1819 or 1820 (the record is unclear) Parkinson was succeeded in the chair by Joseph Hayes.[11] In 1816–17 the Association was successful in opposing an attempt by the College of Surgeons to make its diploma compulsory, on the grounds that the motives of the College were 'too glaringly calculated to benefit the College rather than the Profession'.[12] This was followed by an attempt to persuade Parliament to legislate against irregular practice, but this attempt failed because 'Parliament is very wisely jealous of making enactments at the suggestion of petitioners who may be actuated by motives of private advantage rather than by a desire to benefit the public'.[13]

Thus the Association, failing in the field of medical reform, resorted to the status of a forum for medical men to discuss matters of common concern. As its membership grew after 1815, district committees were encouraged. One such committee in Staffordshire remarked that an incidental result of the Association had been to bring about a medical and surgical library for members living in and around Wolverhampton.[14] The Association became just one of a growing number of societies and associations, some local, some national, which were such a notable feature of the period. Meanwhile, the Society of Apothecaries introduced a series of new examination regulations. Physiology and medical botany were the first to be added in 1816. In 1827 attendance at lectures on midwifery and diseases of children were made compulsory, but a planned examination in midwifery was never introduced on the

[10] The Association, now named the Associated General Practitioners, held a meeting in the Crown and Anchor Tavern on 12 June 1833. *LMG* 12 (1833), 367–8.

[11] An account of the post-1815 period of the Association can be found in the preface to the *Transactions of the Associated Apothecaries*, I (1823).

[12] Ibid., p. lix.

[13] Ibid., pp. lxxiii–lxxiv.

[14] Ibid., p. lxxii.

grounds that no suitable examiners could be found. The time spent at medical schools and hospitals was extended from one to two years, as the curriculum was gradually expanded.[15]

But surely, it is said by those who have praised the Act, at least the Act provided a comprehensive medical education for the first time. In fact the curriculum was in many ways remote from the content of general practice. It is a commonplace of medical education that the teachers will teach what they are most interested in and, implicitly or explicitly, will instil their sense of values as to what is and what is not 'real' and important in medicine by the importance given to certain subjects in the examination. Insufficient Latin was the most common reason for rejecting a candidate for the LSA in the first half of the nineteenth century.[16] Chemistry, *materia medica*, and medical botany were the important things to learn for the examination. The College of Surgeons looked after the surgical side, and detailed questions on operations which the average general practitioner would seldom be called on to carry out formed a major part of the oral examination for the MRCS. Midwifery, the diseases of children, and public health were generally ignored, although these subjects lay at the centre of general practice. Clinical teaching was slanted to an increasing extent on the teaching hospitals. It is a recurrent complaint even today that hospitals are not the ideal place for training medical men whose working lives will be spent in patients' homes and in the community. This was especially true of the nineteenth century where the restrictive rules of the hospitals denied to the students experience of the major problems of general practice—the infectious diseases in patients of all ages, and the whole spectrum of children's diseases. The dispensaries were much better placed to provide a representative sample of all the illnesses of general practice,[17] but the growing power and status of the teaching hospitals predominated, and eventually eliminated the dispensaries as teaching institutions.[18] The relative number of students attending hospitals and dispensaries in London during the three years between 1831

---

[15] Sir Zachary Cope, *Some Famous General Practitioners and Other Essays* (London, 1961).

[16] 'Report of the Court of Examiners to the Society of Apothecaries', *BFMR* 2 (1836), 606–7.

[17] Evidence of John Ridout, *SCME*, part III, Q. 1023 which explains the advantages of dispensaries as teaching institutions.

[18] An excellent account of the growth in power and prestige of the nineteenth-century teaching hospitals can be found in M. J. Peterson, *The Medical Profession in Mid-Victorian London* (Berkeley, 1978).

and 1833 were 678 and 217 respectively, although some students spent part of their time in each type of institution.[19]

It was often said that the Act was remarkably well administered by the Society of Apothecaries. Sir David Barry in 1833 believed 'that the examination established by the Company of the Apothecaries is now by far the most comprehensive examination in London'.[20] To use this as an argument in favour of the Act is to confuse administrative efficiency with educational content. Indeed, immediately after the above quotation, Sir David Barry remarked that the standard of examination must be kept below that required of the physician or 'it will be unattainable by a great many'.[21] While the Act was in existence it was generally conceded that the examination for the Licence was fair and well administered. But there were two aspects of the Act which were the subject of continual criticism. These were apprenticeship and the power of the Society to prosecute unlicensed practitioners.

Apprenticeship

Few had a good word to say for apprenticeship as a system of medical education. Even if it could be defended in theory, the reality was described by a Salisbury apprentice in a letter published within a few weeks of the Act becoming law.

I who am an apprentice, embraced a covenant, two years since, with an ardour that gave confidence to myself. I had then the most flattering hope apparent upon a situation that evinced every possible advantage. But what have these two years shown me. ... where I am likely to continue five years more, behind a counter, dispensing medicines? In this the sole employment of a young man apprenticed to a surgeon-apothecary and man-midwife? ... it is not my lot alone, but the lot of hundreds—the practice is become as general as it is vile—it is become a common practice of masters towards their apprentices. ...[22]

Some critics maintained that apprenticeship was wrong in principle; others that five years was far too long. The evil of apprenticeship was a recurrent theme in the report of the Select Committee on Medical Education. George Man Burrows was almost alone in defending apprenticeship on the pragmatic grounds that country practitioners could not

[19] *SCME*, part III, Appendix, 139.
[20] Evidence of Sir David Barry, *SCME*, part I, Q. 2583.
[21] Ibid., Q. 2585. Dr Neil Arnott believed that the association of the Act with the Society of Apothecaries had deterred well-educated men from taking the LSA. On the continent, he added, the apothecary was excluded from good society, *SCME*, part I, 2471–4.
[22] An apprentice in Salisbury, *LMPJ* 34 (1815), 432.

manage without them. Sir Benjamin Brodie[23] and Benjamin Travers,[24] both eminent surgeons, condemned it. Joseph Henry Green, who wrote extensively on medical reform, believed that it degraded the character of the general practitioner with the public and the profession.[25] The apprentice got nothing out of it but drudgery while the master was handsomely paid.[26] 'Apothecaries' wrote one critic, 'secure a good living automaton in their shops for a period of five to seven years'[27] and apprentices, who as 'medical students' saw themselves a cut above any other kind of apprentice, complained of the indignities that went with their occupation.[28] Nevertheless, many who condemned the five-year period supported a much shorter time—six months or two years at most. G. J. Guthrie, the flamboyant surgeon who was three times president of the College, was one of these, and he emphasized that if four years were spent behind a counter, the last two were 'thrown away'.[29] A number of masters allowed their charges to spend the last two years in hospital studies,[30] and Mr Sankey of Margate suggested a novel system where a general practitioner with a genuine interest in systematic teaching, instead of mere drudgery should be allowed to take four to six apprentices at a time, each at a lower premium.[31]

Under this hail of criticism, those who had been involved in framing the Act entered a disclaimer. It had never, they said, been their intention to include apprenticeship. It had been forced on them, behind their backs, by the House of Lords in the person of Dr Parson, the 'late Bishop of Peterborough'.[32] This was a distortion of the truth. Apprenticeship was included in the Association's Bill from the first, but the clause was removed in the Commons by Mr Rose because of recent legislation which deplored apprenticeship unless there were special and exceptional circumstances. There was no special reason for making the profession

---

[23] *SCME*, part II, Q. 5725.

[24] Ibid., Q. 5823.

[25] Ibid., Q. 6474.

[26] 'Medical Politics and Intelligence', *Medical Quarterly Review*, 5 (1816), 60–1; see also *London Medical Repository*, 16 (1822), 311–25 and *Companion to the Newspaper* (1833), 120.

[27] 'Alexipharmicus', *A General Exposition of the Present State of the Medical Profession* (London, 1829), 2.

[28] *Lancet* (1840–1), i. 327.

[29] G. J. Guthrie, 'Introductory Lecture to Medical Students', *LMPJ*, NS 11 (1831), 444–7. See also *Quarterly Review*, 67 (Dec. 1840), 64–5 where abolition of apprenticeship was advocated.

[30] W. Hempson Denham, *Verba Consilia* (London, 1837).

[31] W. H. O. Sankey in *LMG*, NS 2 (1842–3), 394–6.

[32] 'Omnicron' in *LMPJ*, NS 3 (1827), 566–8.

of surgeon-apothecary an exception. It is, however, true that the Bishop of Peterborough, for reasons best known to himself, decided that the apprenticeship clause should go back in the Bill, and so it did. There was no protest all from the Association at the time.[33]

The most important argument against apprenticeship was its deadening effect on the mind and spirits of a youth at the beginning of his career.

A mind long conversant with trifles will certainly be rendered incapable of using exertions of a higher order, and the young man, after spending five years of his apprenticeship in the usual manner, will enter upon the real studies of his profession under much greater disadvantages than if he had never been apprenticed at all.[34]

'Mediculus' in 1830 believed that insistence on a five-year apprenticeship meant that 'a long and useful season of life has been wasted in the low employment of the shop'.[35] John Davies, physician to Hertford Infirmary, complained that the apprentice 'instead of being allowed to expand his mind ... he is, from the age of 14 or 15, immured for five years behind the counter to acquire a knowledge which he might obtain easily in six months.'[36] Those who defended apprenticeship did so on three grounds—educational, social, and moral. 'Books alone will not put a man in possession of this kind of knowledge ... it is perhaps one of the strongest objections to the abolition of apprenticeship', said one, ignoring the fact that the absence of practical clinical experience was the heart of the matter.[37] More cogently, it was pointed out that apprenticeship, at least in theory, provided practical experience of two very important groups who would not be encountered in hospitals, children and old people.[38] And, of course, there was midwifery. 'Nectemere' of Rochdale—and one wonders what apprentices thought of him—wrote in 1822:

[33] See evidence of G. M. Burrows, *SCME*, part III, Q. 312. 'Mr Rose ... struck this clause [apprenticeship] out of the Bill. When the Bill got into the House of Lords, that clause was restored without consulting us.'

[34] Anon., 'On Medical Apprenticeships', *London Medical Repository and Review*, 15 (1821), 89–101.

[35] 'Mediculus', 'The Physician and the Apothecary', *LMG* 5 (1830), 274–6.

[36] John Davies, *An Exposition of the Laws which relate to the Medical Profession* (London, 1844), 65.

[37] 'Alexipharmicus' (1829).

[38] Guildhall Library London, records of the Society of Apothecaries, MS 8211/1, May 1833, letter to Lord Melbourne.

A country Surgeon-Apothecary's apprentice has a situation well calculated for improving his mind ... he has no manipulation to perform but what he may accomplish in his drawing-room dress. ... As to midwifery, no adequate substitute can be found for a Country Apprenticeship in this department ... pages might be filled with the numerous and ludicrous blunders of those who have attempted it from a full course of lectures.[39]

In the voluminous letters and articles on apprenticeship, the principles of the system were mixed up with the realities. Many would have supported the system had it not been abused so extensively, but even the defenders of the system admitted that the opportunities for clinical experience were necessarily very limited: 'It cannot be expected that many opportunities of teaching youth the treatment of diseases can occur in private practice. But in country practice, especially, attendance on the sick poor often affords this advantage and should never be neglected.'[40] Apprenticeship, therefore, stood condemned on two counts. It did not do what it was meant to do—provide practical clinical experience as well as experience in making up bottles of medicine; and its perpetuation lowered the status of the general practitioner. Sensitivity on professional status was shown by perceptive Elizabeth Gaskell when she made Mr Hall refer to his apprentices as his 'pupils' because it was more genteel, although they were 'bound by indentures and paying a handsome premium to learn their business'.[41]

Why then was apprenticeship allowed to persist? One reason, and whatever we may think of it now it was seen at the time as a compelling reason, was the cost of education. It was argued that those who wanted their sons to follow a career as a general practitioner came from a section of society which would not be able to pay for education past the age of fourteen to sixteen.[42] If they were rich enough to pay for a full education then they would expect a better return for their money than the income of the country general practitioner: they would expect their sons to become physicians.[43] If it was insisted that all medical men should have had a full schooling to seventeen or eighteen you might 'force into practice a body of ill and cheaply-educated irregular practitioners ... because the class of persons who bring up their sons as

[39] 'Nectemere', *London Medical Repository and Review*, 16 (1822), 186–9.
[40] 'Report of the Progress of Medical Science', *London Medical Repository and Review*, 5 (1816), 60–1.
[41] Elizabeth Gaskell, *Wives and Daughters*, (Penguin edn., Harmondsworth, 1969) 64. First published 1864–6.
[42] Evidence of G. M. Burrows, *SCME*, part III, Q. 316.
[43] *SCME*, part I, Q. 2461.

general practitioners cannot afford to keep them at school after the age of 16'.[44] And, of course, sixteen was much too young to turn them loose amongst the temptations of the metropolis. The student of sixteen or seventeen needed firm 'moral control ... which cannot be exercised at any medical school whatsoever'.[45] G. M. Burrows said he had seen many instances when the character of a youth had been ruined by giving him his freedom amongst the vices of London at too early an age.[46]

Critics of apprenticeship could point to the waste of time, but in the end they came up against the practical problem. The physicians were all for apprenticeship. The last thing they wanted was recruitment from a broad social spectrum. They wanted to remain a select band of men and they stressed the social division between the origins of the physician and the general practitioner and the impossibility of parents of the latter finding the fees for full schooling. But there were others who stated just as firmly that a good general education was every bit as important for the general practitioners of the future as for members of any other branch of the profession. Benjamin Brodie was one of these and he expressed his views forcibly in an unsigned review on medical reform published in 1840 in the *Quarterly Review*.[47] Brodie saw apprenticeship as a positive hindrance to a good general education. He found it 'remarkable that twenty-five years should have been allowed to elapse without any attempt having been made to repeal a clause so unjust and mischievous'. An attempt to persuade the legislature to repeal this clause would probably have been successful in the prevalent atmosphere concerning apprenticeship; but it was never put forward by the Society of Apothecaries, the Association of Apothecaries and Surgeon-Apothecaries, or any other body. One can only conclude that apprenticeship with all its evils was so convenient to general practitioners that they made no move against it. To have justified its continuation on these grounds alone would have smelt too much of self-interest, so the usual justification was that apprenticeship served the useful purpose of filling the gap between school and the age at which it was safe to turn the lad loose as a medical student in London. Apprenticeship therefore persisted until it was abolished by the Medical Act of 1858.

[44] *SCME*, part I, Q. 2144.
[45] Guildhall Library, London, MS 8211/1, May 1833.
[46] Evidence of G. M. Burrows, *SCME*,, part III, Q. 316.
[47] (Sir Benjamin Brodie), 'Medical Reform', *Quarterly Review*, 67 (1840), 53–79. Published anonymously.

The prosecution of illegal practitioners

One of the great objects of the Apothecaries Act was clearly stated in section VII of the preamble:[48]

And whereas much mischief and inconvenience has arisen from great numbers of persons in many parts of England and Wales exercising the functions of an apothecary, who are wholly ignorant, and utterly incompetent to the exercise of such functions, whereby the health and lives of the community are greatly endangered: and it is become necessary that provisions should be made for remedying such evils ...

To remedy these evils it was enacted in section XX:

That if any person (except such as are then actually practising as such) shall, after the first day of August, one thousand eight hundred and fifteen, act or practise as an apothecary in any part of England and Wales without having obtained such certificate as aforesaid, every person so offending shall for every such offence forfeit and pay the sum of twenty pounds.

This was the penal clause which placed on the Society the responsibility for prosecutions against illegal practice. General practitioners regarded this clause as the means by which they would be protected against what they saw as the unfair competition of quacks. For a variety of reasons, the penal clause was an almost total failure, and that failure was bitterly resented by general practitioners from the time the Act was introduced.

In 1827 a general practitioner wrote to complain:

I am not factious or querulous, but I fearlessly maintain, that the promised rights, which I naturally expected, as a member of the College and Hall, have no existence, and that those who have never been educated have had as many advantages, and much more, than those who qualified and received diplomas in surgery and pharmacy. As the profession is now constituted a man cannot select a worse mode of life than that of a general practitioner. ...[49]

The operation of the penal clause depended on informers who were usually medical men, sometimes laymen, and occasionally anonymous. Once the information was received, the Society wrote to an 'agent living in the neighbourhood of the individual informed against' who was responsible for collecting the evidence of illegal practice.[50] The Society

[48] The Apothecaries Act is published in full in the *Transactions of the Associated Apothecaries*, 1 (1823), pp. xliv–lvi.
[49] Correspondence from 'General Practitioner', *LMSJ* 3 (1828), 55–6.
[50] Evidence of John Nussey, *SCME*, part III, Q. 105.

then decided whether it was appropriate to take action, and in making that decision it was strongly influenced by the knowledge that every prosecution would cost between £300 and £400 and that the Society itself would have to bear the entire cost.[51] The potential number of cases was legion. The Society was therefore torn between the need to be seen as carrying out its duties and the financial losses involved. The result can be seen in the appropriate register of the Society of Apothecaries for 1825–32 in which every information was entered, together, in the final column, with the decision of the Clerk to the Society.[52] The striking feature of this register is the rarity of any action on the vast majority of the information. Most of the entries in the final column were in the nature of 'evidence not furnished', 'insufficient', 'too trivial', or 'insignificant'. At other times the entry reads 'run away', 'states he does not practice', 'in practice before 1815', 'promises to quit practice', or 'appears to be unworthy of notice'. Sometimes the alleged offence was 'not a case of *medical* practice' if, for instance, the offender was a bone-setter. Other entries included 'The wrong name given and likely not the same person' [sic], and, mysteriously, 'service in the South Seas Service'.

The Society admitted in 1822 that it had received many informations but proceeded on only four cases. In the first the defendant had served his apprenticeship but had not practised before 1815. He took the examination and passed. The third case was similar. The second defendant protested that he had practised as an apothecary before 1815, but his total ignorance betrayed him. The fourth, who pretended to have been both an active apothecary and a wool-card maker before 1815 was clearly lying.[53] In the first seven years, therefore, only two irregular practitioners were prosecuted out of the swarming multitude, if general practitioners were to be believed, that was said to exist in all parts of the kingdom. Those who informed against a person expected a reward (half of the fine) and looked forward happily to the downfall of their antagonist. Nearly always they were disappointed.

Even more unsatisfactory were the successful prosecutions when they were levelled at well-qualified practitioners who by no stretch of the imagination could be described as ignorant or incompetent. The worst instance of this was, perhaps, the case of a Scottish trained practitioner which was mentioned in the Report of the Select Committee on Medical

---

[51] *A Statement by the Society of Apothecaries* (London, 1844) and evidence of G. M. Burrows, *SCME*, part III, 213–98.

[52] Guildhall Library, MS 8238, vol. i.

[53] 'New Regulations Concerning Apothecaries', *LMPJ* 48 (1822), 452–5.

Education, 1834. This man had followed an exceptionally extensive course of study in Edinburgh, had obtained the MD, and worked as assistant to two departments of Edinburgh Infirmary. Four years after matriculation he returned to England and set up in practice as a general practitioner in 1824. He dispensed medicines as part of the routine of practice. He was, moreover, 'unanimously elected medical attendant to the Parish, and Surgeon to the Yeomanry Cavalry'. Information was given (probably by a medical neighbour jealous of his success) and proceedings against him were instituted by the Society which, he said, cost him a total of £400. Then, he said, 'after this action, to enable me to dispense with impunity, I took a partner who was a licentiate of the Society and also a fellow of the London College of Surgeons; and I have now received another notice, that information has been laid against me, and that proceedings are again to be commenced forthwith.'[54] The Society's excuse was that it had 'no alternative but of proceeding at once against a man where the clearest evidence exists of his being an irregular practitioner.'[55] This excuse scarcely rang true when the known tendency of the Society was to avoid prosecution whenever possible. The Select Committee was amazed and shocked that the unforeseen result of the Apothecaries Act was prosecutions of this sort.

The refusal of the Society of Apothecaries to recognize Scottish qualifications as an automatic reason for granting a licence was manifestly unjust. But it was also more complex than appears at first sight. The strongest argument was in favour of recognizing Scottish MDs, but here they came up against the delicate problem of distinguishing between the well-trained Edinburgh and Glasgow graduates and the bought MDs of Aberdeen and St Andrews. That was bad enough, but the LRCS Ed., a popular diploma, presented other problems. It was widely acknowledged even in England that the course for this diploma was closer to the ideal training for the general practitioner than any other medical qualification in existence at the time, for it included an excellent education in medicine, surgery, midwifery, and pharmacy.[56] But recognition of the Edinburgh diploma might upset the English College of Surgeons which

does not possess and does not aspire to, the privilege of granting licences to general practice; the parties know, and feel, that the moment they did so, they

---

[54] *SCME*, part III, Q. 100.   [55] Ibid.

[56] See a comparison of the syllabus of the MRCS (London) and the LRCS (Ed.) in *SCME*, part II, Q. 4845 (table). See also 'A Disinterested Physician' (Dr E. Barlow), *MPJ* 30 (1813), 287: *LMPJ*, NS 11 (1831), 498: *EMSJ* 14 (1818), 11.

would become a College of Apothecaries. ... Such being the case, the question is, whether a privilege is to be forced upon the gentlemen of Lincoln's-Inn Fields which they do not covet; or a jurisdiction to be given to the Edinburgh and Glasgow surgeons over the practice in England, in which the London College of Surgeons does not participate?[57]

The problem was made worse by the atmosphere of jealousy and suspicion between the Scottish medical corporations and their English equivalents. Scottish graduates who applied to take the Licence of the Society were advised to conceal their degrees and diplomas or they would be sure to fail; and an instance was given of such a case when the candidate was told ' "we don't want any of your MDs—it will not serve your purpose here"—and neither it did, for they rejected him.'[58] Yet in spite of this there was a steady movement of opinion towards reciprocity between the two parts of the United Kingdom. But it was slow, and the chief hindrance was the stolid obstinacy of the English medical corporations. In November 1838 the three medical corporations of Edinburgh wrote to the Society of Apothecaries to suggest complete reciprocity between themselves. The letter was simply acknowledged, and there the matter ended.[59]

In the case of the prosecutions and the attempted negotiations, the Society may have followed the letter of the law, but not the spirit. It was no wonder that the *Edinburgh Medical and Surgical Journal* complained in 1845 that:

A doctor or a surgeon may bleed, blister, sweat diureticize and mercurialize patients as much or so long as he chooses if he do not supply the means by which these various functions are performed. The moment he spreads a blister or dispenses a few grains of calomel, or squill and digitalis, he places himself within the fangs of the Apothecaries Company.[60]

The Society also came under criticism when it prosecuted Mr Ryan, MRCS, on the grounds that he had undertaken, as all surgeons did, the treatment of medical cases. Ryan's defence was based on the fact that although he had treated cases of internal diseases and supplied medicines, he had not charged for medicines and therefore had not

    [57] 'Amended Apothecaries Bill', *LMG* 12 (1833), 294–6.
    [58] *Medical Quarterly Review*, 1 (1833–4), 465–7.
    [59] Guildhall Library London, MS 8211, vol. ii.
    [60] 'Leading Article', *EMSJ* 63 (1845), 159–97.

acted as an apothecary.[61] Was this an adequate defence? The views of the *Lancet* were relevant to the answer to this question. Wakley, whose hatred for the Society of Apothecaries ('Rhubarb Hall') was only exceeded by that for the Colleges of Physicians and Surgeons, had, with characteristic vigour, already challenged the Society's right to prosecute, believing that he had driven the coach and horses of pure logic through the deficiencies of the Act.

> Now we defy his Lordship, or any other person, to point out a single sentence in the Apothecaries Act which tends to prove that *visiting* a patient is acting as an Apothecary: that *prescribing* for a patient is acting as an Apothecary; or that dispensing a prescription, even, is acting as an Apothecary, unless that prescription bears the initials of a legally authorised physician. The Apothecaries Act contains *no such clause*: and every conviction, *without exception*, that has occurred under the operation of that Act, has been *illegal*.[62]

While it seems that Wakley may very well have been right, the judiciary were more concerned with the meaning of the Act than with a literal interpretation of such a flawed piece of legislation. Ryan was found guilty on the direction of the judge, albeit rather reluctantly, when it was decided that the province of the surgeon was external diseases and the treatment of internal disease was, in instances such as this, 'acting as an apothecary'.

Other cases against surgeons were to follow, and the anonymous contributor to the *Provincial Medical and Surgical Journal* of 1841 correctly observed that 'a more signal instance of solid supineness could not well be exhibited than the neglect of the Surgeons on this occasion [i.e. when the Act of 1815 was introduced] to protect its own licentiates from the restrictive clauses of the Apothecaries Act'.[63] The absurdity of these cases led to calls for the repeal of the Apothecaries Act. A leading article on medical reform in 1833 pointed out the glaring abuses of the profession. It instanced the London College of Physicians as a 'junta of time-serving, place-hunting intriguing men' and the idiocy of the Society of Apothecaries in its persecution of Edinburgh graduates—'the future medical historian can scarcely believe that this is the State of Physic in 1833'.[64]

---

[61] 'Important to Surgeons', *MCR*, NS 14 (1831), 570–1, and 'Miscellanies', *LMSJ* 7 (1831), 173–5.

[62] 'Leading Article', *Lancet* (1826–7), ii. 514–7.

[63] 'Medical Reform', *PMSJ* 1 (1841), 151–5.

[64] 'Repeal of the Apothecaries Act. Abuses in the Profession', *LMSJ*, NS 3 (1833), 341–2.

All these difficulties formed the subject of a report in 1847 by the clerk of the Society of Apothecaries, Robert Upton, who had been responsible for the administration of the penal clause during the previous thirteen years. Upton believed that the penal clause had been partially effective in the suppression of irregular practice. When Sir James Graham introduced his Medical Bill with its proposal to abolish the prosecution of illegal practitioners, the Society decided to 'put a pause on its police activities'. Instantly it was rumoured that unqualified practice was no longer illegal and there was an upsurge of illegal practice. In response to an open denial by the Society that prosecutions had ceased, informations were laid, and 'actions were afterwards commenced against parties practising in Yorkshire, Nottinghamshire, Leicestershire and Somersetshire, but by far the greatest number of individuals were of necessity left to pursue their practice undisturbed.' This only enraged the general practitioners who protested:

We complain of illegal practice at our own doors—practice which is robbing us of the legitimate reward of a long course of professional study—practice which you have publicly promised to check, but which you suffer to continue undisturbed, and it is nothing to us to know that you are engaged in stopping such practice elsewhere.

The Society replied that the burden of being the sole prosecutor of illegal practice was too great for a single body, and they wanted to inform the profession and the law officers of the Crown that facilities for prosecuting offenders should be opened to others as well as the Society.[65] In fairness, the Society of Apothecaries had never sought, and was constitutionally unfit for, the role of public prosecutor. It was a trading company with no previous experience of such activities, unused to public conflict and public criticism. It was said of the Society that when the Act was introduced they hardly knew 'the important powers and duties that had devolved upon them'.[66] It may be hard to believe, but it would explain why the Society was so inept when it was finally forced to take action on the basis of an imperfect Act lacking a precise definition of illegal practice. Paradoxically, matters got worse when the plans for medical reform included the proposed abolition of the Apothecaries Act and therefore of its penal clauses. While one group of medical men

[65] Guildhall Library, MS 8212, 12 May 1847. This manuscript report is the most comprehensive account of the difficulties of the Society in respect of the penal clause. See also *Gazette of Health*, 9 (1844), 897–9.

[66] *SCME*, part III, Q. 270.

supported the repeal of the Act with its dismal record on apprenticeship and illegal practice,[67] another, which included the Association of General Medical and Surgical Practitioners,[68] called for its preservation on the grounds that, however imperfectly it had performed, at least it had the power to curb illegal practice. Something was better than nothing.

The Society, disturbed from its comfortable if undistinguished existence in 1815, found it was beset on all sides. It could please nobody and was forced to admit its incompetence to carry out the duties conferred on it. The Society's ability to turn out large numbers of licentiates is not disputed. Between 1815 and 1816, 173 candidates passed the examination. This had increased to 381 for the year 1822–3 and 445 by 1825–6. The highest annual number was 535 (in 1836–7) and the number from 1820 to 1844 remained between 300 and 400 a year. At first the pass rate was 93–94%; it fell after a few years to 83–84% but never below 80%.[69] This smooth production line has largely been responsible for the myth that the Act as a whole was a great success.

To assess the Act as a whole from the historical point of view one has to contrast it with some realistic alternative. The main alternative was the original Bill devised by the Association and discussed in the previous chapter. Would it have been an improvement on the Apothecaries Act? It can be argued that the original Bill, which planned the establishment of a 'fourth body' would have been even more divisive by creating a quadripartite rather than a tripartite division when unification rather than division was needed. However, the history of the profession has shown that the multiplication of medical colleges is not in fact divisive. It is also reasonable to question whether there were individuals within the Association capable of forming a nucleus of a 'fourth body' which could regulate the licensing and education of general practitioners. The subsequent history of men such as A. T. Thomson, Burrows, and Parkinson suggests that there was such a nucleus.

In any historical study there is a certain futility in trying to guess what might have been instead of confining oneself to interpreting what actually happened. But the clear plans of the Association of Apothecaries and Surgeon-Apothecaries in 1812–13 formed the basis for a much

[67] 'Medical Reform', *Medical Quarterly Review*, 2 (1834), 233.

[68] See report of the Association of General Practitioners, *LMG* 12 (1833), 367–8.

[69] *A Statement by the Society of Apothecaries on the Subject of their Administration of the Apothecaries Act* (London, 1844).

more satisfactory education for the rank-and-file practitioners than the mangled version embodied in the Act of 1815. If one can postulate that the degraded position of the general practitioner was in large part due to the shortcomings of the Act, then the blame lay fairly and squarely on the Colleges of Physicians and Surgeons whose impenetrable opposition was based on naked self-interest. Neither the medical care of the population as a whole, nor the position of the mass of general practitioners, concerned the Colleges when they considered the supposed threat to their autonomy. Their attitude towards the general practitioner remained unchanged throughout the remainder of the period of medical reform.

9

The Status of the General Practitioner

The profession in a state of confusion

THERE are two separate though connected aspects to the status of the general practitioner. First, his status in the eyes of his fellow practitioners and secondly, in the eyes of society as a whole.

The position of the general practitioner within the medical profession became clear during the second half of the nineteenth century when physicians and surgeons were increasingly perceived as consultants and specialists, and general practitioners were clearly relegated to the 'subordinate grade'. This process of demarcation was, of course, a gradual one. Even in the 1930s in certain provincial towns, the local consultants were accurately defined as local general practitioners who happened to hold an honorary appointment at the county infirmary. But the process of separation had already advanced sufficiently by the last quarter of the nineteenth century to produce a condition of stability, but not contentment, in the medical profession.

The first half of the century was quite different. Open recognition that the tripartite division was obsolete combined with uncertainty about the future to produce an unstable condition within the profession. With the exception of a small minority in London, physicians and surgeons before 1850 did not practise in the modern sense primarily as specialists or consultants. Still less were they specialists within the main division of physic or surgery. Indeed, those who specialized in one organ or system were liable to the scorn of their colleagues who saw them as men who had failed in the general fields of physic or surgery and were forced to set up as specialists in order to attract business.[1] Some of the London consultants believed that in order to know the whole of surgery it had become necessary in the early nineteenth century to devote all one's attention to that subject alone.[2] But this was the view of the

---

[1] *Gazette of Health,* 1 (1816), 84–5. Here, special branches of surgery were condemned as 'partial practice' and 'advertisements for fees'.

[2] Evidence of G. J. Guthrie, *SCME,* part II, Q. 4770. Guthrie, however, used this argument only to justify the restrictive regulations of the College of Surgeons.

celebrated minority, who would usually add the proviso that all medical practitioners, whatever their field, were better doctors for practising as broadly as possible. Specializing in medicine had not become the essential pathway to prosperity or high status.

In 1827 it was pointed out that the 'pure surgeons and consulting physicians are "rarae aves" certainly—to be met with only in very large towns; if we take another step down the ladder of professional distinctions, we find everything mixed and jumbled, brayed [sic] and blended in the pretentions and pursuits of the general practitioner.'[3] It was precisely because everything was 'mixed' and 'jumbled' that opportunities for advancement were open to all ranks of the profession, including the general practitioners. Indeed, the general practitioners with their dual qualification, believed they might well be the leading group within the profession. 'The tendency had continually been to the union of medicine and surgery in practice, and to equalisation of rank: the inferior class pressing upwards to get on a level with the superior and the two classes in continual broils until that level was attained.' The writer of that passage in 1842 believed this 'desirable state of affairs' had 'nearly been reached'.[4]

The blurring of distinctions was emphasized repeatedly by witnesses who gave evidence to the Select Committee on Medical Education in 1834. John Sims, physician to the St Marylebone Hospital, believed the division of the profession into physician, surgeon, and general practitioner was 'more ostensible than real'.[5] Neil Arnott believed that 'at present there are men of nearly equal distinction in all departments of the profession and the whole scheme of distinction is falling to pieces'.[6] Others noted the same tendency.[7] *Punch* made fun of the outdated division between physic and surgery based on 'internal' and 'external' diseases. 'The faculty has decided that the body has an *inside* and an *outside*, just like an omnibus, the laws of nature with respect to each being different.'[8] More seriously, it became accepted wisdom that 'surgeons, considering it impossible to form a line of separation, either on the principle of science or on the grounds of public good, practise not only surgery in all its branches, but medicine also'.[9] One of the reasons

[3] Editorial, *London Medical Repository and Review*, NS 5 (1827), 188.
[4] *BFMR* 14 (1842), 402–11.
[5] *SCME*, part I, Q. 2121–31.
[6] Ibid., Q. 2467.
[7] *BFMR* 9 (1840), 283–4; *PMSJ* 2 (1841), 152.
[8] Quoted in G. Allarton, *Mysteries of Medical Life* (London, 1856), 61.
[9] N. Dickinson, 'On the State of the Medical Profession', *LMPJ* 44 (1820), 470.

was the loss of surgical cases, especially in the provinces, to general practitioners who believed themselves competent in this, as in all, branches of medicine. Sir James Clark noted in 1843: 'Previously those who have been styled "pure surgeons", were alone intrusted with ... the performance of all operations of any consequence ... and patients were brought great distances to London.' But times had changed and 'a considerable part of the practice of the Surgeons as well as of the Physicians, has thus fallen into the hands of the General Practitioners'.[10] Moreover, surgery in the early nineteenth century had moved into a conservative phase. Medical treatments had replaced operation for many surgical conditions, a change which Sir Benjamin Brodie referred to 'as one of the proudest distinctions of English Surgery as compared with that in most parts of the Continent'.[11] The surgeon had to be conversant with medical treatment as well as surgical, so that fashion, financial need, and medical science urged the surgeon constantly to cross the time-honoured division between physic and internal diseases, and surgery and external ones.

Sir Anthony Carlisle, never noted for his modesty, believed himself able to treat medical disorders as well as any physician. In his opinion 'distinctions between what belongs to the physician and what to the surgeon are indefinable. ... Suppose a man has a disease of the lower intestine. If it is out of reach of the finger it belongs to the physician; but the moment it comes down and within reach of the finger, it belongs to the surgeon.'[12] Since most diseases contained an element of common ground the distinction between physic and surgery was essentially false.[13] In 1815 John Yeatman of Frome in Somerset, a general prac- titioner of energy and ability, considered that only by 'unnatural and narrow-minded efforts' could anyone defend the old division, because 'the internal and external parts of the body are governed by the same general laws'.[14] As surgeons encroached on the practice of physic, a few conditions, previously the territory of surgery, were absorbed by the physicians, especially skin diseases and venereal disease.[15]

A physician complained in 1816 about surgeons treating 'phthisical

---

[10] Sir James Clark, *Remarks on Medical Reform* (London, 1843).

[11] 'Report on the Select Committee on Medical Education', *Quarterly Review*, 67 (1840), 53–79. The authorship is attributed to Sir Benjamin Brodie.

[12] *SCME*, part II, Q. 5981–3.

[13] R. Hull, 'On the Division of Medical Labour', *LMG*, NS I (1842–3), 520–3.

[14] John Yeatman, 'Observations on Medical Reform', *MPJ* 34 (1815), 186–93.

[15] Evidence of Dr George Birkbeck, *SCME*, part I, Q. 3533.

and dropsical patients'[16] and others echoed the loss of practice to the surgeons.[17] Not surprisingly, it was the backward-looking physicians who longed for a mythical past when, they believed, every practitioner knew his place and kept within his boundaries. They saw the eighteenth century as an idyllic *ancien régime*: 'Physician, surgeon and apothecary are the ancient, the true, the English arrangement. Interwoven with the very structure of English Society, the medical practice has been tripartite—physic, surgery, pharmacy, or surgery *united* with pharmacy. This adapted, this scientific, this ancient division of labour the medical reformer seeks to destroy.' But they found little sympathy with most of their colleagues. In 1840, in an editorial on medical reform, the *British and Foreign Medical Review* remarked

it is strange that any can be found to regard a renewal of the old system practicable, or even desirable. Yet there are several, chiefly amongst the class of physicians, who, yearning for a return of the good old times, really imagine that the old system could be revived, and whose beau ideal of medical reform would be the re-establishment of the physician, surgeon, and apothecary (i.e. druggist) each restricted to his own special functions, as was presumed to be the case in the earlier period. No reform can have a chance of permanency unless ... it adapts itself to those wants of the public which have been so unequivocally demonstrated; namely, by supplying an adequately qualified class of general practitioners.[18]

Physicians, surgeons and general practitioners were therefore competing with each other in the market for medical care. It was inevitable that in doing so they trod on each other's toes. This overlapping of the roles of the three groups of practitioners is a recurrent theme. It is considered again in chapter 10 in the context of a statistical analysis of the numbers of medical practitioners and their qualifications. It is introduced here not only because it is the key to understanding the period of medical reform, but to underline the uncertain status of the general practitioner.

Because it was an age that admired breadth of knowledge rather than narrow specialization, there was substance in the claim of general

---

[16] *Annals of Medicine and Surgery*, 1 (1816), 514.

[17] Sir James Clark (1843); and evidence of J. Wardrop, *SCME*, part II, Q. 6259–70.

[18] The nostalgic view of the old system of medicine was expressed by Dr R. Hull, a physician, and is quoted by D. O. Edwards in 'Thoughts on the Real and Imaginary Grievances of the Profession', *Lancet* (1841–2), ii. 510–14, 606–14, 742–7, 776–83. The editorial in the *British and Foreign Medical Review*, 19 (1840), 281–7, was presumably the work of its editor, John Forbes, MD (Edin.), FRCP London, consulting physician to the Hospital for Consumption and Diseases of the Chest.

practitioners to a leading position within the profession. On the other hand it was recognized that whatever their position in the second quarter of the nineteenth century it was only yesterday that they were on the lower deck. This was shown by the practice of pharmacy which acted as a constant reminder of the stigma of trade and the image of the shop associated with the apothecary. To make matters worse, that association had evolved to form a new connection between the general practitioner and the druggist. If only the general practitioner could clear this hurdle and free himself from his past associations, it seemed there was nothing to stop him from rising to the top. After all, he had the numerical advantage over his rivals.

The optimism of the early general practitioners

If that was true, it was the physicians who had most to fear. When they heard the 'raw licentiates of the Apothecaries' boast that 'really our education is now so good ... we must supersede the physicians ere long'[19] they could dismiss it as crude youthful arrogance. But it was not so easy to dismiss the flood of papers in the medical press, many by senior and influential practitioners. These said, in essence, the same as the raw licentiates, asserting that the medical education of general practitioners was at least as good as, the physicians'. A senior member of the Metropolitan Society of General Practitioners wrote to the *Lancet* in 1829 to explain:

It is only the general practitioner who, when called upon, does not stop to inquire if the patient is afflicted with a 'surgical' or a 'medical' disorder; he feels himself doubly armed for either emergency and it is upon these grounds we take our stand. ... The title of general practitioner is that, which, more than any other title, is descriptive of what we are ... and we want no other assumption to give us dignity.[20]

'Surgeon Snipe' wrote that 'General Practitioners are strictly *the* Medical Men of this century—Scientific Medical and Surgical Practitioners. Amongst this class of men may be ranked some of the highest names in the annals of Medicine.'[21] Another believed the general practitioner 'is to all intents and purposes a *physician* as truly and unquestionably as ever was Radcliffe himself';[22] while the *Gazette of Health*, always the

[19] 'The State of the Profession—the General Practitioner', *LMG* 6 (1830), 619–21.

[20] Letter from 'Member of the Committee of the Metropolitan Society of General Practitioners', *Lancet* (1829–30), ii. 653.

[21] Surgeon Snipe, *Remarks on Physicians, Surgeons, Druggists and Quacks* (London, 1842).

[22] Editorial, *London Medical Repository and Review*, NS 5 (1827), 188.

extravagant friend of the 'rank and file' and enemy of the physician, believed that 'General Practitioners are years, if not centuries, in advance of the medical graduates of Oxford and Cambridge.'[23] Others with a cooler approach felt the general practitioner might be a physician in the profession's eyes but not in the public's;[24] and the *Medico-Chirurgical Review* devised a new classification of medical men where it was suggested that the general practitioner should be designated as the 'physician-in-ordinary' as opposed to the 'graduate physician'.[25] The title, it was supposed, would lend dignity. In 1831 Dr W. Cooke remarked on the frequency with which the general practitioner of 'intelligence and ample experience' often became 'the consulting physician and surgeon to a wide circle of his brethren'.[26]

By the 1830s, examples of general practitioners could be found in many provincial areas whose practice and reputation seemed to make nonsense of rank and divisions in the medical profession. When this was said publicly, however, it was strongly denied by the medical corporations. The denials were subjected to Wakley's sarcasm in one of his vintage editorials in the *Lancet* which is frequently quoted.

The Royal Colleges have discovered the most extraordinary ground for creating professional distinction that ever entered into the mind of man. With them, the chief qualification for eminence in the healing art is ignorance of one or the other half of it. A physician need not know much of physic; an entire ignorance of surgery will be sufficient to give him a respectable standing; a surgeon need not possess any real knowledge of surgery, but if he be sufficiently ignorant of physic—if he does not know the gout from the measles—that will render him 'pure' and make him eligible to receive the highest appointments; but a general practitioner—a man so preposterous as to understand both physic and surgery—is fit only to become a subordinate.[27]

Many of the witnesses to the Select Committee on Medical Education (1834) stressed the high level of education of general practitioners. One believed 'the education now required ... is of the very highest kind; I should say as good as that of physicians some years ago.'[28] From some that might have been faint praise; but from a Cambridge graduate,

[23] *Gazette of Health,* 11 (1826), 67; ibid. 12 (1827), 906.
[24] 'Mediculus', 'The Physician and the Apothecary', *LMG* 5 (1830), 274–6.
[25] 'Medical Statistics and Reform', *MCR* 20 (1834), 567–71.
[26] W. Cooke, *Separation without Dissension* (London, 1831).
[27] *Lancet* (1842–3) ii. 719–22.
[28] E. J. Seymour, *SCME,* part I, Q. 1060; see also John Sims, ibid., part I, Q. 2124–35, 2150, 2234; Neil Arnott, ibid., part I, Q. 2467; B. Brodie, ibid., part II, Q. 5676; Anthony Carlisle, Q. 5984, G. J. Guthrie, Q. 4902, and ibid., part III, G. M. Burrows, Q. 280.

FRCP, censor of the College of Physicians and physician to St George's Hospital, it was a notable endorsement of growing respect for the education and office of general practitioner. To an increasing extent people were saying that the general practitioner had been created by a public demand for a reliable, education all-rounder, to replace physicians and surgeons who colluded with each other and the apothecary to rob the patient.[29] 'The public stood in need of a general Practitioner— that is, one who could officiate in all departments of the profession and dispense medicines as well as prescribe. This species of practitioner, which had sprung up insensibly, got to such an extent that the formal recognition of this new department became indispensable.'[30] Kerrison had stressed in 1814 that nineteen out of twenty patients were treated by general practitioners alone.[31] The *Edinburgh Medical and Surgical Journal* in 1818 called the general practitioner 'the only full doctor',[32] and 'Alexipharmicus' in 1829 said the general practitioners were 'respectable, useful, upright'.[33] The Regius Professor of Medicine in Oxford in 1842 thought the status of the general practitioner was higher and that he attended all classes of society,[34] while Sir James Clark in 1843 declared that 'upon the skill and judgement of the General Practitioner depends mainly the health of the Community'.[35] Editorials in the *British and Foreign Medical Review* in the 1840s saw the general practitioners as members of a new, essential 'third estate', created by public demand;[36] while the *London Medical Gazette* quoted with approval the view that a supply of adequately qualified general practitioners was a matter of national importance.[37] Likewise, the *Medical Examiner* in 1830 asserted that general practitioners were well educated and thus 'the fittest persons to administer medicine and surgery to the population at large'.[38]

Medical opinion appeared to endorse these laudatory views, at least

---

[29] 'Of Mr Abernethy', *Gazette of Health*, 3 (1818), 96.
[30] 'Medical Reform', *PMSJ* 2 (1841), 151–5.
[31] R. M. Kerrison, *An Inquiry into the Present State of the Medical Profession in England* (London, 1814).
[32] Editorial, *EMSJ* 15 (1818), 8.
[33] 'Alexipharmicus', *A General Exposition of the Present State of the Medical Profession* (London, 1829).
[34] J. Kidd, *Further Observations on Medical Reform* (London, 1842).
[35] Sir James Clark (1843).
[36] 'Medical Reform', *BFMR* 9 (1840), 281–9; and 'Mediculus', *BFMR* 19 (1845), 193–232.
[37] *LMG*, NS 2 (1842–3), 52–3.
[38] *Medical Examiner*, 1 (1830), 105.

in public. What is notable by its absence is a robust counter-claim by hospital physicians and surgeons that superior status lay in consultant practice, or specialization, or in hospital appointments. None of these features had yet acquired the importance with which they would be invested in the second half of the century.

In view of this chorus of praise for the general practitioners, why did they fail so conspicuously to establish themselves in the eyes of the public and the profession as the equals if not the superiors of all groups of medical practitioners? The answer to this question is complex. Some of the reasons will appear later in this chapter and in the next. But there was one factor above all which pointed to the inferior status of the general practitioner; and that was the practice of pharmacy. To a lesser extent midwifery was also regarded as an inferior occupation. For the socially ambitious, upwardly mobile general practitioner, 'the rubbish of pharmacy and obstetricity'[39] was the albatross around his neck.

The practice of pharmacy and the druggists

'Well then,' asked a correspondent in 1836, 'in what consists the difference between the general practitioner and the physician, seeing that in medical education they are perfectly on the level?' And he answered that it was the public image, due to 'the business of selling draughts. . . . So long as the general practitioner vends medicine he is a mere poacher on the manor of the Physician, the Surgeon and the Druggist.'[40] Pharmacy degraded, although it was an integral part of general practice, because it was a reminder of the five-year apprenticeship behind a counter, because it was a link to the old-style apothecary, and most of all, because it blurred the distinction between the druggist and the general practitioner.[41]

Medical men protested that the druggist was way below them, 'a set of small traders, ignorant of the property of medicines, and who have nevertheless, the most perfect confidence in their therapeutic skill',[42] but it was undeniable that 'a great number of apothecaries [were] driven by necessity to become the actual chemists and druggists of the narrow streets and bye-lanes . . . content to receive their pittance in the humblest

[39] W. Cooke (1831).
[40] 'Ille ego qui Quondam', *Lancet* (1836–7), i. 647–8.
[41] For a description of the variety of chemists and druggists in early nineteenth-century London, see Anon. *The Book of English Trades* (London, 1818).
[42] *Medical Examiner*, 1 (1830), 105–7.

coin; while their more dashing rivals the "pharmacopolists" ... take possession of the broadways and line their "tills" with a more noble metal.'[43]

Some of the druggists had become very successful indeed, especially in London. It was a group of such men who, in 1802, formed the standing committee of an association of druggists which successfully opposed the attempt to place them under control when the Apothecaries Act was introduced. Clause 28 of that Act which exempted the chemists and druggists was a tribute to their influence. The committee included amongst its thirteen members men such as Allen, Bell, and Savory, whose names are still associated with pharmacy.[44]

By the 1820s when the dispensing druggist was firmly established, the chemist's shop had become 'a social necessity'[45] and in every new area shops retailing drugs sprang up 'long before the grocer, the butcher, the cheesemonger' and 'put "Doctor" over the door'.[46] Some were 'mere druggists' while others were 'licentiates of Apothecaries Hall or Surgeons forced into retail trade in order to survive.'[47] It was clear that 'so long as the Medical Man persists in identifying himself to the tradesman, he cannot expect the public to draw a distinction'.[48]

The distinction was even more blurred by the allegations that druggists visited patients at home and even practised surgery and midwifery. How much these reports were apocryphal is hard to say, since definite evidence is so often lacking and they often raise the suspicion of mere rumour.[49] But there is at least one report—from Wales—which has the ring of authenticity.[50] The reports, however, stressed the hairbreadth's difference between the druggist and the general practitioner in the eyes of the public, although one had a formal and expensive education and the other did not.

Burrows in his time as chairman of the Association of Apothecaries hated the druggists because they had 'greatly deteriorated the profits' of the general practitioners; but in 1813 he had the intelligence to recognize long before the majority of his colleagues that the druggist was

---

[43] J. Davies, *An Exposition of the Laws which relate to the Medical Profession* (London, 1844).

[44] Jacob Bell, *Historical Sketch of the Progress of Pharmacy* (London, 1843).

[45] D. O. Edwards, *Lancet*, (1841–2), ii. 779.

[46] Leading article, *Lancet* (1833–4), i. 722.

[47] *LMG*, NS 2 (1842–3), 52–3.

[48] *Medical Times*, 19 (1848–9), 594.

[49] *LMPJ* 43 (1820), 500.

[50] Correspondence, 'General Practitioner—North Wales', *Lancet* (1836–7), i. 412.

too firmly established to be dislodged. 'It had indeed become difficult', he wrote, 'to define who was and who was not an apothecary, and I greatly rejoiced when the Chemists and Druggists prepared the twenty-eighth clause because it, in some measure, defined that which before was undefined.'[51] Separation was the only alternative to suppression. Any attempt at legal suppression and 'John Bull would strenuously resist this law as contrary to the spirit and safety of his "CONSTITUTION".' From their position of strength, the druggists then had the impudence (as the general practitioners saw it) to suggest that all dispensing should be in their hands alone; and they argued that when that happened, their 'education ought to be regulated' so that the druggists would become, 'as they were fast becoming, the ci-devant APOTHECARY'.[52] Guthrie, the surgeon, agreed, quoting the absurd experience of a friend of his who was refused a simple bottle of his usual medicine by a nervous druggist in Pall Mall because he had brought no prescription.[53] But if the druggist was educated, examined, and licensed, the difference between the general practitioner and the druggist would be almost invisible. Therefore, if the general practitioner wanted to become a 'physician in ordinary' and a respectable member of the medical profession, he would have to abandon pharmacy and become 'a physician who will take plebian silver instead of patrician gold and pocket half-a-crown without blushing'.[54] There were many who shared this view.[55] Others defended the right of the general practitioner to dispense, arguing that it was a skill best performed by one with a medical education who had the opportunity of observing the effects of his own dispensing. Things should be left as they were for the public good.[56]

The argument, however, was largely academic. General practitioners continued to dispense medicines and, indeed, 'except in a few large towns, every man who practises medicine at all deals in drugs and must

[51] G. M. Burrows, *A Statement of Circumstances connected with the Apothecaries Act* (London, 1817).

[52] G. Crook, *The Proposed Scheme of Medical Reform in Reference to Chemists and Druggists*, reviewed in *MCR*, NS 36 (1842), 162–3. See also *Lancet* (1829–30), i. 711.

[53] Evidence of G. J. Guthrie, *SCME*, part II, Q. 4901.

[54] 'Medical Reform', *Medical Quarterly Review*, 2 (1834), 232–3.

[55] 'Chirurgo-Medicus', *ESMJ* 10 (1814), 128–30; Surgeon Snipe (1842); Dr James Turnbull, *PMSJ* 3 (1842), 321. Correspondence, *Lancet* (1836–7), i. 647–8; D.O. Edwards, *Lancet*, (1841), ii. 779; Sir James Clark (1843); 'Medical Statistics and Reform', *MCR* 20 (1834), 576–71.

[56] *Medical Examiner*, 1 (1830), 105–7; Leading Article, *Lancet* (1833–4), i. 722; see 'Alexipharmicus', *A General Description of . . . the Medical Profession* (London, 1829), where it was stated that 'The Apothecary is the very Keynote of Physic'; A. Banks, *Medical Etiquette* (London, 1839).

do so',[57] at any rate in his early years in practice.[58] Trollope showed this well in his portrait of Dr Thorne who shocked his physician neighbours by dispensing drugs, outwardly oblivious of the social implications of doing so.[59] Others said it was a matter of indifference whether a general practitioner or a chemist supplied the medicine to the patient;[60] but the stigma of 'trade' remained. Whether the general practitioner would have risen in the eyes of the public by depriving them of the convenience of providing medicines, even if it was at a higher price, is doubtful. They were convinced they could not afford to do so, even if some of them yearned to be known as the 'physician-in-ordinary' to the mass of the people. What, then, was the social standing of the general practitioner in the society of early nineteenth-century England? A professional gentleman, a tradesman, or somewhere between the two?

The status of the general practitioner

In a recent paper on the medical profession in Victorian England, Peterson concluded that there was a chasm between the 'liberal professions' of law, the church, and the military—the traditional occupations for the younger sons of gentlemen—and the profession of medicine.[61] Whereas the 'liberal professions' recruited a majority of members from the 'social crème' (defined as the gentry and non-medical professionals), less than 20 per cent of medical practitioners came from this level of society; and a similar social difference was noted in the grammar school/public school divide within these two groups. But Peterson's most important conclusion was that the chasm was unbridgeable. It was only the 'liberal professions' that provided the freedom from outside interference to which the younger sons of gentry were accustomed. Medicine was different. Medical men were ruled by governors of hospitals, by their patients, by sick-club committees and bureaucrats. Because of this, medicine was a subservient profession, the subservience being an inherent quality. It was also, in its close physical contacts, often a menial profession as well. It follows that attempts to improve the status of medicine by recruitment from the 'social crème'

---

[57] 'Amendment to the Apothecaries Act' The Companion to the Newspaper (1833).
[58] Editorial, *EMSJ* 63 (1845), 175.
[59] Anthony Trollope, *Dr Thorne* (London, 1858).
[60] 'A Practitioner', *Is the Practice of Medicine a Degenerate Pursuit?* (London, 1850).
[61] M. J. Peterson, 'Gentlemen and Medical Men: The Problem of Professional Recruitment', *Bulletin of the History of Medicine*, 58 (1984), 457–73.

were bound to fail. The nature of the profession, not the background of its members, determined its position. Reader's view of the Victorian medical profession is different in part. While he does not draw the distinction between medicine and other professions, he broadly agrees with the position of medicine within society as a whole. He summarized his view by saying 'the lawyer and the doctor took the lead amongst the middle classes and could make a claim to gentility in the High Street of Middlemarch, or in the suburbs of London and Birmingham, even if not in the mess of a fashionable regiment, in the ward-rooms of Her Majesty's ships or in the drawing-rooms of great country houses.[62]

Peterson's work is based on London in the second half of the nineteenth century. While there is no reason to suppose that, in point of social origin, the general practitioner of the first half of the century was different from the second half, there may have been a significant difference between London and the provinces and especially between the cities and the market towns. In the latter, the general practitioner may have occupied a higher and more secure social position than many of his urban colleagues. As the sole medical attendant to all social classes, he was not overshadowed by physicians and 'pure' surgeons competing for the better families. Within his own practice area he represented all branches of medicine and took pride in the fact. Moreover, when dispensaries and small local hospitals were established, as many were in country areas, they were nearly always staffed by local general practitioners who were in many instances the moving force in their establishment. Such institutions enhanced the image of the local medical man. The houses occupied by general practitioners in the nineteenth century, and in some cases their family histories, suggest that the local doctor was the equal of other professionals in his area. Here, in most cases, the chasm between medicine and the liberal professions described by Peterson seems not to have applied, or at least, not consistently.

For example, the Beadles family produced between the late seventeenth and the twentieth century twelve medical practitioners as well as a solicitor and a clerk in holy orders. They were also connected through marriage to the law and medicine, the family tree suggesting a tendency to choose (through occupation or marriage) medicine, the law, and the church as equivalent professions. John Nathaniel Beadles (1802–?1876), who practised in the Cotswold village of Broadway for

---

[62] W. J. Reader, *Professional Men* (London, 1966), 68.

forty-two years, recorded some of his cases and also his main interests in his notebook. His interests included shooting and the makes of sporting guns, an intense and informed interest in ornithology, the wood-engravings of Bewick, whist, chess, Beethoven's string trios, and variations in the weather recorded in the greatest detail. This suggests an all-round man, capable of accommodating himself to the interests of both his artistic and his hunting-and-shooting patients and friends.[63]

In an article reprinted from *The Times* of 1851, there is a cameo of the typical country doctor, named 'Dr Camomile', who is 'well with the squire: a sound churchman, and on dining terms with the Rector ... He occupies a square white house neatly slated ... Behind the house is the stable with two stalls.'[64] The market-town and village doctor had his house in the town or village, while the squire had his outside, surrounded by its estate. But of all the houses in the town, the medical practitioner's was often the largest and most respectably solid.

In London, too, there were notable general practitioners in the first half of the nineteenth century. J. F. Clarke in his *Autobiographical Recollections* (1874) recalled Edward Headland (1803–69; LSA 1823) whose

career as a practitioner is identified with a wholesome change in the position and practice of what was called at the time the 'subordinate grade'. He commenced as did all his brethren with 'physicking' his patients ... but he soon became disgusted with this vicious and degrading system. He was one of the foremost, if not the first, to insist on being paid for his services as a 'Physician and Surgeon'.

He was a prominent fellow and one time President of the Medical Society of London when that society was the most prestigious of all the London medical societies. 'In person, Mr Headland was above the middle height, of a fine presence ... He dressed in the Professional style and always wore a white cravat.' He began in a 'comparatively humble abode in

---

[63] Records of the Beadles family in the possession of Mr Simon Beadles, quoted with his kind permission. Dr John Guy of Yeovil has kindly pointed out that the Jolliffe family of Crewkerne in Somerset in the nineteenth century showed a similar scatter of occupations where a predominantly medical family also included a banker and a solicitor. The Carrs of Leeds were a similar dynasty of general practitioners and surgeons and one of the William Carrs in the mid-nineteenth century showed a range of sporting and cultural interests closely similar to that of J. N. Beadles. (Wellcome MS collection—the notebooks of William Carr.)

[64] 'The Income Tax and its Oppressive Effect on General Practitioners', *PMSJ* 11 (1851), 111–12.

Featherstone buildings', but he ended in an 'aristocratic house at the West End'.[65]

In the lay and the medical press, in novels of the early and mid-nineteenth century, and most of all in manuscript sources left by medical practitioners, references to the status of the general practitioner are by no means uncommon. Of course manuscript sources tend to reflect only those practitioners who were sufficiently literate and energetic to write about themselves, their families and their work, and in this sense represent a self-selected sample from the most educated of their kind. Taking all the sources together one finds it increasingly difficult to make useful generalizations, so wide is the variety of men in general practice, and so vivid the contrast between the cultured, widely read practitioners and those who were scarcely able to write and were ignorant of most parts of their profession. As always, in this kind of exercise, quantification is the difficulty. But if one wants a single sentence to describe at least the upper levels of general practitioners it would be hard to improve on Reader's summary of the status of the medical practitioner in Victorian England which is quoted above.

Whatever their position in society, however, there is no doubt that general practitioners were socially insecure to an extent not observed amongst their eighteenth-century predecessors. Reader attributes some of this to the excessive acrimony of the medical profession during the period of medical reform, and remarks perceptively that some of the touchiness is still with us today in the general practitioner.[66] More important, perhaps, is the rise of gentility in the early nineteenth century of which the main feature was the growing chasm between trade and the gentlemanly occupations in the various professions. On this count, certainly, the general practitioner had reason to worry about his position in society as a whole and the socially degrading effect of his trade in pharmacy. But he often worried much more about his position within the medical profession, and to add to his worries, he often felt he had, in a way, been cheated. He and his family had undertaken the labour and expense of medical education, examination, and licensing in the confident expectation of being rewarded by an established position and a comfortable income. For many, this promise proved false. Instead, the

---

[65] J. F. Clarke, *Autobiographical Recollections* (London, 1874), is one of the richest sources on the social history of medical men in London in the mid-nineteenth century.

[66] W. J. Reader (1966), 31. It is an indication of the extent and rapidity of the change in morale amongst general practitioners that the comment on the touchiness of the general practitioner today was appropriate in 1966 but is no longer so in 1985.

general practitioner was subjected, or (which amounts to nearly the same) believed he was subjected, to sneers from patients and colleagues. In Inkster's phrase he was a 'marginal man' with one foot in trade and the other in a profession,[67] described by a practitioner in 1820 as 'the way things are constituted [the general practitioner] finds himself treated rather as a tradesman than a gentleman'.[68]

A critic in 1845 accused the general practitioners of being 'a body of men 99 out of 100 of which are most imperfectly educated, all engaged in the trading, money-making parts of the profession and not one of them distinguished by anything like science or liberality of mind'.[69] That, perhaps, was unnecessarily harsh, but the Professor of Materia Medica in Pennsylvania after a visit to England described the general practitioner of the 1830s as 'a mongrel kind of doctor, man-midwife surgeon and druggist, a true Jack-of-all-trades and master of none ... used by the public yet looked upon by them with a sort of good-natured contempt'.[70] In 1856, Allarton wrote that 'you cannot travel by train without hearing the whole race of country doctors ridiculed and abused'.[71] An 'Old Practitioner' in 1844 grumbled that the aristocracy were 'ready enough' to call in their general practitioner 'immediately they are, or fancy they are, unwell ... but in health they almost always treat the doctor as a menial'.[72] The title or address of the general practitioner was a difficult subject. When it was suggested in 1850 that 'Esq.' should only be used by fellows of the Royal College of Surgeons, not by mere members, the *Medical Times* exploded in anger at the slight on the general practitioner.[73] And there was also the question of 'Mr' as opposed to 'Dr'. It was considered deplorable taste for a general practitioner to call himself 'Dr' even if he was, as a substantial number were, a graduate of a Scottish university.[74] It was therefore quite common for general practitioners to be addressed as 'Mr', even in this century, until by a reversal of values the use of 'Mr' became confined to qualified surgeons, but not their house-surgeons. It is a detail of

---

[67] Ian Inkster, 'Marginal Men. Aspects of the Social Role of the Medical Community in Sheffield, 1790–1850', in J. Woodward and D. Richards (eds), *Health Care and Popular Medicine in Nineteenth-century England*, (London, 1977), 128–63.

[68] 'Medical Education and Rank', *London Medical Repository*, 14 (1820), 123–9.

[69] 'On the Medical Reform Bill', *EMSJ* 64 (1845), 255–6.

[70] *Homeopathic Times*, 1 (1834), 34–6.

[71] Allarton (1856).

[72] 'An Old Practitioner', *The Public and the Medical Profession* (London, 1844).

[73] *Medical Times*, 21 (1850), 343.

[74] R. Hull, *LMG*, NS 2 (1841–2), 917–19.

medical etiquette which, understandably, still puzzles not only foreign visitors but many of the British public.

At the start of a career, degrees and diplomas were, in any case, less important than 'manner and appearance', although 'the manner which is pleasing to one patient is the reverse to another.'[75] But manners were largely a product of social background and it was on this that the general practitioner was so often attacked. His 'low' social origins were visible in his student days when he was supposed to be an uncouth, lazy, hard-drinking, and womanizing hooligan. Dickens's portrait of Bob Sawyer and Ben Allen may have been cruelly unrepresentative but it became the stereotype almost as soon as it was published.[76] The *London Medical Gazette* in 1842 protested that 'The medical student no longer merits that character which it has been his lot to possess, and which was attached to him by a modern writer with no sparing hand.'[77] In a curious way, general practitioners and the editors even of medical periodicals devoted to the cause of the medical underdog, took perverse pleasure in self-abasement. They mocked themselves not with the light touch of modest self-assurance, but with a coarse and snobbish animosity.

In the *Gazette of Health* in 1817, 'Medicus' typified the country practitioner as the farmer's son who 'instead of being brought up to the plough ... must figure away in a profession'. He drinks and wenches his way through a dissolute apprenticeship and a spell in London ('with the help of the *Squire*') where he cuts his lectures to follow low pursuits. Nevertheless, he obtains his certificates 'for having *diligently* attended the Hospitals and Lectures!!' which are 'stuck up in a conspicuous part of the surgery' to impress the neighbours when he returns home.[78]

In 1845 *Fraser's Magazine* produced an article in which the social origins of the profession as a whole were savagely attacked. Physicians included the 'occasional son of a country gentleman' who enters medicine only to find that he is forced to associate with 'a hook-nosed regimental surgeon' and 'an apothecary's apprentice who managed to get a Heidelberg degree'. These were the physicians. When it came down to the general practitioners they were typified as the son of a butcher, 'the scion of the chopper in love with amputations' who marries 'the red-headed daughter of the grocer' after a training spent in

---

[75] 'An Old Practitioner' (1844).
[76] Charles Dickens, *Pickwick Papers*, first published in serial form from 1836.
[77] 'On Medical Education', *LMG*, NS 1 (1842–3), 53–5.
[78] 'Medicus', 'On Practitioners', *Gazette of Health*, 2 (1817), 603–5.

'adultery, drinking, murder and what-not before the age of nineteen ...
such as he is the immense majority of the general practitioners'.[79]

George Allarton, MRCS LSA, deputy coroner for South Staffordshire,
painted a gallery of medical practitioners in 1856 in which the general
practitioners came off worst. The lowest form of general practitioner
was the 'son of an ordinary trader' who practised in 'the low pestiferous
districts where he exercises his functions amongst the dirtiest and most
ignorant'. Next was the 'son of a prosperous trader' who 'delights in
unions and sick-clubs ... attends "low-midwifery" ', and is 'patronised
by the shoe-maker and milkman—the huckster and the greengrocer—
he is in great force with domestic servants, and a great gun with the
stable fraternity'. The third and highest grade, the son of a rich trader,
'assumes a brusqueness of manner and vulgarity of language which
his admirers denominate eccentricity'. He attends the 'better class of
merchants and traders'. Above the general practitioner came the
SCIENTIFIC DOCTOR, much respected but seldom wealthy, and the
FASHIONABLE DOCTOR, always seen at the opera and 'a *darling*
doctor' with 'the gentler sex'. Next was the LITERARY DOCTOR,
eccentrically dressed and with little practice, who spent his time at
meetings or writing for the medical press; and, finally, the PHILO-
SOPHICAL DOCTOR, renowned and eminent through 'giving his
attention to those collateral subjects which the man engaged in practice
cannot give', and he seldom practised at all. But in the end, Allarton
maintained that the physician 'is very inferior in all that concerns the
practice of his profession, to the General Practitioner'.[80]

Throughout the period from about 1820 to 1850, as mentioned
earlier in this chapter, these two contradictory themes run side by side.
On the one hand the general practitioner was praised for the quality
and breadth of his medical education and welcomed as the new medical
man in an age that admired innovation. On the other, he was denigrated
for his association with the drug trade, for his allegedly low social
origins, and for his pretentiousness if he 'abandoned his open shop or
surgery for his silver plate and "ring of bells" on his shut door'.[81] His
low social status was attributed to an 'excess of practitioners'. The
parents of well-educated youths, doubtful of their sons' future in medicine, put them instead into counting houses with merchants or bankers.
'Hence, young men, neither so respectable in education or property as

---

[79] *Dublin Medical Press*, 19 (1845), 205–6.
[80] Allarton (1856).
[81] Dr Black, 'On the Medical Profession and its Reform', *PMSJ* I (1840), 147–9.

they ought to be, have found ready access to the profession.'[82] Rivington, in 1879, devoted a section of his essay on *The Medical Profession* to the low status of medical practitioners compared to the other professions. 'When', he asked, 'did any scion of a noble house become a medical student?'[83]

The ranks of the supporters and the denigrators of the general practitioner were by no means as obvious as one might imagine. On the whole, the denigrators were led by physicians within the profession and by the upper levels of society outside it. But the supporters were often unexpected, including physicians, Regius Professors of Medicine and Members of Parliament. In the electric atmosphere of the period of medical reform, invective and praise were often expressed in the most extravagant terms, as this example from Dr W. A. Greenhill (consultant physician to the Radcliffe Infirmary, Oxford) will show.

In fact, both in a scientific and a religious point of view it seems to me that a *perfect* specimen of a general practitioner would be the noblest member of the whole medical profession ... with his long and weary rides at all hours and in all weathers ... surely we may call him the *Missionary* of the profession.[84]

Why was there such an extremity of opinions concerning the general practitioner? Was it a symptom of the extreme degree of intra-professional conflict, which was such a feature of this period? Many believed it was, pointing to the excessive acrimony that marred the relations between medical men.

Unfortunately for physic, the perpetual wrangling, accusations, acerbity of language, recriminations, etc. [are] the bane of medical society—almost totally unknown in divinity or even the law. ... No men of any other profession are so kind and liberal to each other, in the hour of sickness or distress—but that hour over, they are the thoroughest haters of one another on the face of the globe.[85]

At the beginning of this chapter the instability of the profession in the first half of the nineteenth century was stressed, and the extent to which the clinical practice of the physician, surgeon, and general practitioner overlapped was the main part of that instability. This was obviously part of the reason why the English practitioners were 'the thoroughest haters of one another on the face of the globe'. But relation-

---

[82] 'Observations', *London Medical Repository*, 15 (1821), 498–509.
[83] W. Rivington, *The Medical Profession* (Dublin, 1879), 396.
[84] W. A. Greenhill, *Address to a Medical Student* (London, 1843).
[85] G. Crook (1842).

ships might have been easier if prosperity (and with it, enhanced social status) was readily achieved by all branches of the profession. That it was not, was attributed at the time to an 'over-crowded profession', as we have mentioned more than once. Overcrowding was said to lead to excessive competition, fee-cutting, and ultimately to recruitment from the lower levels of society, lowering the status of medical practitioners in the eyes of the public. In the next chapter, the evidence for over-crowding is considered.

10

The Number of Medical Practitioners, their Qualifications and Appointments

The overcrowded medical profession besieged by an army of irregulars

BETWEEN 1820 and 1850 it was an article of faith that medicine was *the* overcrowded profession. 'The supply of medical practitioners', said one famous surgeon, 'is in fact not only very much beyond what is necessary to ensure a just and useful competition ... [it is] so great as to be actually mischievous.'[1] From 1821, when the excess of practitioners was said already to be 'notorious', assertions of this kind recur regularly.[2] The only question was the cause of the excess. Some, for example, blamed the Apothecaries Act for making a career in medicine too popular, and we noted in chapter 8 the steep rise in the number of licentiates produced by the Society.[3] Almost certainly this rise, which was evidence of the growing popularity of medicine as a career, was a continuation of a tendency already present by the beginning of the century; but reliable figures on the number of students of medicine before 1815 are lacking. There were, however, other reasons for over-production of general practitioners than the thriving medical schools of London.

The Scottish medical schools, especially Edinburgh, whose productivity came to a peak at the turn of the century, continued to produce more practitioners than were needed for practice in Scotland and service abroad.[4] Many settled in England. Moreover, some three hundred

---

[1] Unsigned article by Sir Benjamin Brodie on medical reform in *Quarterly Review*, 47 (Dec. 1840), 53-79.

[2] A. S. Taylor, 'On the Numerical Relation of the Medical Profession to the Population of Great Britain', *LMG*, NS 1 (1844-5), 497-503; 'Medical Reform', *EMSJ* 63 (1945), 188-9; *SCME*, part II, Q. 5722, evidence of Benjamin Brodie; J. H. Black, 'On the Medical Profession and its Reform', *PMSJ* 1 (1840-1), 147-9; 'The Overcrowding of the Profession', *Lancet* (1842-3) i. 795-8.

[3] 'Remarks on the Apothecaries Act', *London Medical Repository and Review*, 6 (1827), 375-8.

[4] D. Hamilton, *The Healers: A History of Medicine in Scotland* (Edin., 1981), see especially chapter 4.

practitioners a year were recruited into the Army and Navy in the latter years of the Napoleonic wars. Most of these were discharged to civilian practice just at the time the Apothecaries Act came into force. There was also, as Dr Black of Manchester remarked in 1840, 'the increasing intelligence and wealth of the middle classes' which led them to choose 'a more liberal education for their sons' with a view to a career in medicine and similar professions.[5]

Musgrove in his review of middle-class education and employment concluded that the expansion of education after 1830 was not matched by a corresponding increase in middle-class employment opportunities. Complaints of overcrowding were therefore commonplace in the professions and other middle-class occupations, and Musgrove warned of the danger of taking such complaints at their face value.[6] Such complaints, of course, expressed the views of the professional classes. From the patients' point of view there was much to be said for an excess of medical practitioners which provided a wide choice and low fees. In an age of liberalism (the belief in the social desirability of maximizing economic competition in the market place) and *laisser faire* (the undesirability of state interference in economic affairs)[7] complaints of an overcrowded profession were unlikely to produce a sympathetic response from the public. Legal restrictions on entry were out of the question. Agreement between the medical corporations on the imposition of a voluntary quota would have been unthinkable when they were competing for students. It was a question of supply and demand for medical care. If the supply of practitioners could not be reduced, demand might be increased by excluding the irregulars, ensuring a monopoly of medical care for the regulars. Believing this was necessary for their very survival, regular practitioners turned the force of their anger on the irregulars. Here, at least, they anticipated the sympathy of the public and legislature. Medicine, they argued, differed from trade and must be treated as a special case in which the overriding principle of the public good outweighed the dogma of *laisser faire*. The irregulars were not open, fair competitors; they were responsible for fraud and injury to the unsuspecting sick, and sometimes for murder. When medical practitioners were 'jostling each other for the merest crumbs

[5] J. H. Black (1840–1), 147.

[6] F. Musgrove, 'Middle-class Education and Employment in the nineteenth Century', *Economic History Review*, NS 12 (1959–60), 99–111.

[7] J. L. Berlant, *Profession and Monopology: A Study of Medicine in the United States and Great Britain* (Los Angeles, 1975), see especially chapter 4, 147–53.

of practice' and 'considerable numbers are worn out by desperate com-petition'[8] the irregulars were the obvious target. If they could have been prohibited from practice, however, would it have made an appreciable difference to the livelihood of regular practitioners?

In the first half of the nineteenth century many practitioners saw the solution to their problems in the abolition of quackery. They believed, and historians have sometimes accepted their view, that the irregular practitioner, through open competition, was invariably employed as an alternative and opponent to the regular. This was discussed in chapter 1 in the context of the eighteenth century, where it was suggested that irregular practitioners often provided an additional rather than an alternative form of care and that their clientele and type of practice were not invariably the same as those of the regular practitioners. The situation was broadly similar in the early nineteenth century. Indeed, the language of quackery was remarkably similar in the mid-eighteenth and early nineteenth century so that, apart from clues from the typeface, it is often impossible to date an irregular's handbill by its style or content.

The pre-Victorian irregular was an entrepreneur, characterized by his individuality and vigorous salesmanship, and usually by the extrava-gance of his claims. Admirers of Donizetti may think Dr Dulcamara in *L'elisir d'amore* a pardonable operatic exaggeration, but he had his equals if not superiors in provincial England.[9] Later in the century the flamboyant entrepreneur tended to give way to groups of serious-minded practitioners whose therapies were based on heterodox systems of pathology or therapeutics. They were a different breed. Some het-erodoxies, for example homeopathy and mesmerism, dated from the eighteenth or early nineteenth century, but their heyday was mainly after about 1830 or 1840. These and similar systems were often con-sidered by their proponents to be intellectually and scientifically as respectable as those of their orthodox opponents, and much less danger-ous. For them, the term 'alternative medicine' is precise; and, as they flourished, so the old-fashioned quack disappeared, as a practitioner noted in 1841. 'This class of practitioner', he wrote, referring to the itinerant irregular, 'is fast coming to a close' and was being replaced by literate and educated empirics who produced, with the druggist, a formidable combination against the regular practitioners.[10]

[8] *Quarterly Review*, 47 (1840), 53–79.
[9] *L'elisir d'amore* was composed in 1831 and first performed in 1832. 'The elixir of love' was one of the products sold by the itinerant quack, 'Dr' Dulcamara. It was cheap wine.
[10] 'Omega', 'Remarks on Quackery', *PMSJ* 1 (1840–1), 418–19.

Were the irregulars of the pre-Victorian period, the itinerants, and other entrepreneurs, few or many? What methods did they use? What did they charge for their services? And, finally, who were the people who employed them? These are extremely difficult questions to answer. It was not the nature of irregulars to keep diaries, write memoirs, form associations, and publish lists of their membership or their views; still less did they keep tidy accounts. What we can see of them is mostly through the jaundiced eyes of the angry regulars. For example, the response to Edward Harrison's survey in 1802 was described in chapter 6 where it was suggested that in many English counties at the time the ratio of irregulars to regulars was as high as 8 or 9 to 1, although many of the irregulars were only part-time healers. Whatever the actual numbers, however, most practitioners would have agreed whole-heartedly with the editor who published a leading article in his journal complaining of 'The vile race of quacks with which this country is infested'.[11] In attempting to answer some of the above questions, an important source is provided by a collection of pamphlets held in the Bodleian Library, Oxford. They provide a picture of the medical sub-culture of Hull and its surrounding towns and villages between 1780 and 1830. This collection is described in more detail elsewhere and only a summary can be provided here.[12]

About half the bills and pamphlets consist of advertisements; the other half consists of irregulars advertising their skills or specialities, but the two were often combined. Few could excel 'Dr' Solomon of Liverpool in the field of patent medicines. He sold the 'Cordial Balm of Gilead' and lived in 'Gilead House'.[13] His Balm was recommended for those 'suffering from shattered constitutions, nervous and bilious complaints and phthisis pulmonalis'. If you were ill the Balm cured you; if down in the dumps, it cheered you up.[14] At half a guinea a bottle, sales were enormous and Solomon made a fortune, spending £5,000 a year

[11] 'On the Patronage of Quacks and Impostors by the Upper Classes of Society', *British and Foreign Medical Review*, 21 (1846), 533–40.

[12] Bodleian Library, Oxford, 'Medical Advertisements', Gough Pamphlets 2919. See I. Loudon, 'The Vile Race of Quacks with which this Country is Infested' in W. F. Bynum and R. Porter (eds.), *Medical Fringe and Medical Orthodoxy*, to be published by Croom Helm, 1986.

[13] 'Is there no balm in Gilead? Is there no physician there? Why, then, is not the health of the daughter of my people recovered?', Jeremiah 8: 22.

[14] Some guests called and took wine with 'Dr' Solomon and then requested a bottle of his Balm, which they drank straight down. Solomon demanded half a guinea and, when his guests protested, replied, 'Gentlemen, I give my wine, but I sell my Balm of Gilead.' I am grateful to Mr Adrian Allan of Liverpool for drawing my attention to this anecdote.

on advertising because, he said, £100 of advertising brought £2,000 of profit. It is hinted that Solomon managed in the end to buy a respectable MD from Aberdeen.[15]

Patent medicines were sometimes named after their inventor ('Squire's Original Grand Elixir, the True Daffy's Elixir, Dr Norris's Fever Drops') or after the famous ('Dr Boerhaave's Red Pill, Dr Radcliffe's Elixir'). Extravagant claims of patronage were common. 'Dr Scott's Bilious Pills' were used with good effect, according to the pamphlet, by 'The Dukes of Devonshire, Northumberland and Wellington, The Marquesses of Salisbury, Angelsea [sic] and Hastings, The Earls of Pembroke, Essex and Oxford and the Bishops of London, Exeter and Gloucester'. Letters from grateful patients (real or composed?) were often printed as well. Most notable was the long list of diseases which were cured by the medicine or practitioner. Certain disorders recurred with special frequency, notably venereal disease, but also deafness, eye disorders, ruptures, and nervous conditions. Conspicuous by their absence were disorders of children and pregnancy. Ann Stanley, noted in chapter 1, was an exception, possibly because of her sex, because no instance has been noted of male irregulars who specifically mention the diseases of women and children. Dr Norris's Fever Drops were recommended for every conceivable type of fever except children's fevers and childbed (puerperal) fever, and one irregular actually boasted of his knack for instant diagnosis of any or every disorder 'except childbed'. The treatment of venereal disease, usually described euphemistically, was often combined with the management of sexual disorders. Dr Natras of 56, Carr Lane, Hull[16] not only treated 'a certain disorder, however inveterate' but also 'seminal weakness, unhappily so frequent and prevalent, arising from early abuse, intemperance, excess of pleasure, mental sympathy or other injurious causes'. Usually, two characteristics in these lists of diseases stood out: first, their comprehensiveness, paediatrics and obstetrics excepted; secondly, the casual mixture of the trivial with the deadly. Rubbing shoulders in the same sentence came the claims to cure 'typhus and corns', 'phthisis and warts'.

Irregulars were well known for their tendency to travel. One group walked the town pushing handbills through doors with the warning to

[15] *Gazette of Health* 8 (1823), 533; 9 (1824), 891; 10 (1825), 173; 11 (1826), 764.

[16] Probably 'John Natras, 56 Carr Lane, Hull, 1838, surgeon, no qualifications' in J. A. R. Bickford and M. E. Bickford, *The Medical Profession in Hull, 1400–1900* (Kingston-Upon-Hull City Council, 1983).

'keep this bill clean until the Doctor calls for it'. For instance, one handbill announced that 'The Doctor who calls for this Bill will tell any person, male or female, their complaint or disorder without any examination or the least resemblance of their countenance, only by the smell of their handkerchiefs or casting their urine.' Another group followed a regular circuit of inns. Their bills specified the day and the time that they would be available to tell, instantly, from the patient or his water, whether they were curable or not. These were mostly bone-setters or water-casters. They included 'Dr Taylor of Beverley' in 1815 who attended the Blue Boar, Beverley, on Saturdays, the Star Inn, Bridlington, on Wednesdays, and the Bell at Driffield every Thursday from ten till four. The real itinerants travelled far and wide, although their bizarre circuits sometimes strain credulity. Dr Lambert ('from his dispensaries at 36 High Street, Borough, London, and 49 Queen's Square, Bristol') regularly visited amongst other places 'The West Indies, the Isles of Scilly, London, Bristol, Birmingham, Nottingham, Leicester, Norwich, Wolverhampton, Stourbridge, etc.'

How much an irregular charged for his services is seldom recorded. Patent medicines, however, were usually sold in two or three sizes, the smallest at 1s. or 1s. 6d., the medium at 2s. 9d., and the family size at up to 7s. Even an ointment specifically called the 'Poor Man's Friend' cost 1s. 1½d. for the small size and 2s. 9d. for the large. There seems little doubt, however, that, for all their claims of royal and noble patronage, the patent medicines and their various purveyors found their ways mainly into the homes of the poor. Only a few of those who advertised in the above fashion were regular paractitioners who cashed in on the customs and methods of the quack. The large majority of quacks, although they flourished their 'Doctors' and 'Surgeons', or claimed to have 'regularly graduated' or had 'attended the principal hospitals of England' (to quote examples from this collection) seem to have had no semblance of regular training of any kind.

There is, therefore, evidence of substantial numbers of irregular prac-titioners, both 'stationary' and 'itinerant', and there is no reason to believe Hull was subject to an unusual invasion. A similar collection of advertisements from London closely resembles the Hull collection.[17] Mr Rumsey, a surgeon from Gloucester who had looked into such matters, confirmed the wide extent of irregular practice amongst the poor in various parts of England. But, although he was able to be specific about

---

[17] Bodleian Library, Oxford, 'Collection of Advertisements', Douce Adds., 138.

the quantity of care provided by druggists in various towns, he was silent when it came to the other irregulars, having no exact figures to go on.[18] It is questionable whether the true extent of the archetypal quack can be determined. More research is needed, especially in the late eighteenth and early nineteenth century when the 'regular itinerant quack' may have reached the zenith of his career. When their numbers began to diminish, alternative medicine seems to have drawn most of its support from an unusual assortment of people including those too poor to employ the cheapest general practitioner, certain branches of religious dissenters, the politically radical, and the aristocracy: strange bedfellows, but numerically only a small proportion of potential paying patients for the general practitioner.[19] The impoverished general practitioner had much greater cause for concern from the competition of his regular colleagues than he had from irregular practice, because there is, in fact, confirmatory evidence of overcrowding and excessive competition in the medical profession during the first half of the nineteenth century.

The evidence of an overcrowded profession

When reviewing the evidence of an overcrowded medical profession, the main theme will be the ratio of medical men to the population. The relative number of nurses, midwives, and druggists will be noted in passing. In the following section of this chapter the qualifications and appointments of different categories of practitioner will be examined.

The author of *An Exposition of the State of Medicine* in 1826 calculated that there were in London 3,174 medical men and 300 'chymists and druggists'. By a complex and largely unconvincing calculation he estimated that London had 2,000 more medical practitioners than it needed.[20] But London, of course, was not representative of England as a whole. A. S. Taylor (MRCS 1830, LSA 1828) published a detailed paper in January 1845 based on an alalysis of the 1841 census.[21] He calculated that 500 new entries to the medical profession were required

[18] Evidence of H. W. Rumsey Esq. Select Committee on Medical Poor Relief, PP 1844, IX, Q. 9121.

[19] J. Pickstone, 'Establishment and Dissent in Nineteenth-century Medicine', in W. J. Shiels (ed.), *The Church and Healing, Studies in Church History* series 19 (Oxford, 1982), 85–97. Here, Pickstone suggests that in a town of 44,000 in mid-19th century, the devotees of 'anti-establishment medicine ... may have numbered only hundreds; those sympathetic no more than a thousand or two'.

[20] Anon, *An Exposition of the State of the Medical Profession* (London, 1820).

[21] A. S. Taylor (1844–5), 497–503.

annually in Great Britain together with a small increment in step with the increase in the population to provide the 'right' number of medical practitioners. But the estimated annual output of the seventeen licensing bodies was between 800 and 1,000 a year, so that 'many more members are annually licensed than can find any profitable occupation'. The ratio of medical practitioners to the population was, he believed, 1 : 1,000, and this, in his opinion was clear evidence the profession was 'overstocked'. This ratio was confirmed by other authors in the same period[22] and by my own analysis of the report of the 1841 census (the first census to include occupational data in detail). The results of the latter are summarized in table 19 and in Appendices IV and V. Comparative data from the census of 1851 are shown in table 20, and the comparison of the numbers of medical practitioners to other professions and selected occupations are shown in Appendix VI.

The ratio of all medical practitioners and of general practitioners to the population in England and Wales in 1841 were 1 : 926 and 1 : 1,243 respectively. In 1851 they were virtually the same. London had a much larger proportion of medical practitioners producing a ratio of 1 : 410 (all medical practitioners) in 1841 and 1 : 419 in 1851. Scotland had proportionately fewer medical practitioners than England (1 : 1,122 compared to 1 : 926) and Wales substantially less with a ratio of 1 : 1,442. Druggists were numerous, about two to every three practitioners in England and Wales, but only two to every five in Scotland. Nurses (categorized as 'Nurses, not Domestic Servants', see Table 20) were also numerous, amounting to almost one per practitioner and outnumbering practitioners in London. The small number of midwives recorded in the census is misleading. Many probably combined midwifery with another occupation, especially nursing.

What was the position in the provinces? Here the striking feature is the relatively even distribution of medical practitioners throughout England. No county could claim to be seriously short of regular medical practitioners although London and Middlesex could claim to have too many. The counties with the largest number of practitioners relative to population followed no predictable pattern. Apart from Middlesex, the counties with the highest practitioner/population ratios included Devonshire, Durham, Gloucestershire, Northumberland, and Somerset; while those with the lowest included Cambridgeshire, Cornwall, Derbyshire, Lancashire, Norfolk, and Staffordshire (see Appendix IV). Flint

[22] 'Medical Reform', *EMSJ* 63 (1845), 188; and *LMG* 2 (1843–4), 784.

Table 19 *Medical practitioners, nurses, midwives, and druggists in Britain, 1841*

	Great Britain	England	London	Wales	Scotland
Population in 1841	18,655,981	15,000,154	1,873,676	911,603	2,560,184
Physicians	1,476	1,063	340	30	364
Surgeons, apothecaries and medical students	18,658	15,422	4,221	602	2,485
Total of medical practitioners	20,134	16,485	4,561	632	2,849
Nurses	13,255	13,060	4,687	126	not recorded
Midwives	1,384	676	127	58	641
Druggists	10,583	9,648	1,806	414	731
Physicians	1,457	1,063	340	30	364
'Pure' surgeons	300	300	200	—	?
Students[a]	3,374	2,472	912	63	569
General practitioners[b]	15,003	12,650	3,109	539	1,916
Ratio to population:					
Medical practitioners[c]	1:926	1:909	1:410	1:1,442	1:1,122
General practitioners[b]	1:1,243	1:1,185	1:602	1:1,691	1:1,336[d]
Druggists	1:1,762	1:1,554	1:1,037	1:2,202	1:3,502

[a] On the basis of the age of medical practitioners as a whole it was calculated that the proportion of students was likely to be about 20% of the total in London and Scotland, 15% in England, and 10% in Wales. This assumption was used for the numbers of students. The number of 'pure' surgeons is based on a number of different sources which generally agreed there were about 200 in London and 100 in the provinces.

[b] Calculated by subtracting physicians, 'pure' surgeons, and students from the total of all medical practitioners.

[c] This includes medical students.

[d] This calculation included all physicians in Scotland as general practitioners because the nature of their practice closely resembled the English general practitioner. (See Report of the Select Committee on Medical Registration, PP 1847–8, XV, Q 1758–62).

Source: 1841 census. Parliamentary Papers (1841), XXVII, pp. 31–44. 48–51.

Table 20   *Medical practitioners, nurses, midwives, and druggists in Britain, 1851*

England and Wales		
Population in 1851	17,927,609	
Physicians	1,771	
Surgeons (including general practitioners)	13,470	
Other medical men[a]	3,949	
TOTAL	19,190	
Nurses (not domestic servants)	23,571	
Midwives	2,204	
Druggists	14,307	
Ratio: Medical practitioner to population		1 : 934
Druggist to population		1 : 1,253
Scotland		
Population in 1851	2,888,762	
Physicians	511	
Surgeons	1,576	
Other medical men[a]	923	
TOTAL	3,010	
Nurses (not domestic servants)	1,543	
Midwives	815	
Druggists	1,227	
Ratio: Medical practitioners to population		1 : 959
Druggists to population		1 : 2,345
London		
Population in 1851	2,362,236	
Physicians	552	
Surgeons	3,407	
Other medical men[a]	1,672	
TOTAL	5,631	
Nurses (not domestic servants)	7,807	
Midwives	190	
Druggists	2,370	
Ratio: Medical men to population		1 : 419
Druggists to population		1 : 996

[a] Mostly medical students because most under 20 years of age.

Source: 1851 census. Parliamentary Papers (1852–3), LXXXVIII, Part 1.

Table 21 *The proportion of general practitioners to physicians and surgeons in London and the provinces, 1847*

	London	The provinces
General practitioners	680	853
Physicians	155	94
Surgeons	165	53
TOTAL	1,000	1,000

Source: Medical Directory (1847). Random sample of 2,000 entries.

Table 22 *The proportion of different types of medical practitioner in London, 1847*

	No.	%
1. Consulting physicians (including physician-accoucheurs)	301(30)	12.0
2. 'Physician general practitioners'[a]	133	5.5
3. Consulting surgeons (including the leading dentists)	176	7.3
4. Practitioners holding only the MRCS[a]	468	19.4
5. Practitioners holding only the LSA[a]	275	11.4
6. Practitioners holding both the MRCS and the LSA[a]	990	41.0
7. In practice before the year 1815[a]	70	3.0

[In addition there were 360 practitioners with no assigned qualifications]

[a] The general practitioners of all grades consisted of groups 2, 4, 5, 6, and 7. These amounted to 80% of the total.

Source: Evidence of John Ridout to the *Select Committee on Medical Registration*, PP 1847–8, XV, Q. 493–5.

was the only exception to the under-supplied counties of Wales. Industrial cities of the Midlands and the north of England tended to have fewer practitioners per unit population than the non- or semi-industrial cities of the south, but the difference was inconsistent and not significant. Druggists had increased in number so much faster than medical practitioners since the beginning of the century that in most towns they had achieved parity with medical practitioners.

Broadly speaking, therefore, in England and Wales in the 1840s there was one medical practitioner and one druggist to every 900–1,000 people, and one general practitioner to every 1,100–1,200. How does this ratio compare with subsequent decades? The answer is provided in Appendix VII, but there are difficulties which make comparison uncertain (see footnotes to the appendix). Methods of classification of medical practitioners were constantly changed, and the apparent fall in the number of practitioners between the census of 1851 and that of 1861

Table 23   *The qualifications of provincial general practitioners, 1847*

	No.	%
MRCS/LSA	451	53
MRCS alone	138	
LSA alone	146	
TOTAL	735	86
'Gen. pract. pre-1815'	24	
General practitioner: no qualification	2	
In addition the following qualifications were held, either alone or with the MRCS and/or the LSA:		
MD Edin.	26	
LRCS Edin.	10	
Glasgow qualification	6	
MD Aberdeen	1	
MD St Andrew's	3	
GP accoucheur LRCS Edin.	1	
LRCS Edin. and MD Heidelberg	1	
TOTAL with Scottish qualifications	48	6
FRCS Eng.	14	
MD: university not specified	6	
Foreign MDs	3	
LRCP London and MD	1	
Extra-licence RCP London	1	
MB London	3	
Irish qualification	2	
MD Munich, FRCS England	1	
GP Accoucheur, MD London	1	
The remainder described themselves as:		
Physician in general practice	2	
Surgeon in general practice	10	
TOTAL (for all groups)	853	

Source: *Medical Directory* (1847). Random sample of 2,000 entries.

is an artefact associated with registration. After the introduction of the Medical Act of 1858, 'medical practitioner' became 'registered medical practitioner'. In 1851 a substantial number of men, most of whom probably regarded themselves as regular practitioners, either held no formal qualification or, if they did, chose not to register in 1858. These technical difficulties, however, only disguise slightly the differences in the practitioner/population ratios which have taken place in the last one and a half centuries.

If one compares the medical profession as a whole between 1841 and 1971, the most obvious difference is the larger number of consultants

Table 24 *The origin of university medical degrees recorded in a sample of 2,000 medical practitioners, 1847*

	General practitioners	Physicians	Surgeons
Scottish universities	67	96	6
English Universities	9	38	1
Cambridge		23	1
Oxford		8	
London	9	7	
Irish Universities		1	1
Foreign Universities	10	13	3
MD Erlangen	3	1	1
MD Paris	1	2	
MD Vienna	1	1	
MD Berlin		1	
MD Tübingen		1	
MD Giessen	3		
MD Heidelberg		1	
MD Munich	1		
MD Univ. of France [sic]			1
Grad. in Med and Surg, Univ. of Heidelberg	1		
MD Jena		1	
MD Pavia		1	
MD Modena		1	
MD Catania, Rome, and Paris		1	
MD Geneva and Cologne		1	
MD Bonn			1
MD Frieborg		1	
MD (university not specified)	8	17	
TOTAL	94	165	11

Source: *Medical Directory* (1847).

and specialists today. Most of the increase is in fact recent, having occurred since the introduction of the National Health Service. Hospital medical staff in England and Wales (measured as whole-time equivalents) increased from 11,735 in 1949 to 23,806 in 1971: consultants, from 3,488 in 1949 to 8,655 in 1971. The number of general practitioners, however, remained virtually unaltered at about 20,000 (unrestricted principals) in England and Wales throughout the same period. The ratio of general practitioners to population in the 1970s was therefore approximately 1 : 2,500 compared with 1 : 1,000 in the 1840s and 1850s. This appears to be confirmatory evidence that the medical

Table 25 *Honorary appointments at hospitals or dispensaries held by various categories of medical men, 1847*

	Hospitals	Dispensaries	Both	Total
General practitioners				
London	13	52	5	70 (10%)[a]
Provinces	31	35	10	76 (9%)
Physicians				
London	46	30	17	93 (60%)
Provinces	19	10	12	41 (44%)
Surgeons				
London	44	28	4	76 (46%)
Provinces	19	3	3	25 (47%)

[a] The percentages refer to the total numbers in each group of practitioners, e.g. 10% of all the London general practitioners in the sample, and 9% of provincial, held appointments at hospitals, dispensaries, or both.

Source: Medical Directory (1847). Random sample of 2,000 entries.

profession as a whole, or at least general practice, was indeed over-crowded in the 1840s, but is the comparison valid?

It can be argued that morbidity in general, and especially morbidity from infectious diseases, was very much higher in the first half of the nineteenth century than it is today. Measured as work for the general practitioner, illness, both as new cases per unit population and as total consultation rates (because many of the illnesses were prolonged requiring frequent visits) was much greater, occupying more time and bringing potentially greater profits. A higher birth rate, too, meant a larger number of obstetric cases. Referral to hospital was rare before 1850 and medical and surgical cases as far as private practice was concerned were managed at home. It is easy to argue, therefore, that an average of 1,000–1,200 patients provided a full workload for the early nineteenth-century general practitioner. On the other hand, the general practitioner today is occupied by many activities which were uncommon or unknown in the 1840s. These include such obvious activities as the treatment and follow-up of conditions unknown in the 1840s (hypertension, for example), immunization, routine screening (including ante- and post-natal care) and sickness certification. Consultations for emotional and social problems are probably more common today. The outcome of any attempt to balance these two very different patterns of general practice must be conjectural. But the ratios given above are crude medical practitioner/population ratios. The population able to employ and pay a general practitioner in 1841 was substantially smaller than the total population. The alternative care provided by the irregulars probably represented only a small loss of income to general practitioners. But the numbers attending the dispensaries and hospitals as a source of primary care (they were not, as today, cases referred from general practice) ultimately became very large indeed. The largest increase was in hospital out-patients in the second half of the nineteenth century. Here, the increase was spectacular. At the London Hospital, Whitechapel, for example, annual out-patient attendances averaged 3,000–7,000 cases a year between 1750 and 1840 and then began to rise steeply. In 1870 there were 52,000 attendances and by the end of the century 200,000 new cases were attending a year and a similar pattern seems to have occurred at most voluntary hospitals in London and the provinces.[23] the system of letters of recommendation was

[23] See especially Robert Bridges, 'An Account of the Casualty Department', *St Bartholomew's Hospital Reports*, 10 (1878), 167–2. The statistics quoted here are published in further detail in I. Loudon, 'Historical Importance of Out-Patients', *BMJ* 1 (1978), 974–7.

intended to ensure that patients who attended hospitals and dispensaries were only those who were unable to pay a medical practitioner. In practice there appears to have been some abuse of the system, and, in the suspicious opinion of the general practitioners, it was abuse on an enormous scale. Complaints of this kind were a feature of late nineteenth-century general practice, but even in the first half of the century some of the population who would have employed a general practitioner and paid at least a small fee, were treated at medical institutions.

Meanwhile, the well-to-do, fewer in number perhaps, but an important source of revenue, sometimes employed a physician and 'pure' surgeon as their regular family attendants. Taken together, the reduction of the total population available as regular patients for the general practitioner as a result of irregulars, hospitals and dispensaries, and physicians and surgeons, could amount in some towns to as much as 10–20 per cent. Moreover, the available income for general practice was seldom spread evenly. 'In the same locality we can see two general practitioners—one driving furiously from square to square—from nobleman to nobleman, the other ekeing out a wretched revenue by selling matches, cold cream and Morrison's Pills; yet the rank and education are the same.'[24] Allarton described the situation in 1856 in suburban areas. 'Thousands of wealthy people congregate in the villages round our large towns—doctors by dozens follow in their wake, and—although many are talented experienced men—yet we never find more than two in each village or small town are enabled to support the respectability of life.'[25] The possession of the apothecaries' licence and the surgeons' diploma was not a guarantee of a life of professional prosperity. It was only the first step in an uncertain career.

The ranks, qualifications, and differentiation of medical practitioners within the profession

If one imagines a provincial town in the 1840s with a population of 20,000—larger, then, than Gloucester or Cardiff, but smaller than Oxford or Exeter—it probably would have contained some twenty-five medical practitioners. Two would probably have been physicians, two or three, surgeons, and the remainder general practitioners. Conventional wisdom suggests that the physicians would have held a university MD, usually from Oxford or Cambridge, as well as the licence or extra-licence

---

[24] 'Medical Statistics and Medical Reform', MCR 20 (1834), 567–71.
[25] G. Allarton, *Mysteries of Medical Life* (London, 1856).

of the Royal College of Physicians of London. They would have been expected to be the most prosperous practitioners, living largely by consultant practice but also by acting as the primary care physicians to the richest inhabitants. The surgeons would have held the diploma of membership or, after 1843, the fellowship of the College of Surgeons. They would have confined themselves to surgery, mostly in a consultant capacity. The general practitioners would have been clearly distinguished on three grounds. First, by the nature of their practice which included all four branches of medicine, physic, surgery, pharmacy, and midwifery; secondly, by their dual qualification of 'College and Hall', the MRCS and LSA; and thirdly, by the level of their income which would, on average, have been substantially lower than those of the physicians and surgeons. This is the conventional picture of the medical profession after 1815 in which the original tripartite division was replaced by a division into general practitioners and consultants, clearly defined and separate from each other. It is a picture that readily appeals since it is, in broad essentials, the British medical profession of today.

The profession, however, was not so clearly defined before 1850 as it was in the second half of the nineteenth century. The process of differentiation was slow and the boundaries between groups of medical men blurred. London was atypical, the division into general practitioners and consultants with hospital appointments being more clearly defined at an earlier stage than in the provinces; but even in London, differentiation was incomplete in the first half of the nineteenth century. The point is of some importance. Absence of clear distinctions was partly responsible for the instability of the period of medical reform. The position of the general practitioner of the profession was still uncertain and the future of the physician was threatened most of all.

The conventional assumptions described above were tested by an analysis of a random sample of 2,000 entries in Churchill's *Medical Directory* for 1847.[26] In this edition, but not in later ones, the practitioner defined himself in terms of the divisions of medical men as 'physician', 'surgeon', or 'general practitioner', indicating his own sense of belonging to one or another group within the profession, and how he wished to be recognized by his colleagues. One thousand of the

---

[26] Tunbridge Wells, for example, had a population of 10,587 in 1850 and supported 19 practitioners, two of them physicians—a ratio of 1 practitioner to every 557 inhabitants. W. D. Foster, 'Dr William Henry Cook', *Proc. of the Royal Soc. of Medicine* 66 (1973), 12–16.

entries were provincial practitioners, 1,000 were from London.[27] The results are shown in tables 21 to 25[28] and the important features of the analysis can be summarized as follows:

1. By 1847, the terms 'apothecary' and 'surgeon-apothecary' were to all intents and purposes obsolete.
2. In London, 68 per cent, and in the provinces 85 per cent, of the sample consisted of general practitioners.
3. Surgeons conformed to their stereotype in holding either the MRCS or FRCS; 3 per cent held an MD in addition, usually from a Scottish university.
4. Physicians varied widely in their formal qualifications. In London, 21 per cent were graduates of English universities, 28 per cent of Scottish ones. In the provinces only 4 per cent held English university degrees and 55 per cent were graduates of a Scottish university, the largest group by far being graduates of Edinburgh University. Half the London physicians were licentiates or fellows of the London College of Physicians, but only 7 per cent of provincial physicians had any formal connection with the College. While the London connection with the College was weak, in the provinces it was almost non-existent. It would only verge on caricature to suggest that in this period—the first half of the nineteenth century—the Royal College of Physicians of London was little more than a club for the élite London physicans.
5. Appointments at voluntary hospitals and dispensaries were not confined to physicians and surgeons. In fact, only about half the physicians and surgeons held an honorary appointment at an institution, and, conversely, between 9 and 10 per cent of general practitioners held an honorary appointment, mostly at a dispensary. This was equally true of London and the provinces.
6. The blurring of distinctions was emphasized by practitioners who described themselves as 'physician in general practice' or 'surgeon in general practice'.
7. General practitioners, like the physicians, did not always conform to the stereotype. Those who held the dual qualification, MRCS LSA, and no other qualification amounted to 53 per cent of the sample of

---

[27] An account of this analysis was published in I. Loudon, 'Two Thousand Medical Men in 1847', *Bulletin of the Society for the Social History of Medicine*, 33 (1983), 4–8.

[28] Table 22 is based on the report of Dr J. Ridout to the Select Committee on Medical Registration, PP 1847–8, XV, Q. 493–5.

general practitioners. Another 33 per cent practised on either the MRCS or the LSA alone. The remainder, apart from those whose entry read 'in practice before 1815', held a wide variety of qualifications including foreign MDs, but the most common were the Edinburgh MD and other Scottish qualifications.

A number of practitioners whose appointments and qualifications would appear to suggest a higher grade nevertheless described themselves as general practitioners. Edward Stephens of Manchester, LSA (1825), MD Leyden (1827), FRCS by examination (1845), D. Chir. Berlin (1828), Lecturer in pathology and morbid anatomy at the Royal School of Medicine and consultant surgeon to the Manchester Lying-In Hospital is an example of a practitioner who possesed a wide range of qualifications and appointments but described himself in 1847 as a general practitioner.[29] Nevertheless, the most common of all entries in the medical directory was that of a general practitioner who held the dual qualification and often an appointment as medical officer to a union of parishes under the new poor law.

Perhaps the most apt description of the three divisions of medical practitioners is that they resembled three overlapping circles, the degree of overlap being greater in the provinces than in London. This overlap applied to their formal qualifications, their appointments to institutions, and also to the nature of their practice. Movement by an individual from one circle to another through the area of overlap was comparatively easy in the first half of the nineteenth century as it had been in the eighteenth. The supposed distinction in social class of patients as between the physicians and the general practitioners was exceptional. In 1841 Dr Charles Cowan, MD, physician to the Royal Berkshire Hospital and the Reading Dispensary, described his extensive non-consulting private practice. Most of his patients were described as housewives, followed by 'domestics, labourers, sempstresses, carpenters, shoemakers, smiths, iron-founders, shopkeepers, publicans and bricklayers'.[30] A typical provincial physician, he was, in effect, a 'physician in general practice' who happened to hold honorary appointments at both a hospital and dispensary.

Such details as these underline the point which was stressed in the last chapter, namely, that the medical profession in the first half of the

---

[29] *Medical Directory* (1847), provincial volume.
[30] C. Cowan, 'Report of Private Medical Practice for 1840', *Lancet* (1841–2), ii. 358–62, 395–401, 433–9.

nineteenth century was in a transitional state in which everything in the way of professional distinctions was 'mixed, jumbled, brayed and blended'[31] as the general practitioner rose to 'get on a level with' the 'superior classes of the profession'.[32] In the modern sense, the consultant is a specialist whose occupation is dependent on the referral of patients by general practitioners who require the consultant's expertise for their patients. In that sense the idea of the consultant certainly existed before 1850. Indeed, John Gregory defined the physician (see chapter 1) as 'the final arbiter in cases of difficulty and danger' in 1772. But, before 1850, the number of physicians and 'pure' surgeons whose practice was largely—let alone wholly—consultant practice, was very small indeed. It is therefore misleading to describe the medical profession in clear terms of a division into consultants and general practitioners in the period with which we are concerned. Had there been such a division after 1815 there would have been less intra-professional conflict. Instead, the physician and 'pure' surgeon were distinguished from the general practitioner not by consultant practice, nor even necessarily by special expertise; they were distinguished by their refusal to undertake what they saw as the degrading side of medical practice, pharmacy, and to a lesser extent midwifery.

When areas of clinical practice in physic and surgery were so ill-defined, the status of an individual practitioner depended greatly on his income and class of patient. One could say he was known by the company he kept—socially and professionally. For this reason the role of the general practitioner as poor-law medical officer played a very important part in identifying the position of the general practitioner within the profession. The poor laws and the general practitioner form the major part of the next chapter.

---

[31] *London Medical Repository and Review*, NS 5 (1827), 188.
[32] *BFMR* 14 (1842), 402–11.

11

Practice and Income:
The Poor Law Medical Services

Sources of income

PRIVATE practice was, of course, the main source of income for most general practitioners. But there were other sources of great importance, and these included appointments as medical officers to medical benefit clubs, provident dispensaries, factories, mines, and other industrial concerns. Much the most important, however, were appointments under the old and the new poor laws as 'parish surgeons' before, and 'union surgeons' following, the Poor Law Amendment Act of 1834. Established practitioners often shunned such posts after 1834, but they remained an important source of income for the young practitioner at the beginning of his career, and for those who failed to make an adequate living from private practice.

While a great deal has been written on the politics and administration of the old and the new poor laws, the comparison of the medical services under the two systems has received relatively little attention. The evidence suggests there were substantial changes not solely as a result of legislation, but rather as a reflection of changing ideas on poverty. Here it will be suggested that by the mid-eighteenth century poor law appointments were not only numerous, but, in terms of the amount of work involved, well paid. They seem, moreover, to have been undertaken as a routine, respectable, and even prestigious part of general practice. The new harsh attitudes to poverty, however, whch disfigured the early nineteenth century, produced profound changes in the payment and status of the poor law medical service, even before the Act of 1834. Medical officers were paid less in actual terms, and much less in real terms, for looking after a larger number of the sick poor. The status of the poor law medical officer was degraded and general practice as a whole suffered in consequence. In many instances the general practitioner accepted a post as union surgeon only out of necessity, knowing he would be poorly paid and subservient to Boards of Guardians. The evidence for this is presented later in this chapter. First, however, it is necessary to consider the changing standard of living between 1750 and 1850 as the background to levels of income.

Costs and inflation

The continuing debate on the standard of living in the industrial revolution is remarkable for its longevity and the passions it seems to arouse. Agreement between the 'optimists' and the 'pessimists' may be rare but most economic historians would probably agree that to maintain a real income in the decade 1810–20 equivalent in purchasing power to that between 1760 and 1770, actual earnings would need to have risen by 60–80 per cent. Tucker, for example, in a survey of the wages of artisans, suggested that between 1770 and 1820 a rise in actual or money wages of 60 per cent represented a fall in real wages of 17 per cent.[1]

Recently, Lindert and Williamson have estimated the rise in nominal earnings for eighteen occupations between 1755 and 1851.[2] The cost of living doubled between 1781 and 1812, but rapid deflation between 1812 and 1820 reduced this to a 42 per cent increase. Earnings generally increased in line with costs, so that real wages remained constant until 1810 for both labourers and professionals. Then the incomes of the 'white-collar' workers and the labourers began to diverge as the professional classes became increasingly prosperous. According to table 26, 'surgeons and doctors' improved their financial position to a greater extent between 1781 and 1819 than other professional groups. I am inclined to distrust the figures shown in this table as far as medical practitioners were concerned. The suggested earnings for 1819 and 1851 may well be accurate, but the figure of £88 for 1781 is probably too low, and incompatible with the evidence presented in chapter 5. There it was shown that ordinary country surgeon-apothecaries with no special skills or reputation could earn £300 to £400 or more, and do so consistently over many years. It seems more likely that, at least as far as the rank and file were concerned, average actual earnings at best stayed level and more probably fell between 1780 and 1820, and then failed to rise between 1820 and 1850. In terms of real income, therefore,

---

[1] R. S. Tucker, 'Real Wages of Artisans in London, 1728–1935', in A. J. Taylor (ed.), *The Standard of Living in Britain in the Industrial Revolution* (London, 1975).

[2] P. H. Lindert and J. G. Williamson, 'English Workers' Living Standards during the Industrial Revolution: A New Look', *Economic History Review*, second series 36 (no. 1) (1983), 1–25.

Table 26 *Nominal earnings of various occupational groups in current pounds,
1781–1851*

Occupation	Year		
	1781 £	1819 £	1851 £
Farm labourers	21.09	39.05	29.04
Non-farm common labourer	23.13	41.74	44.83
Clergy	182.65	266.65	267.09
Solicitors and barristers	242.67	447.50	1,837.50
Engineers and surveyors	170.00	326.43	479.00
Surgeons and doctors	88.35	217.60	200.92

Source: P. H. Lindert and J. G. Williamson, 'English Workers' Living Standards during the
Industrial Revolution', *Economic History Review*, second series, 36 (no. 1) (1983).

the eighteenth-century surgeon-apothecary was more prosperous than
the nineteenth-century general practitioner. This, incidentally, was the
opinion of that acute contemporary observer of medical men and their
incomes, Richard Smith junior of Bristol.[3] The decline in prosperity was
due to the fact that not only was there a substantial rise in the cost of
living as noted, but there were substantial rises in professional expenses
and, of course, increasing competition for patients.

In the late eighteenth century £300 was usually enough to cover the
cost of apprenticeship and starting in practice; between 1815 and 1850
it was nearer £1,000.[4] Parents, choosing a career for their sons, would
balance initial costs against expected income in middle age. Such an
equation in the eighteenth century was usually: initial costs = one year's
income; in the mid-nineteenth century, it was often four or five years'
income. In this respect, medicine compared badly with other nineteenth-
century professions, at least at the level of the average general practitioner.

It will be recalled that in 1747 the business of the apothecary was
singled out as exceptionally desirable; initial costs were low and profits
'unconceivable'. By 1842 a guide to parents warned them: 'there is no
profession in which it is so difficult to make a beginning that that of

[3] BIBM 2. 164.

[4] This included the apprenticeship premium, the cost of hospital training and examination fees, board and lodging in London, drugs and instruments and, for those who
could afford it, the added cost of buying a partnership was ofen £500 or more. See I.
Loudon, 'A Doctor's Cash-book', *Medical History*, 27 (1983), 249–68. For further details
see *SCME*, part III, Q. 5739–41, 5827–8, 5908, 6486; *London Medical Repository*, 15
(1821), 499; *LMPJ*, NS 10 (1831), 534–43; H. B. Thompson, *The Choice of a Profession*
(London, 1857); J. L. Mann, *Recollections* (London, 1887), 72–3.

medicine; and there is much truth in the saying that by the time when a physician earns his bread and cheese he has no longer the teeth to eat them with.'[5] The contrast is striking and there is little doubt it reflects a real decline in the prosperity of medical practice. Why did this occur when, it seemed, medicine was advancing rapidly? Could it have been due to a fall in the demand for orthodox medical care? There is little to support this possibility. Was it due to the rapid increase in the hospitals and dispensaries? This was said to be an important factor for general practitioners in the last quarter of the nineteenth century, but it was not of much significance before 1850. Even if there had been an 'abuse' of charity before 1850 in the sense of medical charities accepting patients able to pay a medical practitioner, the scale of hospital and dispensary admissions was too small to make an appreciable financial difference to private practice. This possibility can be dismissed. The most likely explanation was the influence of an excess of medical practitioners on market forces. Excessive competition for patients affected all sources of income. It affected the salaries paid under the poor laws which are considered in this chapter, as well as the income from other sources, which are considered in the next.

Poor relief under the 'old' poor law

Under the old poor law based on the famous 43rd Act of Elizabeth, 1601, relief was administered at the level of the parish. Care was provided mainly on an outdoor basis (i.e. at home) and poor law infirmaries were few. The general tendency in the mid- to late eighteenth century seems to have been in favour of paying the medical officer, in the terminology of modern general practice, on an 'item of service' basis, paying him separately for visits, medicines, surgical procedures, midwifery, and (in the early nineteenth century) for vaccination; each parish was free to negotiate levels of payment with the parish surgeon. As we saw in chapter 4, however, fees charged and payments approved by overseers were, more often than not, the same as in private practice. The poor may sometimes have been treated with less finesse and courtesy than the paying classes but the level of payment was an incentive to high standards of care.

Crowther in her paper on the Poor Law Medical Service before 1914, suggests that the reputation of the parish surgeon, both for skill and

---

[5] R. Campbell, *The London Tradesman* (1747), and J. C. Hudson, *The Parent's Handbook* (1842).

benevolence, seems to have have been low, and that vestries probably employed the lowest bidder since they did not require any qualifications from their medical men.[6] Sometimes this may have been true, but the evidence from the eighteenth century and the first decade of the nineteenth points largely in the opposite direction. The small scale of the parish system of medical relief had advantages and disadvantages. It was open to local petty abuse with no hope of redress from a higher authority; but the same, in practice, was true after 1834. The main advantage was that parish work was not despised by medical practitioners, was usually paid at the same level as private practice, and the parish surgeon was the familiar local doctor whose concern for his reputation in his community would have made him generally careful and considerate towards the poor. Here and there, the surgeon and the patient may have found themselves at the mercy of a parsimonious vestry or a brutal overseer, but the worst feature of the old poor law medical system was probably its patchiness. G. C. Lewis in his evidence to the Select Committee on Medical Poor Relief in 1844 believed the systematic provision of medical care by the parish dated back no further than the latter half of the eighteenth century and, even then, was confined largely to the Midlands, the south, and the west.[7]

Under the old system, sometimes a parish surgeon was responsible for a single parish, sometimes for several. In Bedfordshire, for example, in the first decade of the nineteenth century, Mr McGrath of Biggleswade was surgeon to seven parishes but the work was not arduous. The total population was only 3,429 and 10 per cent were eligible for poor law relief, but in 1811 he received £106 5s. for his work in the seven parishes.[8] Frederick Seagram of Warminster, surgeon to the parish of Deverall Longbridge (population 1204 in 1811), was paid on an item of service basis from 1822 to 1824. His average annual payment for parish work was £64 and ranged from £35 to £129 p.a.[9] These were considerable sums.

Table 27 shows the payments made to a number of parish surgeons in Bedfordshire in 1811. It shows several typical features: the generous scale of payment when measured against population, the mixture of payment by salary and payment by 'bill' (i.e. by item of service given),

[6] M. A. Crowther, 'Paupers or Patients?' *Journal of the History of Medicine and Allied Sciences*, 60 (1984), 33–54.

[7] *Select Committee on Medical Poor Relief* Q. 2, 8, 13.

[8] Bedfordshire CRO, Bedford, the Whitbread correspondence, W/773.

[9] Wiltshire CRO, Trowbridge, Wilts, overseer's records, ref. 1020/107.

Table 27 *Payments under the old poor law to several parish surgeons in Bedfordshire, 1811*

Parish	Population	Surgeon	Stipend (£ s. d.)	Bill (£ s. d.)
Biggleswade Hundred				
Astwick	88	Mr Hicks		1. 7.0
Biggleswade	1,895	Mr McGrath and Mr Gaylland alternately	45. 0.0.	
Cockayne Hatley	110	Mr Verrall		2.15.0
Dunton	303	Mr McGrath		7.16.0
Edworth	88	Mr McGrath	4. 4.0	
Eyworth	96	Mr V. Payne	11.17.0	
Langford	469	Mr Layman	8. 0.0	1. 1.0
Potton	1,154	Mr Verrall	15. 0.0	
Sandy and Girtford	937	Mr Gall	18. 0.0	
Sutton	301	Mr McGrath		19. 0.0
Tempsford	475	Mr Saunders	5. 5.0	9. 2.0
Clifton Hundred				
Arlsey	464	Mr Hicks	12.12.0	1. 1.0
Campton	324	Mr Layman	3. 3.0	
Henlow	601	Mr Layman	3. 3.0	
Shifford	536	Mr Layman	3. 3.0	
Shillington	500	Mr Gay	20. 0.0	
Wixamtree Hundred				
Cardington and Eastcott	1,034	Mr Short	18.18.0	
Warden	492	Mr McGrath	10.10.0	
Willington	249	Mr Dowsett	7. 7.0	

Source: The Whitbread correspondence, W/773, Bedfordshire County Record Office, Bedford.

and the tendency for many surgeons to compete for and obtain the post of parish surgeon to several neighbouring parishes.

From the late eighteenth century through to the new poor law system of the 1830s there was a gradual change. Item of service payments were largely replaced by salaries although certain services such as midwifery were usually paid separately. Vestries found it easier to control expenditure through a salaried system than an open-ended one. Salaries, however, were still on the generous side in the late eighteenth and early years of the nineteenth century, as table 27 demonstrates. For example, the small parish of Stour (Stower) Provost in Dorset (population 600), paid an annual salary of 5 guineas in 1786, £8 in 1788, and 12 guineas in 1803 while allowing separate payments for 'broken bones', midwifery and vaccination.[10] One typical parish in Bedfordshire paid 11 guineas a year for a small population in 1803 and raised it in 1812 to 14 guineas.[11] Another parish, Henlow, paid 10 guineas a year in 1812 to the parish surgeon although the population was only 601.[12] Likewise, the parish surgeon of Sandy, Bedfordshire (population 937), had his salary raised progressively from £10 to £18 p.a. between 1790 and 1810.[13] In other words, payments in relation to populations at risk were not only generous by mid-nineteenth-century standards, but were usually raised in line with inflation. The sums may seem trivial, and the matter unimportant; but it suggests that a value was put on the services of the parish surgeon which allowed, as Lane has expressed it, for the care provided for the regular and occasional poor to be no worse than that enjoyed by other villagers.[14]

The first three decades of the nineteenth century show such variation in the level of payment to parish surgeons, however, that it is difficult to be certain about trends. Agricultural parishes paid a salary varying from £10 to £40 p.a. and towns from 40 to 60 guineas. Chichester paid 80 guineas and each of the two districts of Brighton carried a salary of £100 p.a.[15] But one senses a deterioration in levels of payment and status of parish medical work in the twenty or so years before 1834, as parishes farmed out the parish sick to the lowest bidder regardless of

[10] Dorset CRO, Dorchester, Dorset, P 354/OV, 4, 5.
[11] Bedfordshire CRO, Bedford, DDP, P/30/8/1 and DDF 23.
[12] Ibid., the Whitbread correspondence, W1/783.
[13] Ibid., W1/780.
[14] J. Lane, 'The Provincial Practitioner and his Services to the Poor, 1750–1800', *Bulletin of the Society for the Social History of Medicine*, 28 (1981), 10–14.
[15] *Commission on the Poor Laws*, PP 1834, XXVII, Q. 536A.

his experience or qualifications, if any.[16] Cynically, parish surgeons were encouraged to supplement their incomes by 'high charges to non-parishioners since through a settlement order, they may be paid elsewhere and thus the parish "winks" at the custom'.[17]

If one looks at the poor law system of parish surgeons in the late eighteenth century and, comparing it to the poor law medical service in the 1840s, notes the decline in salaries and quality of medical care, it seems natural to lay the blame on the Poor Law Act of 1834. It would simply be driving another nail into the coffin of an Act already despised for its inhumanity. Attitudes to poverty, however, were changing rapidly before the commissioners met in 1832. To some extent, although it is difficult to measure, the poor law service under the old poor law had probably deteriorated in the one or two decades before 1832. Overseers were more parsimonious in their payment of the parish surgeon and were able to be so because of increasing competition of medical men for public and private practice. The commissioners were primarily concerned with what they saw as wasteful expenditure and they sought to introduce economies in an already reduced system of medical poor relief mainly by the attempted reduction in domiciliary care. Believing the poor got what they deserved, they were determined to ensure that costs were at worst kept level, or better still, reduced; and reduced they were, in fact. One must, of course, enter some obvious provisos in this story of degenerating poor law relief. There was wide variation in the quality and liberality of poor law care before and after 1834. No doubt there were callous parish surgeons in the 1790s just as there were able and conscientious, although poorly paid, union surgeons in the 1830s and 1840s. But the general trend in the first half of the nineteenth century seems to have been, slowly at first, and then more rapidly, in a downward direction, both from the patients' and from the practitioners' points of view. The Poor Law Amendment Act of 1834 reflected and contributed to this degradation of the medical care of the poor.

The poor law medical officer after 1834

In general, the Poor Law Amendment Act of 1834 stands condemned for its harsh inhumanity. So much has been written on the Act and the

---

[16] J.C. Yeatman, Sick and Hurt Poor', *LMPJ* 38 (1817), 364–6; 'Remarks on the Medical Care of the Parochial Poor', *LMPJ* 39 (1818), 331–4; 'Regulations suggested for the Treatment of Sick Paupers', *Lancet*, (1830–1), ii. 151–4.

[17] *Commission on the Poor Laws*, PP 1834, XXVII, Q 662A.

attitudes to poverty which shaped the legislation that it would be superfluous to attempt to review the relevant literature.[18] The underlying conviction that the old poor law system had encouraged pauperism and the equating of pauperism with indolence, vice, and crime led to the cardinal principle in the reform of the poor laws—the principle of less eligibility, which laid down that the condition of recipients of relief should always be made less enviable than that of the lowest paid labourer. Priority was given to preventing potential abuse of poor relief, rather than the provision of adequate relief to those in genuine need. The principle of less eligibility led to a drastic reduction in outdoor relief, which only continued at all because it was impractical to abolish it altogether. The same principle led to the establishment of the first non-psychiatric public hospitals (apart, of course, from the voluntary hospitals) in England, the workhouse infirmaries. A few existed before 1834, (St Peter's Hospital in Bristol, for example) but the new poor law made them a national institution.

While there is no doubt that poor law legislation was designed to make life unpleasant for the able-bodied pauper, it was never intended that the conditions for the sick, the aged, and the infirm should be any harsher than they had been previously. Indeed, the commissioners in 1834 paid a back-handed compliment to the old poor law medical system by stating that on the whole it had been 'adequately supplied and economically, if we consider only the price and the amount of attendance'.[19] If poor relief had been abused, it was the able bodied who had been guilty, not the sick. But the problem of the independent labourer who had been turned into a pauper by sickness was a problem which the commissioners refused to grasp, and this refusal led to continual ambiguity in the application of poor law medical relief. The authorities tried to limit poor relief to the pauper, when harsh treatment could, in their view, be justified.

As Himmelfarb has stressed, the emphasis on previous poor law abuse was already to some extent out of date by 1834, and thus the new legislation was by no means popular, especially in the many parts of the country where the prospect of central control from London was hated not just by the potential recipients of poor relief but also by those who

---

[18] Amongst the most notable recent works (which has influenced the writing of this chapter) is G. Himmelfarb, *The Idea of Poverty: England in the Early Industrial Age* (London, 1984).

[19] *Commission on the Poor Laws*, PP 1834, XXVII, p. 25.

had administered the old system and thought it adequate and fair.[20] What, then, was the attitude of medical practitioners to the whole question of poor relief? They were middle-class citizens, and it is not surprising that they reflected many of the middle-class attitudes of the period. But at least they took a reformist stand on medical care.

In 1835, a committee of the Provincial Medical and Surgical Association was established to consider and report on the Poor Law Amendment Act. It did so with admirable thoroughness, especially the Gloucester surgeon, H. W. Rumsey, whose notable contributions to the concept of state medicine date from this time. The committee's conclusion on the poor law in general was in line with the commissioners' report. They believed the old poor law was 'bad in principle, worse in practice ... spreading idleness, vice and destitution'. The principle of 'less eligibility' was right and proper in its application to the able-bodied pauper but the committee questioned whether it should apply to the sick pauper. Medical relief 'is always expensive ... a luxury beyond the poor man's reach'. Without being wholly explicit about it, the Association's committee was nudging its way towards the proposition that poor law medical relief should be available to all who could not pay for medical care. This was to be the only criterion.[21] This may sound obvious enough today, but for the commissioners it was opening the door much wider than they had intended. Such a criterion which said nothing about the indefinable grades of pauper, undeserving poor, deserving poor, and independent poor, opened up the possibility of increased medical costs on a huge scale.[22] The poor law authorities, locally and centrally, refused to adopt such criteria for access to poor law relief.

This difference of opinion underlines a matter of central importance. The pretence that a clear distinction could be made between the undeserving pauper and the deserving poor did more than anything else to limit and degrade the new poor law medical service. The sick poor were inevitably, if unintentionally, subjected to a harshness for which no excuse can be found, and which persisted into the twentieth century. In the *Report of the Royal Commission on the Poor Laws* in 1909 a witness stated:

[20] Himmelfarb (1984), 147–76.

[21] 'Reports of the Poor Law Committee (of the Provincial Medical and Surgical Association)', *PMSJ* 1 (1840), 166–8, 184–6, 197–9, 212–14, 228–30. The first committee was established in 1835 and reported in 1837, the second established in 1838 and reported in 1840.

[22] M. W. Flinn, 'Medical Services under the New Poor Law', in D. Fraser (ed.), *The New Poor Law in the Nineteenth Century* (London, 1984).

The tradition of the service is that every pauper is to be looked on as being such through his or her own fault, and the tendency is to treat the case accordingly ... I believe that the tradition, as to the pauper, is that he is a shade only from the criminal ... Now, to this tradition the Medical Officers tend, like all other officers, to become a victim, and the tendency is that the case of sickness is treated as a 'pauper' and not as a patient'.[23]

In the 1830s, moreover, this attitude coincided with an increasing crisis in the health of the poor. The well-known demographic, social, environmental, and occupational changes associated with the industrial revolution were recognized then, as now, as being accompanied by increasing amounts of sickness.[24] What was needed was an expanded and much more efficient system for administering medical relief. But:

The truth of the matter was that a health service of the degree of com-prehensiveness attempted after 1834 was simply not compatible either with the underlying ideology of the New Poor Law, or with the willingness, let alone the capacity, of the ratepayers to pay it. Finance and ideology, in other words, stood between the Poor Law Medical Service and efficiency.[25]

Under the new law some 2,500 unions of parishes were created out of the nine to ten thousand parishes which existed. The replacement of the parish surgeon by the union surgeon led to a reduction in the number of posts as medical officers to the poor. The exact extent of the reduction is unknown as the number of parish surgeons under the old system is not recorded; but all the evidence suggests that the reduction was substantial.

In Derby five parish surgeons were replaced by one union surgeon, and even in 1840, when, over the previous six years, population had increased by one third, no extra appointment was made.[26] The reduction in poor law medical posts after 1834 was from sixteen to three in Lincoln, from sixteen to seven in Bridgewater, from sixteen to three in Aylesbury, from eleven to eight in Epping, from eight to three in Eton, from ten to two in Shipston, and from twelve to six in Newbury. These reductions allowed economies to be made. In the Shipston Union the population of 19,000 had, before 1834, been served by ten local prac-titioners who shared a payment of £500 p.a. After 1834 first two,

[23] M. A. Crowther (1984).
[24] M. W. Flinn (1984), and R. Hodgkinson, *Origins of the National Health Service: Medical Services of the New Poor Law, 1834–1871'* (London, 1967).
[25] M. W. Flinn (1984).
[26] J. Jones, *Observations on the Self-Supporting Dispensaries* (London, 1844).

and then only one—an outsider specially brought in—acted as union surgeon to the same population for £200 p.a.[27] The degradation in the provision of medical care for the poor is obvious. There were many similar examples.

In 1844 the number of available posts as surgeons to a union in England was about 2,400. The average salary was £69 p.a. When this is compared to the salaries paid to parish surgeons at the end of the eighteenth century it can be seen at once that payment per unit of population was much lower. The union surgeon had, on average, about four to five times as many patients for whom he was supposed to care as the old parish surgeon had treated for the same salary; when inflation is taken into account the poor pay of union surgeons is even worse than apparent at first sight.[28] Nevertheless, after 1834 poor law work was still much sought after when any extra source of income was important in such a competitive profession as medicine.

A random sample of two hundred entries in the provincial section of the *Medical Directory* (1848) showed that 19 per cent of general practitioners held appointments as surgeons to a union of parishes, 3.5 per cent were union surgeons and also held an appointment at a hospital or dispensary (or both), 7.5 per cent held an appointment at a dispensary only, 5 per cent held a hospital appointment only, and 65 per cent appeared to hold no appointments but confined themselves to private practice. It should be remembered, however, that a post as a union surgeon was often held for a brief period by young practitioners who, when they had established an adequate private practice, resigned from the poor law medical service. Therefore, the number of general practitioners who at one time or another were surgeons to a union was possibly twice the above number.

The grievances of poor law medical officers were many and genuine. Low salaries were bad enough; even worse was the rule (nearly, but not quite, universal) that the surgeon should provide drugs and dressings. The temptation to withold treatment was obvious.[29] As a result of the union of parishes, practitioners in country areas were often required to travel long distances, and were often complete strangers to some of

[27] Poor Law Committee Report, *PMSJ* 2 (1841), 266–71, 292–5, 304–10, 334–8, 354–7, 372–4, and *PMSJ* 1 (1840), 229.

[28] H. W. Rumsey, *Select Committee on Poor Law Medical Relief*, PP 1844, IX, Q. 9173. Higher fees were paid on average to poor law medical officers in London and the South and East than in the North and the South-West and Wales. Details can be found in R. Griffin, *The Grievances of the Poor Law Medical Officers* (London, 1859).

[29] H. W. Rumsey, Q. 9157.

the outlying areas they visited. The old parish doctor might or might not be popular with the parish poor; but at least he was the devil they knew. Under the new poor law, patients were reluctant to send for the union surgeon because he was unknown, lived far away, and might well refuse to attend. Rumsey described how the Whitminster Union in Gloucestershire included the parishes of Brookthorpe and Harescomb, six and eight miles respectively from Whitminster where the union surgeon lived. To get to Brookthorpe he had to cross the Severn valley and mount the Cotswold range, often impassable in winter, although this parish was only four miles from Gloucester and Stroud, and two miles from Painswick. The union officer was, as it happens, a 'superior and indefatigable practitioner' so that it was the union system, not the medical officer, which was to blame for the impossibility of the poor in some distant areas receiving poor relief when they needed it.[30] Mr John Fox, union medical officer to Cerne in Dorset, told the same committee that he attended 857 poor law cases a year in a union of twenty parishes. The total population was only 8,000, but he travelled 2,000 miles a year on horseback, much of it over bleak country where, in winter, he frequently had to dismount and lead his horse. His poor law payment averaged 1s. 6d. per case, but this was reduced to 7d. after deduction of expenses.[31] Boards of Guardians in cases like this did not have a free hand in applying the obvious remedy—that of appointing extra surgeons. It was the assistant commissioners from London who had the final responsibility for deciding which parishes should be joined in a union, how many surgeons should be appointed, and what they should be paid. If local surgeons offered their services (and many had long experience of treating the poor in their district) but jibbed at the salary, they were told there were 'plenty in London' willing to take the job. One of the penalties of an overcrowded profession was the acceptance of very low salaries by inexperienced young outsiders over the heads of local, experienced, and known practitioners.[32]

The old system of medical poor relief had its faults, but it was dismantled with a singular scorn and brutality towards the general practitioners of the country and their poor patients, and an extraordinary indifference to the size of the populations to every union surgeon. In Exeter in the 1840s, there were four union surgeons. The most senior

---

[30] H. W. Rumsey, Q. 9150.

[31] Ibid., Q. 5784–95.

[32] There are numerous instances in the reports of the poor law committee of the Provincial Medical and Surgical Association in the *PMSJ* 1 (1840).

had the least arduous job of looking after the union infirmary. The others looked after the three districts of the town. The total population was 10,400 and each surgeon received £40 p.a. with £15 in lieu of drugs. This was generous. In Leeds, two union surgeons cared for a total of 75,000 and each received £80 p.a., but at least in this instance the city employed a dispenser and supplied the drugs. This was unusual.[33] In Hull, with a population of 41,000, there was only one surgeon who was paid £100 p.a. from which he had to provide medicine,[34] and Huddersfield provides a vivid example of the exploitation of the union surgeon by the local Board of Guardians.

Mr Tatham was appointed medical officer to the northern division of the Huddersfield union in 1843 at a salary of £40 p.a. In his first year, besides 1,633 journeys and visits, he supplied medicine at a personal cost of £37. 18s. 7d., reducing his profit for his work to just over £2 p.a. He applied to the Guardians for an increase in salary to £70 p.a. He was allowed £50, and some time later this was increased to £80. In 1847, however, a fever hospital was opened owing to the prevalence of typhus in the locality. Cases were sent to the hospital from adjoining unions but Mr Tatham had the sole responsibility for the fever hospital cases, and there were, on average, twenty-seven admissions each week. For treating these, Mr Tatham not only had much more work to do, but he was 'more than out-of-pocket'. On applying to the Guardians for an extra salary, he was refused any addition to his income, and he therefore sued the Board. Through a technicality he lost, and costs were awarded against him, although the judge and jury were indignant at the wrong perpetrated against Mr Tatham.[35]

Manchester provided evidence of the way two adjoining unions could differ. In the densely populated township of 160,000 people, five union surgeons had an easy life. Although they attended on average eight hundred patients a year each for a salary of £50, two-thirds were only seen at the surgery for certification of fitness to work. All serious, acute, and chronic case were sent to the union hospital (for which the union surgeons were not responsible), fevers to the House of Recovery or fever hospital and injuries to the Infirmary. Vaccination was paid extra at 1s. 6d. a case, and, by scrutinizing the birth registers, and employing men at 2d. a case to 'search out and bring up cases of vacination', an

[33] H. W. Rumsey, Q. 9103.
[34] Ibid.
[35] 'Working of the Poor Law for Medical Relief in England', *Dublin Medical Press*, 19 (1848), 286–7.

easy profit was made. Next door, so to speak, in the out-townships of
Manchester with a widely scattered population of 30,000, two union
surgeons travelled long distances, were forced to keep a horse and were
rarely able to send their serious cases to an institution. Their annual
salary of £50 was almost totally eroded by the costs of drugs and a
horse.[36]

Liverpool was unusual, the whole town being a single parish where
the dispensary was partly funded from the time of its establishment in
1778 by the parish authorities, and there was no parish surgeon under
the old poor law. The annual payment of the parish to the dispensary
had risen by 1834 to £500 p.a. but this payment was promptly stopped
in 1834. Instead, six surgeons were appointed under the new poor law
medical services at a salary of £100 each. The poor, however (and
Liverpool had more than its fair share), continued to attend the hospitals
and dispensaries of the city in preference to the poor law medical officers.
In 1834 25 per cent of the population received some form of medical
poor relief, 2 per cent from the district surgeons appointed under the
poor law and 23 per cent from the medical charities.[37]

Liverpool was not alone in this respect. A careful estimate was made
of the number of sick in 1843 in the town of Newark and a radius of
eight miles. The total population included in this area was 25,000 and
the estimated number of sick people that year 12,500. Of these, about
60 per cent were treated privately. The remaining 40 per cent were the
sick poor who received 'gratuitous treatment' as follows: 1,400 obtained
free advice from physicians, 2,200 from other practitioners, 660 from
the Newark Dispensary, and 890 from the union officers. Thus 'legal
medical relief reached little more than one-sixth of the destitute sick,
nearly five-sixths being left to the charitable feelings of a profession
which certainly does not luxuriate in the marrow of English opulence.'[38]

In Bristol, the poor had traditionally come under the care of St Peter's
Hospital, founded in the late seventeenth century. Here, the existing
system was used to provide poor law medical care, the house apothecary
being the poor law medical officer. Outdoor care seems to have been
left to the Bristol dispensary, but the house apothecary treated 2,600
cases of sickness amongst the Bristol poor each year.[39]

These examples from Exeter, Hull, Huddersfield, Manchester, Liver-

[36] H. W. Rumsey, Q. 9104.
[37] Ibid., Q. 9103.
[38] Ibid., Q. 9119.
[39] Ibid., Q. 9103.

pool, Newark, and Bristol show how haphazard and unco-ordinated were the systems and institutions established for the medical relief of the sick poor. The conventional picture of medical care in this period suggests three clearly defined levels at which medical care was available. For the lowest layer, the paupers, there was the poor law medical service: next came the 'hospital class' of patients, mainly the labourers and their families, for whom the hospitals and dispensaries were established; and finally the third and top layer for everyone else which was private practice supplemented by various medical benefit clubs or similar private schemes. Although this was broadly true, local variations in the way that medical care was administered led to considerable blurring of the boundaries between the three layers. An itinerant bricklayer or carpenter who had the ill fortune when travelling around the country to suffer a series of illnesses and accidents would have experienced some of the variety of medical aid in different areas. Here, he would have been directed to a hospital or a dispensary; there he would find nothing but the private practitioner; and in another place he might be fortunate and persuade the relieving officer to sanction treatment by a union surgeon. Towns and villages in the south and east of England and to a lesser extent the south-west, tended to have the most extensive provision of poor law medical care, treating more cases of sickness than the charities.[40] In the industrial North, however, medical services for the poor were, very often, so inadequate that it was generally recognized the majority received no medical care at all but 'allowed indisposition to go without calling a medical man'.[41] There is no doubt of the truth of this.

If the definition of the sick poor is used in the sense that H. W. Rumsey used it, namely, any family which, although able to purchase the necessities of life, could not pay a medical practitioner,[42] various sources indicate that in the first half of the nineteenth century the annual number of episodes of major serious sickness and injuries amongst the poor amounted to at least half of the total number of poor persons. Since the poor as so defined amounted to at least two-thirds of the

[40] H. W. Rumsey, Q. 9117.

[41] Ibid., Q. 9111.

[42] Ibid., Q. 9125–45. To his eternal credit, Rumsey argued firmly, (1) in favour of applying poor law medical services to all who could not pay, and not just the paupers, and (2) in favour of abolishing the letters of recommendation demanded by hospitals and dispensaries. No one, he said, not overseers, relieving officers, or subscribers to medical institutions, should be allowed to interfere between a sick person and the medical attendant.

total population in an industrial town, the annual number of sickness
episodes amongst the poor can be estimated as amounting to a figure
equal to one third of the total population. Yet in Bradford in the 1840s
(total population c.132,000) the annual number of cases of illness
treated under the poor law system amounted to less than 1 per cent of
the population, and those treated by the charities to less than 3 per
cent.[43] Only one in every six of the sick poor in Bradford received any
form of medical poor relief and the total number of sick poor was
probably about 40,000 cases a year. Leeds in 1843 had 63,000 people
judged as belonging to the working classes. The thriving medical benefit
clubs had some 10,000 members, but it was estimated that at most
one-third of those in the working classes who were not club members,
received any kind of medical poor relief.[44]

Why was the medical poor relief of the new poor law system so
inadequate and apparently ineffective? A major reason, for which we
have provided abundant evidence, was the low incentive in financial
terms to provide a good service; another was the ratio of union surgeons
to population, so that some union surgeons, even if they had been paid
generously, would have found it impossible to cope with the medical
problems in their appointed areas. Another and important reason was
the stigma of pauperism and the resistance of the poor to applying for
relief. This existed even before 1834. In 1832, in his evidence to the
Poor Law Commission, Dr Calvert opened his evidence with a story of
the fate of the independent poor man when struck by sickness which
might have been the subject of a series of prints by Cruickshank. The
victim avoided the parish doctor 'not only from an idea that he is
inferior, but to prevent its being supposed he himself is a pauper'.
Frequently he 'fell into the hands of quacks', a category which included
the druggists, and they demanded 'ready money'. When all his money
had gone a regular practitioner might be called in. The patient's debts
mounted and the bill to the regular practitioner was 'soon equal to a
large part and often to the whole of a patient's annual income'. Debts
to tradesmen were paid off first, to medical practitioners last, and the
practitioner sometimes put his debts 'into the hands of an attorney'.
The last picture in the series sees the patient incarcerated in 'the poor
house or gaol'.[45] In theory this was just the kind of sequence which

---

[43] H. W. Rumsey, Q. 9109.
[44] Ibid., Q. 9120.
[45] *Commission on Poor Laws*, PP 1834, XXXVIII, Appendix C.

medical poor relief should have prevented, but the stigma of pauperism was, and remained throughout the nineteenth century, a powerful disincentive for those in need of medical poor relief.

To the medical officers, as to the recipients, the poor law medical service after 1834 was on the whole a miserable, degrading system. Low pay and the system of tendering (officially but not in fact abolished by the medical order of 1842)[46] headed the lists of complaints by medical officers, followed by the system of annual appointments which placed medical officers in perpetual servile dependence on the Boards of Guardians.[47] Populations served were, as we have seen, often absurdly large. Rumsey suggested there should be a union surgeon and a deputy to stand in for him in his absence (paid by the union surgeon) to every 4,000 inhabitants, with adjustments according to local circumstances. This, however, would have required at least twice as many appointments, excluding the deputies.

Recognition of the poor levels of pay by the commissioners in London was followed by recommendations that pay should be increased. Being recommendations, not orders, they were often ignored. in 1844 Mr Robinson of Newbury received £20 p.a. for work which should, by the recommendations of 1842, have been paid at a level of £100 p.a.[48] Charles Goodwin in Bethnal Green attended six hundred persons a year as union surgeon, nearly all of them attended at their homes. Under the old poor law system he received £100 p.a. Under the new, he received only £70 p.a., he was 'never paid a farthing' for midwifery, and the cost of medicines severely eroded his salary. If the recommendations of the commissioners had been put into effect he would have been paid £200 p.a.[49] Two country surgeons in Suffolk who received £30 and £40 p.a. respectively, claimed this did not cover the cost of the horse, let alone drugs.[50] Yet union posts were competed for in spite of this, simply because 'there are many members of the medical profession who have a very hard fight to live, who are needy men',[51] and the service was often staffed by penniless and inexperienced youths.[52]

When Henry Peart, aged twenty-two, settled in Feckenham in Wor-

[46] 'New Poor Law Regulations', *PMSJ* 3 (1842), 515-20.
[47] Dr George Webster, *Select Committee on Medical Poor Relief*, PP 1844, IX, Q. 9021-71.
[48] Ibid., Q. 6848-85.
[49] Ibid., Q. 1299-1436.
[50] Ibid., Q. 7547-80.
[51] Ibid., Q. 487-503.
[52] Ibid., Q. 8-22, 882-1008, 9021-71.

cestershire in 1830, his total earnings from private practice in the first six months were £4. 18s. A contribution of £183 from his family kept body and soul together. A year later hs six-month accounts showed a rise in private fees, but only to £16. 9s. 9d. An appointment as parish surgeon at £50 p.a. provided him with a reliable income, paid every quarter, and he survived to spend the rest of his life as the general practitioner to the small town and surrounding villages.[53] Mr Bloomfield, surgeon to the Poplar union in London, who found his salary did not even cover his expenses, took the post because 'as a young man it was important to be seen occupied and to be talked about'.[54] Others accepted an appointment as union surgeon to keep competitors out who might take away private practice.[55] J. P. Watkins of the Carmarthen union 'visited up to 7 miles' and covered a population of 17,000 with many poor. He had to keep two horses, but took the post 'because I love practice, and to prevent an interloper'.[56]

Once the post as union surgeon had been accepted, it was sometimes retained by a practitioner, even when he was established, for one of the above reasons. Mr J. G. Leete of Thrapston in Northamptonshire (LSA 1829, MRCS 1830) became a very prosperous practitioner, earning between £1,800 and £2,000 a year by the 1860s. But he remained the local union surgeon, showing that they were not always the young and inexperienced. His union accounts survive for the year 1850 (see table 28). They amounted in all to only £43, but they are quoted here as an illustration of the method and level of payment to the poor law medical officer in the mid-nineteenth century.[57]

The deficiencies of the poor law medical service were recognized, but persisted through the second half of the nineteenth century.[58] Richard Griffin was the chairman of the Poor Law Medical Reform Association which produced three highly critical reports in 1857, 1858, and 1859. In 1868 the Poor Law Medical Officers Association was formed to improve the conditions of service. But there was, even in the 1840s, a general level of pessimism about reform. Instead, many practitioners suggested that the state system should be abandoned in favour of a system of relief based on the provident dispensaries. The popularity of

[53] I. Loudon, 'A Doctor's Cash-book', *Medical History* , 27 (1983), 249–68.

[54] *Select Committee on Medical Poor Relief*, PP 1844, IX, Q. 882–1088.

[55] Ibid., Q. 4277–4300.

[56] Ibid., Q. 8534–8615.

[57] Northampton CRO, Northampton, day-books of Dr Leete of Thrapston, ref. Leete VII/7, IX/1.

[58] M. A. Crowther (1984), and R. G. Hodgkinson (1967).

Table 28 *Payments to Dr Leete for his services as surgeon to the Thrapston union,*
1850

	Payment (£ s. d.)
Paid for attendance on District	21. 3.6
Paid for attendance on Union House	6. 6.6
Midwifery at the Union House	
Difficult case	1. 0.0
3 ordinary cases	1.10.0
Midwifery (outdoor), 2 cases	2. 0.0
3 trusses supplied at 10s. 6d.	1.11.6
Elastic stocking	15.0
Reduction dislocated shoulder, 2 cases	2. 0.0
Reduction fractured leg	3. 0.0
Reduction fractured thigh	3. 0.0
Reduction fractured arm	1. 0.0
TOTAL	43. 6.6

Source: Day-books of Dr Leete of Thrapston, Northampton County Record Office,
Northampton. These accounts can be found at the very end of book: 'Leete IX/I'.

these was rapidly increasing in the 1840s and 1850s,[59] and those who
were appointed to them as medical officers not only applauded the
underlying philosophy of the provident principle, but found they provided a considerable income.[60] Others believed that the free and the
provident dispensaries combined could provide the nucleus of a system
of poor relief, free from central control and the obvious deficiencies of
the state system.[61] Some method of care was needed which did not
require the medical officer to spend as much time as possible in private
general practice in order to survive. Such plans were widely discussed,
but it is doubtful whether a dispensary-based system could ever have
been adequate for medical poor relief. The importance of such plans is
the tacit admission not only that the poor law medical service was
deficient and degrading, but that it was beyond reform or repair.

The best that can be said in extenuation was that the system was

[59] This suggestion was made in 1834 in the *Report of the Commission on the Poor Laws*,
PP 1834, XXXVIII, Appendix C, and was taken up again by many, especially J. Jones,
Observations on the Self-supporting Dispensaries (London, 1844). In his evidence to the *Select
Committee on the Poor Laws*, PP 1844, IX, part III, Q. 5759–83, the Duke of Rutland
described the 'Independent Labourers' Self-Aiding Medical Club extending over the same
district as that comprised in the Grantham Union' as a preferable alternative to the state
system.

[60] W. D. Foster, 'Dr William Henry Cook: The Finances of a Victorian General Practitioner', *Proceedings of the Royal Society of Medicine* 66 (1973), 46–50.

[61] H. W. Rumsey, Q. 9162–5.

defeated by the problem of numbers. It can be argued that the problems of the poor in the eighteenth century were manageable at the parish level; those of the mid-nineteenth century were not. The rate of sickness attendant on the demographic explosion was sufficient to overwhelm such a mediocre system of medical poor relief. On the other hand, the process of centralization should have produced economies of scale and increased efficiency of administration. As Flinn pointed out, however, in the passage quoted above, ideology and economy together prevented a bold and imaginative system of medical poor relief although there were more than enough general practitioners to undertake the care of the poor in a properly organized system in the years following 1834. The new poor law medical service stands condemned for insisting on gross understaffing with medical officers and consequent neglect of the sick poor, at the very time when everyone recognized the profession was overprovided with general practitioners anxiously seeking employment.

Practice and Income: Private Practice and other Sources: Total Income

Income from private practice

MEDICAL bills from private general practice in the first half of the nineteenth century were often long and detailed and, at first sight, confusing. But they were based on quite simple principles which were followed closely by the majority of general practitioners. By far the greatest part of the bill usually consisted of medicines, itemized as draughts, mixtures, pills, boluses, etc. Charges were also made for 'visits' or 'journeys', especially in country practice where the distance travelled by the practitioner was over one or two miles. 'Advice' as such was seldom an item in a general practitioner's bill, being, by custom, the prerogative of the physicians. In addition, separate charges were made for surgical procedures, including venesection and dental extractions, etc., and for midwifery. It is rare to find separate charges for anything else.

In all these instances, fees, as in the eighteenth century, were nearly always kept within surprisingly narrow limits, regardless of the class and wealth of the patient. This can be confirmed by examining a series of practitioners' ledgers. For instance, Mr Sabin, a general practitioner in Towcester, included amongst his patients in 1831, the Earl of Pomfret, the Revd Dr Butler, Mrs Hurst, Lord Southampton, a Mr Gibbs, and Thomas Lovell, a carpenter. There is no difference in the detailed charges he entered in his book for each of these patients. Draughts were charged at the standard rate of 1s. 6d. to the Earl and to the carpenter, and charges for 'journey' were standard throughout.[1] In fact in this, as in other examples of fees and charges, there is a monotonous similarity between the bills throughout the whole period 1750–1850. Charges rarely varied, and medicines amounted to not less than 80 per cent of

[1] Northampton CRO, Northampton. The account books of Mr Sabin, surgeon of Towcester, for the year 1831, pp. 11, 12, 13, 14, 25, and 26 of ledger 688. (This was probably Charles Heath Sabin of High St, Towcester.)

the cost in the large majority of bills. Much the same medicines were dispensed in much the same way and the time-honoured system of sending out small individual amounts very frequently was as much a feature of the early Victorian general practitioner as it was of his forebears in the 1750s. If a practitioner or dispenser who died in 1750–70 was resurrected and re-employed in the same practice in 1830–50 it is difficult to believe that he would detect any important difference in the general custom of dispensing or the book-keeping of the practice, and very little difference in the medicines dispensed.

A single example can serve for a typical medical bill of the mid-nineteenth century.[2] It covered the years 1844–9 and it contained fifty-six items, nearly all items of medicine. Draughts were charged at the standard price of 1s. 6d. (remember, they were a single dose of medicine), a dental extraction 2s. 6d., vaccination 5s. The total bill was £25. 10s. 6d. and the practitioner rounded this off to £30 by adding £4. 9s. 6d. for 'visits'. Note that the charge for 'visits' is added almost as an afterthought to bring the bill up to a round number. This is characteristic of the general practitioner's bills, even, as in this example, from a well-established practitioner in a well-known Somerset medical family. Such methods of charging were traditional, although after 1830 they were no longer required by law, because an important case was heard in 1830 which should have altered the general practitioner's method of payment; it was the case of Handey v. Henson.

James Handey was a surgeon and apothecary in London.[3] He treated the Henson family over a period of seven weeks from July to September 1829. Mrs Henson was suffering from an eruption on the face, and one night Handey was called to see one of the children. Medicine was sent in on twelve occasions, visits were paid on fifteen. Reversing the usual custom, £2. 10s. was charged for the medicines and £4. 10s. 6d. for the visits. Mr Henson, an attorney, refused to pay the charges for visits, basing his case on the Rose decision (see chapter 1). Mr Handey sued successfully for full payment, the judge, Lord Tenterden, commenting: 'I cannot see, if a medical gentleman pursues the same honourable plan of not sending in large and useless quantities of medicine, how he is to be remunerated but by being paid for his attendance.'[4] General

---

[2] Bill presented to Mrs Danithorpe by her general practitioner Mr Jolliffe of Crewkerne, Somerset. I am grateful to Dr J. Guy for drawing my attention to this bill which is in the possession of the Somerset CRO, Taunton, Somerset.

[3] James Handey of Upper Stamford St, London: 'The first to try, and successfully, the legality of charges for visits from General Practitioner', *Medical Directory* (1848).

[4] 'Intelligence', *LMPJ*, NS 7 (1830), 183–6.

practitioners hailed this as a great victory and arranged a celebratory dinner in London. Petitioners in Leamington Spa (Dr C. Loudon in the chair) voted Handey a piece of plate,[5] and Wakley devoted a special, ecstatic leading article to the case.[6] The case was therefore widely known in the profession, but it was only the *London Medical Gazette* which forecast correctly that it would be a long time before habits were changed.[7] Knowing the expectations of the public and the danger in a competitive world if, suddenly, large charges for attendance appeared on medical bills, general practitioners stuck to their old ways and vast quantities of useless medicine continued to be sent out. It was a custom that was criticized at the time, but it continued all the same.[8]

Income from private practice depended, therefore, not on large single fees such as those charged by the most successful physicians and surgeons, but almost entirely on the accumulation of a very large number of small separate items, mostly of medicines. Even the most successful owed their success not to an ability to charge substantially higher fees than their colleagues (although a few exceptionally successful London general practitioners were able to do so) but on the number of patients they could attract and persuade to accept large quantities of medicine and frequent attendances. In a highly competitive profession, therefore, the fine—and to us today seemingly trivial—details of the cost of draughts, mixtures, powders, and pills, played a large part in the business of general practice. To achieve prosperity, a general practitioner needed at least three things—an average of fifteen to twenty visits a day, an efficient pharmacy run by his apprentice or assistant, and the minimum of 'bad debts'.

Other sources of practice and income

Before the introduction of National Health Insurance in 1911, it is often assumed that the general practitioner made his living entirely by private practice, and that other systems of payment were few and unimportant. This is far from the truth. Various systems of providing care for the poor existed. There were numerous sick clubs. There were also the provident

---

[5] *Lancet* (1829–30), i. 711.

[6] Ibid., 539.

[7] 'Remuneration of General Practitioners', *LMG* 5 (1830), 665–7.

[8] 'Medical Renumeration', *MCR* 5 (1824), 509–10; 'The College of Physicians', *Gazette of Health*, 11 (1826), 673; W. Cooke, *Separation without Dissention* (London, 1831); R. Hull, 'On the Division of Medical Labour', *LMG*, NS 2 (1841–2), 71–2; Anon., *Whom to Consult*, 2nd edn (London, 1865); I. Ashe, *Medical Education and Medical Interests* (Dublin, 1868).

dispensaries where an average payment in the mid-nineteenth century of 1d. a week from the breadwinner, and 1s. 2d. from each member of his family was collected, and most of it handed on to the practitioner chosen by the family from those attached to the dispensary. The provident dispensaries were intended primarily for the lower and middle-range earners, and they received much support from the popular belief that self-help maintained the dignity and independence of the subscriber, removing the stigmas of charity and pauperism.[9] Many of the sick clubs catered for the same group of patients, mainly the skilled or semi-skilled labourers, as they had done from their origin in the early eighteenth century; but other clubs recruited from the class of 'small tradesmen and shopkeepers, persons in offices and the higher sort of artificers'. The Odd Fellows was an example.[10]

The hospitals and dispensaries catered in theory for those above the level of the pauper, but below the ability to pay any medical fees at all. In practice they treated a broader spectrum than their rules laid down. In addition there was a very wide range of special medical and paramedical charities. Lying-in charities were often large and clinically important, and there were charities for relieving the sick poor at their own homes, truss societies, and charities for the blind, the deaf and dumb, the aged and infirm, destitute females, and so on.[11]

In other words, there was a wide range of institutions and agencies for the sick, infirm, and lying-in poor, dotted sporadically around the country. As we saw in the last chapter the part played in any area by one type of institution rather than another had no basis in need or in rational planning. It was a matter of chance, local tradition, and local philanthropy. In the 1840s, for example, 19 per cent of the population in healthy Exeter received poor law medical relief and 9 per cent were treated by hospitals and the dispensary, so that 28 per cent of the population received medical poor relief from one agency or another. Contrast this with unhealthy Leeds at the same time, where only 1.4 per cent received poor law medical relief and 3.6 per cent were treated at charities—a total of only 5 per cent of the population.[12] This might be interpreted as an example of the well-recognized tendency for the northern industrial areas to be poorly provided with medical care com-

[9] On the poor laws and provident dispensaries, see John Calvert, 'On Dispensary Associations', Appendix C in the *First Report of the Commissioners on the Poor Laws*, PP 1834, XXXVII.

[10] Report of the *Select Committee on Medical Poor Relief*, PP 1844, IX (531), Q. 9078.

[11] Robson's London directory for 1831.

[12] H. W. Rumsey, in the *Select Committee on Medical Poor Relief*, PP 1844, Q. 9103.

Table 29   *Rates per head of population spent on poor law medical relief*

Farnham, Surrey	£4 3s. 4d.	Canterbury	£1 1s. 2d.
Shrewsbury	£4 1s. 2d.	Oxford	1s. 2d.
Alverstoke and Gosport	£3 1s. 2d.	Hull	1s. 2d.
Knarestone, Yorks	£2 3s. 4d.	Stoke Daverell, Devon	3s. 4d.
Chichester	£2 1s. 2d.	Oldham	1s. 4d.
Bristol	2d.	Rochdale	1s. 4d.
Brighton	2d.		

pared to the southern non-industrial ones, and there is some truth in this in the 1840s; but the division was by no means clear cut. See table 29 for examples of the rates per head of population spent on poor law medical relief.[13] The wide differences were obviously important from the patients' point of view, but they also affected the prospects of the local practitioners. Farnham, Exeter, and Shrewsbury would have provided better opportunities than Oldham, Hull, or Oxford, for general practitioners unable to break into the middle-class market of private practice.

Appointments as medical officer to charities and clubs, parishes and unions of parishes, were often the determining factor in a decision on a place to settle in practice. All of them provided benefits for a young practitioner, either tangibly as income, or intangibly as prestige and introductions which would, perhaps, lead to private practice. The intangible benefits were sometimes exaggerated, or outweighed by the disadvantages of charitable appointments. The surgeon to a dispensary

must be regular in his attendence, or his absence is recorded; he must sacrifice his private concerns to his public duties. If he is a dispensary physician or surgeon in London, he must sit for hours prescribing for the afflicted poor, and then go to visit others in the filthiest situations ... or his task-masters, the governors, or their committee, will sit in judgement upon him with as much gravity as one of the judges would display during a trial for felony ... He is expected to do all this unpleasant and laborious duty ... because, quoth the governors, it makes him known and will ultimately serve him.[14]

This perhaps was an extreme view. John Taunton, when he settled in London as a young surgeon, had no doubts of the value of appointments to his future career, as he explained when he wrote to his uncle saying why he was yet unable to repay the money he owed.

[13] G. C. Lewis in Ibid., Q. 846.
[14] 'Duties and Privations of Medical Practitioners', *LMG*, NS 1 (1832), 633–5.

Dear Uncle,

Reflect upon the situations I hold, and those I am looking up to. I am surgeon to the City Dispensary, one of the most public and respectable institutions in the world, I am lecturer at the London Philosophical Society Leicester Square, am principal lecturer to the London Anatomical Society held at my house, I am Honorary Member of the Physical Society, Guy's Hospital, I am Fellow of the London Medical Society and am now making preparations to give a course of public lectures on anatomy, these things tho' likely to be highly advantageous in the end, have been obtained at no small labour or expense, for I assure you I have worked as hard since I have been in London as ever you did in the Country in your life ... I shall make a very large Fortune in a few years as I am doing quite as much business as can be expected from the time I settled.[15]

He may not have made a fortune, but John Taunton became a well-known and sought-after surgeon in London, continuing with his appointment at a dispensary.

Medical benefit clubs and sick clubs

Private health insurance in the form of the sick clubs seems to have been on the whole unpopular with both members and their medical officers, at least in the first half of the nineteenth century. Payment, usually two to three shillings per head per year[16] was considered expensive by the members and too little by the surgeons who were expected to find the cost of drugs and dressings out of their salaries.[17] The member of the sick club was covered, but not his family.[18] Higher rates were paid by the members of the Odd Fellows and other 'superior' clubs, usually four shillings a year;[19] but, although the committee members enjoyed the power of electing their surgeon, they did not always trust him. 'They expect him to walk in their annual processions and they thank him for his services at club feasts, but individually they often complain [for] their consciousness that their medical contractor is underpaid makes the members naturally suspicious about the due fulfilment of the contract.'[20]

[15] Gloucester CRO, Gloucester. Letter from John Taunton, surgeon, to his uncle, James Hancock, Broad Campden, Glos., 16 Dec. 1801. Ref. 2857/2/7/24.

[16] The evidence of H. W. Rumsey, a Gloucester surgeon, to the *Select Committee on Medical Poor Relief*, PP 1844, IX, Q. 9072–9177, has been used extensively in this section. Rumsey was selected by the Provincial Medical and Surgical Association to represent their views as his knowledge of the subject was unusually extensive.

[17] Ibid., Q. 9080.

[18] Ibid., Q. 9088.

[19] Ibid., Q. 9078, and 112.

[20] Ibid., Q. 9086.

Nevertheless, many people joined sick clubs, although the proportion in a population depended on the nature of the occupations of the working classes. In 1830–40 the proportion of the population which belonged to sick clubs was between 8 and 10 per cent in Liverpool, Wolverhampton, Gloucester, Rotherham, Wakefield, Chester, Hull, and Southampton; in Stroud and Lincoln it was about 5 per cent and in Bath, Cheltenham, Shrewsbury, and Worcester about 3 per cent.[21] Clubs were of greatest importance in heavy industry areas such as mining communities where it was common for medical payments to be deducted from wages; for example, 1*d*. in the pound for accidents, 2*d*. in the pound for full medical attendance on the whole family.[22] Often whole communities were covered by what was in reality a system of compulsory insurance. In heavy-industry areas such as mining communities it was said that some surgeons derived a large income from this system and 'saw a great deal of very important surgical work'; but when wages were lowered or members unemployed the surgeon's salary was similarly affected.

In most sick clubs the members, conscious that unlike the parish poor they had paid for medical attendance, expected value for money and complained readily to the committee about their surgeons. Frequent complaints, subservience to the committees, and low pay, made the post of medical officer to a sick club understandably unpopular. Stratford-on-Avon, for example, had a large and active medical club with 2,600 members from 39 parishes. In 1842 60 per cent of the members received medical relief. The medical officers were paid £240, but, as there were '15 or 16' of them they averaged about £16 each per annum and had to find out of this the cost of medicines.[23] A practitioner put up with such payments and conditions only because it was a means of introduction to the families and friends of club members. It was a way of getting known.

Poyntz Adams, whose time as a medical student was mentioned in chapter 2, went into practice in (Chipping) Sodbury in Gloucestershire in February 1811. He felt optimistic because 'There is a club which I have no doubt but Mr Hetling will get me', Mr Hetling being a local and influential surgeon. A year later he wrote:

---

[21] Ibid., Q. 9087. Matthew Boulton in Birmingham and Josiah Wedgwood in N. Staffs. seem to have been amongst the first to introduce such schemes (personal communication, Dr Charles Webster).

[22] Ibid., Q. 9088.

[23] Ibid., Q. 9090.

I belong to a Friendly Society established in this town and after Whitsuntide next I expect to be the Surgeon which, from the number and respectability of many of them I consider as likely to afford me considerable benefits, more from the connections which it must necessarily create than the amount of the salary attached to the situation.

For Poyntz Adams as for so many of his contemporaries, becoming established was a hard, worrying time. At the end of his first year he had received £20 and was owed £110 in unpaid bills. But he himself owed £45 to his mentor Mr Hetling and £60 to his druggist.[24] The possibility of introductions to private practice was thus so urgent and important that he accepted a low salary from a club without a moment's hesitation.

Having considered all the potential sources of income available to general practitioners, in the next section we consider estimates of the total income of general practitioners in the first half of the nineteenth century.

The income of the general practitioner, 1820–50

It is not surprising that economic historians usually deal tentatively and briefly with medical incomes in the eighteenth and early nineteenth century. Data are not easily obtained, and quoted estimates are often based on the calculated average of all type of practitioner, although the range of incomes was so wide that such averages tend to be as informative as statements about the average speed of athletes or the average size of dogs. The exceptional incomes of celebrated London physicians and surgeons always attract attention. They have been mentioned in a previous chapter. No more need be said of them except to note the warning of J. F. Clarke that they were usually 'overrated'. He quotes Samuel Merriman who said bluntly: 'I do not believe in these enormous incomes.'[25] Merriman was at the top of the obstetric tree, but he never earned more than £4,000 in a year and was sure that Brodie never exceeded £13,000, Abernethy £10,000 or Liston £7,000. Nevertheless, the exceptional opportunities in London ensured that many physicians and hospital surgeons earned substantial fees, even if they seldom approached the level of the Abernethys. A good example was C. J. B. Williams, a successful but not a celebrated physician who succeeded Elliotson in 1834 as professor of Medicine at University College London

[24] Northamptonshire CRO, Northampton, Ref. ZA 6291.
[25] J. F. Clarke, *Autobiographical Recollections* (London, 1874) 115–16.

after Elliotson's contretemps with mesmerism.[26] Williams qualified (MD Edin.) in 1824, and had a hard time at the beginning. In 1830 he earned only £100 from practice. By 1842, however, he earned £1,043, and in 1848, £3,600. Teaching brought in about £400 p.a., the rest being private practice of a consultant kind which included travelling 100 miles or more from London to difficult cases.[27]

Consultation fees varied widely, from one to twenty guineas or more. Journeys were usually charged at a certain rate per mile. Sir Anthony Carlisle in 1806 charged a guinea a mile and 'for every day he might be detained at any place he should charge Ten guineas a day, or Seventy guineas a week.'[28] Walter Rivington in 1879 stated that the usual physician's fees were 3 guineas for the first visit and the mileage fee was two-thirds of the distance in guineas; thus 6 miles was charged 4 guineas.[29] Consultants, therefore, not only used a totally different system of medical fees from general practitioners, but a system that was much more flexible, allowing the increasingly successful to raise their fees substantially, and earn incomes well into the upper range of the upper middle classes.

What were the levels of middle-class incomes in the mid-nineteenth century? Musgrove suggests that incomes of over £1,000 were usually earned by the upper middle classes, men at the heads of their professions, the higher clergy, and successful merchants and manufacturers. Incomes of £200–£1,000 were found amongst the middle ranks of the middle classes, while incomes of £60 to £200 were earned by routine clerks, elementary schoolteachers, some skilled mechanics, bank clerks, etc.[30] For a way of life which included domestic servants, private education for the children, and the necessary standards of house, furniture, and dress, Musgrove suggested £200 p.a. as the minimum although the accounts of one London general practitioner in the mid-nineteenth century with moderate rather than excessive social ambitions suggests the minimum may have been closer to £400 p.a.[31]

General practitioners saw themselves as firmly established in the

[26] J. Miller, 'A Gower Street Scandal', *Journal of the Royal College of Physicians of London*, 17 (4) (1983), 181–91.

[27] C. J. B. Williams, *Memoirs of Life and Work* (London, 1884).

[28] James Greig (ed.), *The Farington Diaries, 1793–1821*, 8 vols. (London, 1922–8), iv. 35.

[29] W. Rivington, *The Medical Profession* (Dublin, 1879), 52.

[30] F. Musgrove, 'Middle-Class Education and Employment in the Nineteenth Century', *Economic History Review*, NS 12 (1959–60), 99–111.

[31] W. D. Foster, 'Dr William Henry Cook: The Finances of a Victorian General Practitioner', *Proceedings of the Royal Society of Medicine*, 66 (1973), 46–50.

centre of the middle classes. They would have regarded a gross income in the upper range of £200 to £1,000 as fair. In one respect, therefore, the physician Neil Arnott, although generally sympathetic to the cause of general practitioners, was out of touch when he suggested in 1834 that the general practitioner wished to be recognized as belonging to 'an honourable body, as the curate who receives £80 to £90 a year belongs to an honourable body and is satisfied with being marked as a gentleman so would the medical man be satisfied with a much smaller income on the same condition. Much of the reward in many cases would be the station which the profession gave in society.'[32] Arnott was right to emphasize the yearning of general practitioners for respectability and the belief of all the 'Dr Joblings' that it was owed to them. They took the College and Hall for that, and their place in society was determined by it.[33] But status and income, in all except a few occupations, were inseparable. To imply that respectability in medicine was obtainable at £80–£90 a year would have seemed sheer nonsense.

The wide range of incomes, even amongst general practitioners, permits only a few confident generalizations. Amongst these are the following. Real income levels of general practitioners in the mid-nineteenth century were generally lower than those of their predecessors in the late eighteenth century. From 1800 to 1850 it became increasingly difficult to become established in general practice, and income for the first few years was often very low indeed. Buying a partnership in a successful practice, or succeeding a father or uncle in a family practice, was the surest way to success; capital or family connections were much more advantageous than social or educational background, or higher medical qualifications. Country practice was generally poorly paid; higher incomes could only be achieved in towns and cities, the highest (and possibly the lowest as well) in London. The poverty of the general practitioner in Scotland was proverbial,[34] and Wales ran it a close second. In England, general practice in the Midlands and the South was usually more prosperous than in the North.

The poverty of country practice was stressed by John Dunn in 1818,[35]

[32] *SCME*, part I, Q. 2480: Neil Arnott, MD Aberdeen, LRCP London, well known for his work with Chadwick and Southwood Smith on fever in London.

[33] Charles Dickens, *Martin Chuzzlewit* (first published 1843–4), chapter 8.

[34] John Brown, 'Medical Reform', reprinted from the *Edinburgh Medical Journal* for December 1857 and published as a pamphlet. Royal Society of Medicine, Tract A7. For manuscript evidence of the low charges made by Scottish compared to English practitioners see the account books of James Steedman of Kinross, Wellcome MS 4702.

[35] J. Dunn, *London Medical Repository* (Jan.–June 1818), 234–6.

by others in later periods,[36] and most convincingly by the histories recorded by Richard Smith of a number of ex-pupils and apprentices at Bristol Infirmary who entered general practice in the 1820s and 1830s. Before 1850, it should be remembered, more than half the total population and more than half the general practitioners lived in rural areas. The general practitioner of the village or market town whose practice involved long journeys on his horse to cottages, farms, and villages was the rule rather than the exception. Many who entered practice in this period hovered for years between bare subsistence and bankruptcy. Some moved from place to place, driven out by competition. Valentine Webb, for example, failed to make a living in Bristol in 1825, or Bath in 1826, and moved to Maesteg in South Wales where he accepted a post as medical officer to a colliery at £50–£60 p.a. In 1836 he moved to Bibury and in 1837 to Cirencester. Failing in both he abandoned medicine as a career.[37]

James Monday, who, like Webb was a capable pupil at Bristol Infirmary, went to South Petherton in Somerset in 1820, but the competition was intense, he earned only £40 p.a., and he was squeezed out. In 1822 he paid £100 to the widow of a general practitioner in Olveston for the goodwill of the practice, and, sensibly, married her a year later.[38]

Charles Price settled in Congersbury *c.*1820 and died there in 1841. He was popular and busy, but in his first twelve years when he claimed to have delivered 3,000 midwifery cases, he averaged only £120 p.a.[39]

Some went to London after failing in the country and generally failed there too. Francis Dwyer[40] and William Seagram[41] were two such. James Pidding, the son of a clergyman, abandoned medicine in London to set up a lottery office in Charing Cross.[42] Several others, unable to make ends meet, came to grief through crime, bankruptcy, or drink.[43] Charles Perry, born in 1788, after teetering on the edge of bankruptcy for years, was finally appointed house surgeon to the Tunbridge Wells Infirmary and Dispensary at the age of forty-seven.[44] Often it seemed that only a hair's breadth separated success from failure.

[36] See, for example, the account of country practice in *LMG* 2 (1841–2), 918.
[37] BIBM 12. 384 and 434.
[38] Ibid., 12. 206.
[39] Ibid., 11, 416.
[40] Ibid., 11. 348.
[41] Ibid., 10. 644.
[42] Ibid., 6. 78.
[43] Examples being Harry Fry, BIBM 10. 42 and 82; Thomas Tutton, ibid., 10. 202; George Weaver, ibid., 9. 242; John Danvers, ibid., 6. 84.
[44] BIBM 8. 265.

Trevor Morris, the son of a sailmaker in Chepstow, obtained his MD in Edinburgh *c.*1820. He returned to his home town in 1830 although there were two surgeons there already as well as 'one in Monmouth and one in Usk who came into his beat.' But he prospered, earning a steady average of £400 p.a.[45]

Richard Edgell stayed in Bristol and struggled on. At the age of forty-two he was earning £380; then his luck turned. By the age of forty-seven he was earning £1,500 a year.[46] Thomas Wade Smith also prospered because he had the capital to buy a half-share in a partnership in Stroud worth £1,200 a year.[47] Edward Phillips settled in Pontypool and with two other practitioners they divided the Usk-Monmouth-Pontypool triangle between them, visiting the various towns on market days and charging 5*s.* for seven miles and midwifery at half a guinea; cheap by Bristol standards, but not in Monmouthshire and South Wales.[48]

John Charlton Yeatman was a member of a well-known Bristol medical family. His father had been an apothecary, and his uncle (a surgeon), finding that his son did not intend to become a practitioner, promised Yeatman that he could join him instead. Then the son changed his mind and there was no vacancy for Yeatman in Bristol who settled instead in Frome in Somerset in spite of the fact that the opposition in that town was especially strong. Against all odds, however, Yeatman prospered, adding to his income by taking pupils for a year as well as apprentices for the usual period; something which his medical neighbours considered an outrageous affectation. But Yeatman was an enterprising and vigorous practitioner who published some good papers (which have been quoted in this book) and he became 'Surgeon Extraordinary' to the Duke of Gloucester, to the fury of his colleagues no doubt.[49]

James Bedingfield left Bristol for Stowmarket, having published a *Compendium of Medical Practice* while apothecary to Bristol Infirmary from 1810 to 1815. He established a 'Medical Academy' in Stowmarket and became a noted local figure as well as a successful practitioner.[50] Teaching helped towards success. J. B. Estlin sought practice and notoriety, not altogether successfully, by establishing an eye dispensary in

[45] BIBM 9. 468.
[46] Ibid., 6. 350.
[47] Ibid., 11. 320.
[48] Ibid., 6. 564.
[49] Ibid., 8. 281.
[50] Ibid., 9.2.

Bristol.[51] But the easiest way to succeed modestly in the country as a writer, tongue in cheek, pointed out in 1834, was for the apprentice to marry the master's daughter and 'succeed to a practice of £150 p.a'.[52]

The most common income of general practitioners who achieved a fair degree of success between 1820 and 1850 seems to have been between £150 and £250 in the country and £300 to £500 in the larger towns. In 1851 the *Provincial Medical and Surgical Journal* republished from *The Times* a cameo of a country practitioner, 'Dr Camomile', who, 'by the most unceasing labour ... is earning £500–£600.' The writer 'gave him every possible advantage': surgeon to the union, medical officer to both the local grammar school and the 'ladies' establishment', and an exceptionally busy practice requiring one horse for the day, another for the night, amongst the clergy and the gentry in the district. It was considered that this practitioner would have to struggle to make ends meet.[53]

In 1841 the *Dublin Medical Press* carried an advertisement for a two-partner Liverpool practice in which it was claimed the receipts were £800 p.a. Partnership could be purchased from Patrick Kelly (MRCS 1837) for £400 cash.[54] The medical periodicals carried many warnings of fraudulent claims of a practice's prosperity, and the demand for cash raises suspicions in this and in similar advertisements. H. B. Thompson in his guide to parents in 1857 wrote confidently that London physicians earned from £800 to £3,000 p.a., and provincial or country physicians from £500 to £1,800: but he was conspicuously unhelpful on the average incomes of general practitioners except to say it was difficult to get started, and he warned against setting up a plate as a single-handed practitioner in a strange area.[55]

The relative sparsity of data on general practitioners' incomes raises the suspicion of an element of deliberate concealment. Income tax, imposed from 1799 to 1816 by Pitt (except during the peace from 1802–3) was reimposed by Peel in 1842 for incomes over £150, may have been the motive for reticence. The general practitioner came under Schedule D and could deduct all expenses incurred wholly in the course of his work. General practitioners were quick, possibly too quick, when their average incomes were mentioned, to say that they were far too

---

[51] BIBM 8. 315.

[52] *Medical Quarterly Review*, 2 (1834), 391–3.

[53] 'The Income Tax and its Oppressive Effects on General Practitioners' *PMSJ* 15 (1851), 111–12.

[54] *Dublin Medical Press*, 5 (1841), 80.

[55] H. B. Thompson, *The Choice of a Profession* (London, 1857).

high and that accusations against general practitioners of tax evasion were unjust.[56] Even in the country, general practitioners were sometimes at least as prosperous as physicians, earning well over £1,000 a year. John Leete of Thrapston in Northamptonshire has been quoted above.[57] Thomas Hodson, a general practitioner surgeon in Lewes until his death in 1842, made £2,000 a year at the height of his career.[58] He could, said the *Lancet*, have made five or six times that figure in London, but London was always different.

To become a fashionable West End practitioner in London, whether physician, surgeon, or apothecary/general practitioner, opened the way to enormous incomes. The wealth of 'Mahogany Fuller' (so called from the magnificent mahogany of his shop-front), an apothecary who, with his partner, 'doctored half the nobility in the West End' in the early part of the nineteenth century, was notorious.[59] Likewise, Robert Battiscombe was provided with exceptional opportunities by his appointment to the Royal Household from 1799, being 'Apothecary in Ordinary to His Majesty' from 1805, for which he received a retainer of £300 p.a. He also treated the Court, and although his notebooks do not reveal his annual income his exceptionally lavish way of living, more in the style of a country landowner than an apothecary, suggests that he prospered on an income probably measured in the thousands rather than hundreds.[60] R. R. Pennington was in his day the most celebrated of all London general practitioners, boasting an income of £10,000 a year and claiming he had treated every member of the Cabinet and every judge upon the Bench. Typically, this was not achieved by excessive charges, but by working to a manic extent. He was reputed to spend all day visiting his 'town patients' and, after a warm bath and some supper, he set out in a post-chaise to visit his country patients all night. He also insisted that his patients kept on indefinitely with their medicines and 'his dispensing department was a regular manufactory of physic'. Having acquired a fortune he sold his practice. He was a 'thorough man of business with no great acquirements' and active in medical

[56] 'Medical Incomes', *Medical Times*, 20 (1849), 13–14.

[57] Northamptonshire CRO, account books of John Leete of Thrapston, Leete VIII/7. In 1863 he 'booked' £1,800–£2,000; in 1864 he received £1,462. Such a discrepancy between 'business booked' and payment received was by no means uncommon, the difference often being from 1/4 to 1/3.

[58] 'Biographical Notice of the Late Mr Hodson', *Lancet* (1840–1), ii. 312–14.

[59] C. J. B. Williams (1884), 278.

[60] Dorset CRO, Dorchester, the notebooks of Robert Battiscombe, D293/F3.

politics throughout the whole of the period of medical reform.[61] He will be mentioned again briefly in chapter 13.

The account of a Victorian GP, Dr William Henry Cook, as well as being one of the most complete descriptions of the economics of general practice, underlines the main features we have discussed.[62] Cook set up in practice in over-doctored Tunbridge Wells (one practitioner to every 557 persons) in 1851. After three years his annual income was only £174. In 1856 he left, took his Edinburgh MD, thinking, incorrectly, that it would enhance his chances of practice considerably, and in 1859 settled in St John's Wood in London. His income after professional expenses in 1859 was £370, his household expenses, £430. By 1863 his income was £576 a year, £100 as union medical officer for Hampstead, £40 for attendance at the workhouse infirmary, £135 as public vaccinator, and the remainder from private practice. In 1874 he tried but apparently failed to obtain an appointment at a provident dispensary. Cook had qualified as an MRCS and LSA in 1847. His father was a naval officer. His wife, an excellent manager, came from a family of modest distinction which had included a surgeon and a Master of the Rolls. They had servants, a carriage, and a respectable house. Cook worked hard and took every step he could to supplement his income from private practice; but life was a continual struggle to make ends meet.

A Leeds practitioner in 1854 blamed the troubles of general practitioners on fair and unfair competition. The upper classes employed physicians at an annual salary and the lower classes employed the druggist. The middle classes also used the druggist and, although well able to pay private fees, belonged to clubs 'for $7\frac{1}{2}d$. per quarter'.[63] The general practitioner was therefore squeezed out, and his bills from private practice were often unpaid.

Complaints of bad debts and underpayment were endemic, not only in Britain but also in other countries. Usually overproduction of medical practitioners was held to be the cause. In the 1830s in Boston, USA, 'there are dozens of doctors who scarcely see a patient from Christmas time to Christmas time ... as a general rule there is not a broken bone apiece in a twelvemonth.'[64] In France in the 1840s most practitioners, it was said, were forced to follow a second occupation in order to

---

[61] J. F. Clarke (1874), 353–7.
[62] W. D. Foster (1973), see note 7.
[63] *Lancet* (1854), i. 458.
[64] George Rosen, 'Fees and Fee-Bills', supplement no. 6, *Bulletin of the History of Medicine* (1946).

survive.[65] We may suspect that grumbling was part of the routine of general practice, and temper our sympathy for the general practitioner. But it is difficult not to feel angry at the exploitation of medical assistants. The problems of the assistant became known when a series of letters were published in *The Lancet* from 1851. It was clear that the abuse was long-standing. Assistants were sometimes unqualified, sometimes qualified but just beginning their careers, and sometimes established practitioners who had fallen on difficult times. They were all treated in the same way.

Samuel Warren wrote in 1838 of outdoor assistantships in London where continuous work day and night was rewarded by an income of £80 p.a.[66] In 1851 an assistant complained that working as an assistant for a master 'with an extensive union practice' meant that the assistant did all the work amongst the 'paupers' (midwifery at night followed by 'a surgeryful of patients' each morning) as well as the dispensing. He was on call all day, every day, for £25–30 p.a.[67] Dr Spong of Faversham was unwise enough to reply that it was all good experience for young men, and practitioners could not afford a higher salary.[68] Another assistant ('experienta') replied that he was paid £30–£40 by a series of practitioners whose receipts amounted to £2,000, £1,200, £800, and £600 annually.[69]

Another assistant ('an Irish Anguis in Herba') wrote to say it was not only the low pay. He was a qualified practitioner, yet, as an assistant he was 'ordered by the lady of the house to leave the dinner-table with the cheese' and 'ordered by his *honourable* master to give no medicine to paupers', to 'send out all mixtures as draughts', to 'use the lancet but spare the leech', and to 'enter slight injuries as fractures to attract the poor law fee'.[70] Another assistant claimed that at one of his posts he was called out at night 'ninety times in seven months'.[71] Paltry salaries, it was said, were offered by 'your union and club doctors who ... think to get low midwifery and the dispensing portion of their business performed by someone who will consider board and lodging and a footman's stipend equivalents for services'.[72] A college or

---

[65] 'Poverty of Medical Men in France', misc. notes, *MCR*, NS 39 (1843), 207.
[66] Samuel Warren, *Passages from the Diary of a Late Physician* (Paris, 1838).
[67] *Lancet* (1851), i. 133.
[68] Ibid. (1851), i. 357.
[69] Ibid. (1851), ii. 404.
[70] Ibid. (1851), ii. 451.
[71] Ibid.
[72] Ibid. (1853), i. 528.

Table 30   *Scale of fees of an association of general practitioners*

For every mile travelled	1s. 6d.
For every attendance on a pauper	1s.
Ditto on a labourer, not a pauper	1s. 6d.
Ditto for a small tradesman	2s. 6d.
Ditty for a grade higher	3s. 6d.
Ditto first class [*sic*] within 3 miles	5s.
Ditto between 3 and 5 miles	7s. 6d.
Extraordinary attendance: at the rate per hr.	7s. 6d.
For first class over 5 miles	10s.

association of assistants was mooted, but there is no evidence of its existence.[73]

Associations of general practitioners, however, were common and are mentioned briefly in the next chapter. One of their activities was to devise scales of fees with a view to reducing the evils of 'under-cutting'. Several such scales were published; table 30 shows an abbreviated version of a typical scale.[74] Suggestions that a standard fee of either 5s. or 2s. 6d. to 3s. a visit should be charged, where made in the 1820s,[75] and a scale of fees closely resembling the above was published in the *Lancet* in 1830 by the Newcastle and Gateshead Association of General Practitioners of Medicine and Surgery.[76] But these scales represented an ideal rather than a realistic scheme to which all general practitioners would agree. Fees, in fact, were determined by custom and competition, and Peterson's work shows that the financial circumstances of the majority of general practitioners in London did not improve appreciably in the second half of the nineteenth century.[77] What was true of London was probably also true of the provinces in the late nineteenth century. What is remarkable is that most of the generalizations about the incomes of general practitioners which have been mentioned in this section, remained as true in the late nineteenth and early twentieth century as they were in the first half of the nineteenth century. For a substantial number, if not the majority, of general practitioners throughout the

[73] *Lancet* (1852), i. 114–15. amd (1853), i. 550–1.

[74] 'Ways and Means of General Practitioners', *PMSJ* 3 (1842), 166.

[75] 'Medical Jurisprudence', *MCR*, NS 2 (1825), 246–8.

[76] *Lancet* (1830–1), i. 536. There is evidence that similar scales of fees were current in America at an even earlier date, and that they were adhered to. See M. S. Blomberg, 'Medical Society: Regulation of Fees in Boston, 1780–1820', *J. of the History of Medicine and Allied Sciences*, 39 (1984), 303–38.

[77] M. Jeanne Peterson, *The Medical Profession in Mid-Victorian London* (1978), chapter 3.

nineteenth century, general practice was a hard, wearing, and poorly paid occupation; a fact which, as shown in the next chapter, was recognized by the public and the profession in the stereotype of the family doctor.

13

The General Practitioner as Family Doctor: Medical Societies and Associations

The physician, the general practitioner, and the provision of primary care

IN the first half of the nineteenth century general practice as a whole was thriving. Individually, general practitioners often complained bitterly of the difficulties of their profession. They complained about the expense of medical education, the difficulty of establishing a practice, poverty due to excessive competition of their too numerous colleagues, and the flourishing condition of the druggists and other irregulars; and they were sensitive to a fault about real or imagined slights from wealthy patients, or physician and surgeon colleagues who labelled them 'the subordinate grade'. Nevertheless, by the second quarter of the century they were firmly established, as an anonymous practitioner explained in 1850.

The Countess of A, or Mrs B the city millionaire's wife, has a physician for one complaint, a surgeon for another, a physician-accoucheur for a third; and an apothecary, probably, provides the medicines and attends the children and servants. But how is this possible for a person in ordinary circumstances? ... It is, therefore, absolutely necessary that, to supply the wants of the middle and lower classes in the metropolis and of nearly all ranks in the provincial towns and villages, there should exist a branch of the profession, the members of which must be competent to undertake the management of all diseases. Whether this branch of the profession do, or do not supply their patients with medicines is, in our opinion quite immaterial.[1]

---

[1] 'A Practitioner', *Is the Practice of Medicine in 1850 a Degenerate Pursuit?* (London, 1850). N. Parry and J. Parry in *The Rise of the Medical Profession* (London, 1976), 131, state that the Medical Act of 1858 'was the major landmark in the rise of the apothecary and the surgeon ... and their assimilation into a unified profession with the higher status physicians'. There is little to support this view, and the evidence of this and previous chapters shows clearly that the general practitioner regarded himself as a member of a unified medical profession well before 1858. Moreover, the Medical Act did no more for the general practitioner than confirm his status as a member of the medical profession, but also of a subordinate grade. See chapter 14, Postscript.

This seems to have been the majority view. Even those who despised the general practitioners as an inferior breed and a set of upstarts, were forced to concede that they dominated the practice of medicine. As we have seen, before 1850 consultant practice scarcely existed outside London and a few large centres.[2] Physicians, 'pure' surgeons, and general practitioners were all largely or wholly engaged in what is now called primary care. That is, most of their consultations were initiated by patients, not by other medical practitioners wanting a second opinion; and, as we have stressed more than once, this was especially true of the provinces. At a time when more than half the population of England still lived in rural areas, the provincial general practitioner had a virtual monopoly of medical care. What is more, the rise of the general practitioners led to a decline of the demand for the physician. This, which has often been overlooked, was noted in a review in 1822 in which, in the author's opinion, the physician was 'not of a very extensive utility or much in demand'.[3] Sir Benjamin Brodie held the same opinion, remarking in 1840 that physicians were much less in demand than formerly because of the rise of the general practitioner;[4] and the author of 'A Plea for Physicians', published in *Fraser's Town and Country Magazine* in 1848, maintained that 'towns in which three physicians formerly lived in comparative affluence cannot now give more than a miserable pittance to one … [their] average income does not exceed a couple of hundred pounds a year.'[5] Dr John Simpson of Bradford, a young physician, kept a diary in 1825 from which it is clear that he saw few patients and survived only because of private means. Indeed he wrote in February 1825 that

there are in Bradford three Physicians and ten Surgeons, besides most of the villages in the vicinity have one Surgeon and some of them two. I don't believe that there is full employment for more than one Physician and six Surgeons … We are surrounded by towns filled with Physicians and these at no great distance. Halifax is eight miles off where there are four Physicians, Wakefield fourteen miles and five Physicians, Skipton twenty miles and one Physician, Harrogate twenty miles and one Physician and also one at Knaresborough.

[2] By the mid-nineteenth century railway travel had enabled London consultants to extend their practice to the detriment of provincial ones. For example, see C. J. B. Williams, *Memoirs of Life and Work* (London, 1884).

[3] *London Medical Repository*, 16 (1822), 311–25.

[4] 'Medical Reform', *Quarterly Review*, 67 (1840), 68–9.

[5] 'A Plea for Physicians', *Fraser's Town and Country Magazine* (Mar. 1848), 286–98.

He thought that attorneys fared better because 'medical men are ill paid here and liable to numerous bad debts. If I had a son to bring up to a profession I certainly should make the choice of law.'[6] Even in large cities physicians found it hard to make a living. William Budd, who qualified MD (Edin.) in 1838, settled in Bristol in 1841 at the age of thirty. In spite of his considerable attainments, patients were few, his income 'a paltry three or four hundred pounds a year'. As he was unable to afford a horse and carriage, his feet were weary with tramping around the city. It was an exceptionally good week when he saw four new patients.[7] Likewise, Sir George Lefevre wrote that the young physician in London could expect to earn nothing in his first two years, and even then many were forced 'to put their diplomas in their pockets and go into the country to practice as an apothecary'.[8]

All this was exactly what Dr Barlow had forecast (see chapter 6) as early as 1813; namely that as the general practitioner rose, so the practice of the physician would diminish until eventually only a few in large urban centres would be needed. Moreover, there was no reason at this time to see the decline of the physician as only a temporary affair. Hospitals were not yet the dominant feature of medical practice, and few foresaw the change whereby specialization would be seen not only as inevitable but also as desirable. Physicians and their London College were a diminishing asset and were subject to a number of blistering attacks in the columns of the medical periodicals. The *Lancet* led the field, reflecting Wakley's passionate hatred of the teaching hospitals and the medical corporations. The *Gazette of Health* published a series of scurrilous attacks on the integrity of physicians, accusing them, amongst other things, of colluding with druggists and receiving 'haunches of venison' in return,[9] of pomposity and pretentiousness,[10] and of ignorance of their profession.[11] The *Medico-Chirurgical Review*[12] and the *London Medical Gazette*[13] joined in the attack. Few had a high opinion of the medical skills of physicians, who were advised to cultivate the social graces to obtain practice. To be successful they had to endure

---

[6] *The Journal of Dr John Simpson of Bradford* (City of Bradford Metropolitan Council, Local Studies Department, 1981).

[7] Library of the Wellcome Institute, London. The letters of William Budd (1841).

[8] Sir George Lefevre, *The Life of a Travelling Physician*, 3 vols. (London, 1843) i. 15–18.

[9] *Gazette of Health*, 4 (1815), 53–4.

[10] Ibid., 8 (1823), 571.

[11] Ibid., 5 (1820), 631.

[12] *MCR* 19 (1833), 567–9.

[13] *LMG* 6 (1830), 112–14.

'the tedium of the card tables and feline tameness of bowling',[14] and cultivate the social tricks of the trade which included not only keeping a carriage and being seen at the opera, but the need 'to keep company with all old women, midwives, nurses and apothecaries.'[15]

An intelligent observer of the profession in the 1840s would have guessed that surgery, which had made such enormous progress in the previous century, would continue to expand and recruit new members. Even so, a great deal of surgery was, and would continue to be, carried out by general practitioners. Looking at the physicians, however, and allowing for their role as the genteel attendants of the aristocracy, he could have been forgiven for suspecting they would dwindle in number.[16] Their great strength, however, was centuries of the tradition of seniority; they were the titular leaders of the profession. But this tradition had grown stale, and the Royal College of Physicians was largely to blame. It set the tone for the practice of physic. Even its warmest admirers (and Sir George Clark, historian of the College, was one) concede that during this period the College was apt to be stuffy, pompous, and backward-looking. The exclusive Fellowship, confined to graduates of Oxford and Cambridge and therefore to Anglicans, was only one of the reactionary features of the College; and it is significant that when a petition demanding a number of reforms was presented to the College in 1833, it was signed not by a group of young and impetuous radicals, but by senior and well-known physicians (most of them Edinburgh graduates), whose anger and shame at the College's reactionary attitudes came out in full force.[17] The attempt by the College to perpetuate an élite of men of good family background and 'liberal' education, who could dine and converse with the highest families in the land, was self-destructive not only for its blatant snobbery, but also because it placed more weight on social graces than on medical knowledge.

The decline of the physician and of the influence of the London College coincided with the nadir of medicine in the older universities. For example, in the twelve years from 1822 to 1834, Oxford produced only fifteen MDs and twenty-eight MBs. In the first thirty years of the

---

[14] H. B. Thompson, *The Choice of a Profession* (London, 1857), 162.

[15] Winslow Forbes, *Physic and Physicians*, 2 vols. (London, 1839), i, chapter 8.

[16] 'The mere physician is a character required principally for the higher ranks of society to uphold the dignity and literary reputation of the Profession ...', *London Medical Repository*, 16 (1822), 311–25.

[17] 'Petition of Physicians Practising in london', *MCR* 19 (1833), 567–9. See also 'Medical Reform', *Quarterly Review*, 67 (1840), 68–9.

nineteenth century lectures on the theory and the practice of physic, founded in Oxford by Dr Aldrich, were rarely given as there were not enough students. Even for the Doctorate of Medicine the candidate was only required to read six 'lectiones', and this had become so much a matter of form they were read to the sole audience of the 'bedel'.[18] It was largely Edinburgh and Glasgow, the source of well-trained physicians (and, as we have seen, of the vast majority of provincial physicians), that prevented the image of the physician from sinking even further than it did; a fact never acknowledged by the London College.[19]

What can be learnt from novelists about the public's perception of medical practitioners, and what is the value of such information? Too great a use of fiction can easily become a self-conscious literary exercise, and fiction has certain obvious limitations. Samuel Squire Sprigge, for example, was a stern critic of fictional medicine on several occasions, pointing out that 'Some of our very best novels contain bad medicine and some of the silliest, good medicine.'[20] His quarrel, however, was with descriptions of illnesses and diagnoses. When one is concerned with the character of medical practitioners and especially with what their patients thought of them, then fiction is undeniably a useful source. Not always, but generally, it is fair to assume that a novelist is writing from experience and reflecting the attitudes of his or her time. If one accepts this with due reservations, then the striking feature of practitioners in nineteenth-century fiction is the contrast between the adulation of the general practitioner as family doctor and the unsympathetic view of the physician, especially the celebrated London physician. There were, of course, exceptions. No one could deny that George Eliot's Dr Lydgate[21] and Trollope's Dr Thorne[22] are outstandingly perceptive and well-informed portraits; and both are almost wholly sympathetic. Both, however, were atypical. They were provincial physicians, and professionally they stood somewhere between the physician and the general practitioner. Dr Thorne dispensed medicines for

[18] Evidence of John Kidd, Regius Professor of Physic in the University of Oxford, *SCME*, part I, Q. 4434–4649.

[19] Between 1826 and 1835 Oxford and Cambridge produced annually about 15 MDs and MBs while Edinburgh and Glasgow produced 160 MDs and 104 surgical diplomas. The annual average of those taking the LSA was 383, *British Annals of Medicine*, 1 (1837), 122.

[20] Samuel Squire Sprigge, 'Medicine in Fiction', *Cornhill Magazine*, NS 31 (Dec. 1911), 822–33. Sir Samuel Squire Sprigge (1860–1937) was editor of the *Lancet* and wrote an oustanding biography of Wakley.

[21] George Eliot (Mary Ann Cross), *Middlemarch* (London, 1871–2).

[22] Anthony Trollope, *Dr. Thorne* (1858).

demanding his fee. His old-fashioned colleagues hated him for breaking the rules and for being successful in the process. They were examples of the 'new men' of medicine, impatient with the traditional attitudes associated with the London College. When Trollope wanted to portray the typical physician he drew Dr Lamda Mewdew, Dr Fillgrave, and Sir Omicron Pie, whose names alone tell all. In line with this, a now forgotten novelist, Amelia Edwards, created a memorable portrait of a famous physician, twin brother to Trollope's collection of pompous and greedy asses. He was described as 'a very stout and pompous gentleman who saw the patient for about ten minutes; offered no opinion one way or another, dined enormously, drank two bottles of port, slept in the best bedroom and went off next morning by early coach with a fee of fifty guineas in his pocket and an air of utmost condescension and unconcern'.[23] Perhaps the cruellest (and in some ways the most crude) picture of the nineteenth-century physician was Dickens's Dr Parker Peps in *Dombey and Son*, the society physician-accoucheur in front of whom the family doctor grovels as he is treated to a display of appallingly snobbish name-dropping by the senior member of his profession.[24]

It would be surprising if such virulence had not produced some sort of backlash. In 1866 Mrs Gascoigne wrote a novel in which the main character, a London physician, was every inch the perfect doctor, invariably polite, well-dressed, elegant, kind, and clever, and given to treating the poor gratis. He was also, of course, successful, kept a carriage and pair, and was driven by a coachman. The most interesting feature of this rather dull saint is that the author made him the son of a very ancient family, who was originally destined for the Church. When he took up medicine instead, his family cast him out and never forgave him.[25] So much, in her opinion, for the equality of the professions.

In general, however, the physician seems to have been an unpopular figure, and this, together with the contrast with the good old family doctor, can not fail to arouse our curiosity about the image of the mid-nineteenth century practitioner, and the ideal demanded by the public; this image, of course, had a profound bearing on the outcome of the competition for patients; for, as emphasized in chapter 10, the physician, surgeon, and general practitioner competed with each other not in just

[23] Amelia Edwards, *Barbara's History*, 2 vols. (London, 1864), i. 114.
[24] Charles Dickens, *Dombey and Son* (1846–7).
[25] Mrs Gascoigne, *Dr. Harold*, 3 vols. (London, 1866).

exactly the same markets for medical care, but certainly in closely overlapping ones.

The market for medical care

Rivington in his essay, *The Medical Profession*,[26] described the variety of general practitioners that existed in his lifetime. At the lowest end of the scale were those who kept open shop and sold articles of toilet as well as medicines; at the upper end the non-dispensing general practitioner merged imperceptibly with the physician. Yet, in spite of the imperceptible merging, a great deal was made within the profession of the differences between the ranks. The differences, however, were based on points of professional etiquette and traditions of practice; such matters, for example, as whether medicine should be prescribed or dispensed, how fees should be charged and received and, of course, the possession of a university degree. The public, however, seldom knew or cared about such matters except in so far as they might affect cost or convenience. University degrees and the extent to which they varied in prestige did not impress them. How could the public assess the merits of an LSA or an MRCS against an MD obtained from Edinburgh, Aberdeen, or a continental university, or a medical qualification from Dublin? They might be weighty matters amongst medical men, but they were not criteria on which the choice of doctor was based. The straightforward competition for patients between the general practitioner and the physician, much greater than is usually allowed, was profoundly affected by two considerations in the front of the minds of medical practitioners; and the two often came into conflict. First, there was the need to attract patients in order to survive; secondly, there was the need to follow the traditional codes of behaviour in order to perpetuate the higher status of the physician. This conflict can be illustrated by imagining that the physicians and their London College, instead of remaining aloof and restrictive, had abandoned traditional attitudes and taken to dispensing medicines, bleeding their patients, and adopting obstetrics as an integral part of the practice of physic. They could have argued, tit-for-tat, that surgeons and general practitioners were increasingly trespassing on the practice of physic, so why not reciprocate? Had they done so, the physician would have been a general practitioner; but he would have been a *graduate* practitioner and, as

---

[26] W. Rivington, *The Medical Profession* (Dublin, 1879).

such, could well have captured the great mass of the middle-class market. Meanwhile the non-graduate LSA, with the label 'apothecary' rusting round his neck, might well have ended up simply as the grossly underpaid doctor for the poor. Of course this is only speculation; but it is speculation with a purpose. If we wish to understand the forces that shaped the development of the medical profession in the nineteenth century it is not sufficient to look for them solely in terms of the growth of medical education, medical registration, the development of the hospitals, and the growing importance of medical science and laboratory medicine. All these were, of course, important, but they were factors which were superimposed (for the most part) in the second half of the century on a structure built in the first; and the latter arose primarily from the struggle for patients and the struggle for rank and position in a changing profession and a changing society. These struggles had little to do with scientific advances and the medical care of the population, but they had a great deal to do with the ideals of class and social position, and the growth of gentility. They were symbolized by a word (now debased) which appears again and again in speeches, articles, and letters from general practitioners about their aspirations—'respectability'. General practitioners yearned as much for the accolade of respectability as they did for prosperity; and they were perceptive enough to appreciate they could never have one without the other.

Perkin has argued that in English society between 1780 and 1880, the origins of class were associated with what he described as a struggle for ideals.[27] These ideals, which shaped the class consciousness and class structure of society, occurred in three main groups: the aristocratic, the entrepreneurial, and the working-class ideals; on all three market forces had a profound influence. Beyond these, however, was the non-capitalist, professional, middle-class ideal, usually seen just as a part of the middle-class values 'tout court'. But, Perkin argues, the professions were different in their relative immunity from the effects of market forces. The Church, the law, and medicine were the prominent examples, and Perkin instanced the clergy whose 'living' was a guaranteed income provided by the laity for the performance of their office. There is no denying the validity of the argument with respect to the Church, but it may be suggested that the Church and medicine were different. It is true that medical care was not a commodity like corn or coal, subject to unpredictable fluctuations in price or overseas compe-

[27] H. Perkin, *The Origins of Modern English Society, 1780–1880* (London, paperback ed., 1972).

tition. Medicine was, nevertheless, profoundly affected by market forces within a broad market embracing all classes. As we have seen, a substantial part of that market was satisfied by the dispensing druggists, and an unmeasurable but probably smaller market by the irregulars; both operated primarily in the poorer end of the market. At the other end, the wealthy and the aristocracy on some occasions stuck firmly to the celebrated physicians and surgeons, paying high fees. But the middle ground was occupied fairly and squarely by the general practitioner, and it was a ground embracing more than is usually understood by definitions of the middle classes, since it ranged from domestic servants and labourers to the minor gentry and professional people. For these, the general practitioner had become, by the second third of the nineteenth century, the family doctor in effect and even in name. Why was he chosen so firmly? If that question could be answered, it would tell us something about the medical profession from the patients' point of view. It is unlikely, of course, that the public as a whole had a single coherent ideal for their family medical attendant; but a surprising degree of coherence emerges from the general practitioner of fiction. It is not an exaggeration to say that the family doctor became a fictional stereotype, like the dashing hussar, the flowery romantic poet, and the pale but interesting young curate. No one takes these stereotypes as literal descriptions of reality, but all are revealing; and if a stereotype contains an element of flattery, there is an inevitable tendency for reality to model itself on fiction.

The origin of the family doctor[28]

Probably the main consideration in preferring the general practitioner was cost. Medicine in the late eighteenth century had, with reason, the reputation of being expensive. The growth of the dispensing druggist, as we have seen, was due to the lowness of his prices. The regular medical attendant, therefore, had to be inexpensive. In addition, however, great weight seems to have been given to a family doctor who was familiar, friendly, and able to deal with all except a few rare medical occasions. In addition, the all-purpose general practitioner should not be too young. He was, in fact, allowed to be old or even ancient provided he was the familiar figure who had attended successive generations of the families in his area. Mr Grimes of 'Grundy's Green' in a novel

[28] The characteristics and consequences of the concept of the family doctor described in this section have been explored in greater detail in I. Loudon, 'The Concept of the Family Doctor', *Bulletin of the History of Medicine*, 58 (1984), 347–62.

published in 1852, was presented as a typical old-fashioned family doctor.[29] He was valued because he had 'brought scores of matrons safely through their confinements, vaccinated hundreds of infants, drawn countless teeth, and physicked, cupped, bled, blistered and clystered generations upon generations'. Likewise, Mr Hall in *Wives and Daughters* was old, blind, and deaf, but 'he was still Mr Hall, the doctor who could heal all their ailments'.[30] The point was emphasized in an article entitled 'Hints for choosing a Doctor' (1832) where the reader was advised 'Let not your doctor be too youthful ... and avoid the man whose dress and demeanour indicate puppyism.'[31] Not surprisingly, a family doctor was popular simply for being a bit old-fashioned in his ways. Mr Mellidew in *Paid in Full* (1864–5) 'was a rising man in his little way. He was old-fashioned though a youngish man and prescribed very much the same remedies which his late employer ... had been in the habit of prescribing.'[32] In the same way he was expected to be a bit shabby. 'Be not averse to him if he is slovenly in his apparel.'[33] Indeed, 'Mr Mellidew wore a cheap·heavy hat which was brown from many showers and always carried a stethoscope. He enclosed his feet in clumsy half-wellingtons which were patched and mended until they lost all semblance of their original shape ... There was generally a button missing from his waistcoat, and an obtrusive pin or two visible here and there about his garments.'[34] This was not a flattering image for a man who was 'compelled to unite the acquirements of a physician with those of a surgeon. Impossible to be more highly educated, impossible to be worse remunerated ... He may enjoy the confidence of his patients; he may possibly be admitted to the tables of the higher classes in the neighbourhood, but his family holds an uncertain and slippery position ... No gentleman ought to enter the profession.'[35]

He might be poor, shabby, and old-fashioned, but the family doctor was expected to be able to deal with every medical emergency at any time of the day or night. In a memorable novel called *A Doctor of the Old School*, published in 1895, the Scottish hero Dr Maclure of

[29] John Mills, *The Belle of the Village* (London, 1852).

[30] Elizabeth Gaskell, *Wives and Daughters* (first published 1862, paperback edn., Penguin Books, 1969).

[31] 'Hints on Choosing a Doctor', *Doctor: A Penny Magazine*, 1 (1832), 309–10.

[32] Henry James Byron, 'Paid in Full', *Temple Bar Magazine*, 13 (1864–5), 246–7.

[33] 'Hints on Choosing a Doctor' (1832).

[34] H. J. Byron (1864–5).

[35] Ellen Wallace, *Mr Warenne, the Medical Practitioner: A novel*, 3 vols. (London, 1848), i, chapter 1.

Drumtochty had all of these qualities and was adored throughout the glen.[36] He resembled Mr Gregory, the 'principal Hilltown practitioner', in *Loved at Last* (1864) who 'bore with noble courage and patient bearing ... broken rest ... long rides through darkness, rain, snow and searching winds' as he exercised 'a skill and knowledge acquired by years of study and acute observation'.[37] On top of all this, the family doctor was expected to sit at the bedside through long and tedious labours, and to listen patiently to matters of doubtful medical importance. Some would say that the essence of the family doctor was his combination of a clinical and a pastoral role, a combination which was implicitly recognized in 1831 by the practitioner who wrote that '[a practitioner] has often to soothe and satisfy where no disease exists' and to advise 'on phenomena little subject to medical treatment'.[38]

In an acid account of the medical profession in Birmingham, written in 1863, which must have made the doctors blush, the writer singled out the family doctor as an exception: 'I know that the family doctor is deservedly esteemed. I know when the father is stricken with fever, or the mother is in danger, or the child is dying, with what anxious suspense his footfall is listened for, how piteously his face is scanned. I know what consolation there is in his kindly assurance, what comfort in his smile.'[39]

The concept of the family doctor was, and continues to be, highly valued by the public because it combines a broad clinical approach with continuity of care and, for want of a better term, a pastoral role.[40] General practitioners in the first half of the nineteenth century were divided on the question of whether they were to be non-graduate

[36] Ian Maclaren, *A Doctor of the Old School* (London, 1895). The author John Watson was a Presbyterian minister at Sefton Park, Liverpool, who wrote fiction under a pen-name.
[37] Mark Lemon, *Loved At Last*, 3 vols. (London, 1864), i. 8.
[38] W. Cooke, *Separation Without Dissension* (London, 1831).
[39] 'Scrutator', *The Medical Charities of Birmingham* (Birmingham, 1863), 36.
[40] Ann Cartwright in 1967 referred to the family doctor as 'one of the sacred cows of general practice which no one except McKeown had dared to criticise', in *Patients and their Doctors* (London, 1967). The recurrent myth that the old type of family doctor, like hot summers, is a thing of the past, can be traced back at least to the 1850s. That the myth is resuscitated at regular intervals is a tribute to the strength and longevity of the concept rather than evidence of decline. See John Brown, *Rab and His Friends and Other Essays* (1858–61), introduction; J. F. Clarke, *Autobiographical Recollections* (London, 1874), 66; Lindsey W. Batten, 'The Medical Adviser', the James Mckenzie lecture of the Royal College of General Practitioners for 1960, *Practitioner*, 186 (1961), 102–12. All deal with the anxiety concerning the imminent disappearance of the old type of family doctor.

physicians or 'physicians-in-ordinary', surgeons, or successors to the apothecary bent on maximizing profits through the sale of medicines. The role of the family doctor had the merit of providing general practitioners with a new identity which did not carry the stigma of being inferior versions of the physician and surgeon. It can, of course, be argued that all the characteristics of the family doctor must have been present to some degree in the medical practitioners of villages and small towns in the eighteenth century. Richard Kay was, in practice though not in name, an ideal family doctor. What was new from about 1830 onwards was the increasing and open recognition by the public and by the profession that the role of the general practitioner should be defined in terms of the ideal of the family doctor. It was an ideal that provided more than patient satisfaction; it conferred on the general practitioner clinical advantages over the physicians and surgeons in their role as consultants.

Professor Thomson of London University (who, as a general practitioner was active in the foundation of the Association of Apothecaries and Surgeon Apothecaries) spoke in 1836 in glowing terms of the replacement of the old, narrow, apothecary by the new general practitioner. The new general practitioners, he said, whose 'genius, observation and industry have advanced the practical side of medicine in a remarkable degree' were now as well educated as the physicians with the added advantage of a surgical training. Their greatest asset, however, was their intimate knowledge of 'the hereditary constitutions, habits, and temperaments of their patients'.[41] Public demand was more important than professional initiative in creating the family doctor. Unfortunately the stereotype of the family doctor has suffered on numerous occasions from an excess of sentimentality in the memoirs and after-dinner speeches of doctors, in novels, and in plays and serials on radio and television. This may have deterred historians from giving it the attention it deserves. In practice the ideal of the family doctor is a demanding one, but it is and has been an ideal of enormous power in shaping the nature of medical practice in Britain. The general practitioner of the nineteenth century ignored it at his peril. Those who set out determinedly to be no more than impassive clinicians and hard-headed businessmen, however efficient in these roles, were likely to fail. The concept of the family doctor, moreover, strengthened the sense of

[41] A. T. Thomson, 'Lecture at London University', *Lancet* (1836–7), i. 77.

corporate identity amongst general practitioners which found expression in the growth of medical societies and associations.

Medical societies and associations

Groups of medical men often met regularly during the late eighteenth century and formed societies. Some were famous, but many were informal societies meeting, for instance, at an inn to eat and drink, exchange ideas on their cases, argue about fees, and sometimes to set up small medical libraries. Some examples were given in chapter 5; probably many small provincial medical societies were ephemeral and faded away leaving no trace. But there was a remarkable proliferation of medical societies and associations in the first half of the nineteenth cetury, and the medical associations founded after 1812 were, for the most part, quite different, meeting for medico-political purposes. The Association of Apothecaries and Surgeon Apothecaries, established in 1812, was perhaps the most important (see chapter 7). Others, though mostly ephemeral, are historically important as evidence of the climate of medical opinion. For example, in the enthusiasm generated by the celebratory dinner following the case of Handey *v.* Henson (chapter 12), the Metropolitan Society of General Practitioners was established in 1830 and took rooms at 4 Regent Street. Its primary purpose was to set up a protection fund and a benevolent fund and to improve the state of general practice 'by altering existing laws'. It also intended to encourage social intercourse between general practitioners. The society was widely reported in the medical press. Predictably it was welcomed by the *Gazette of Health*,[42] the shabby but loyal friend of the general practitioner, and scorned by the *Lancet* because of Wakley's hatred of the term 'general practitioner'.[43]

Wakley himself attempted to form a new medical institution in 1830 calling it the London College of Medicine. The attempt was a product of Wakley's anger at being ejected forcibly at the Royal College of Surgeons when he attempted to disrupt one of the meetings of Council. The avowed purpose of the College was 'A new medical college founded upon the most enlarged and liberal principles and in which all legally qualified practitioners, whether physicians, surgeons or apothecaries will be associated upon equal terms, will enjoy equal rights and will be recognised by the same title.'[44] Joseph Hume was persuaded to chair

---

[42] *Gazette of Health*, 15 (1830), 15.
[43] *Lancet* (1829–30), i. 807; (1829–30), ii. 451, 652, 690.
[44] Ibid. (1830–1), i. 797.

the first meeting at which it was estimated that 1,300 'members of the profession and other gentlemen' attended.[45] Offices were opened at 9 Lancaster Place, The Strand.[46] Although it was Wakley's intention that the College would ultimately become a teaching establishment, it had to be content throughout its short life with issuing diplomas of fellowship for a fee. The diplomas, large and ostentatious, must now be quite rare objects, although many were provided. One which still exists was purchased in 1834 by Daniel Gingell (MRCS 1834, LSA 1834, and MD St Andrews) who, after service in the East India Company settled in Brecon as a general practitioner.[47] It is uncertain when Wakley abandoned his College, but it probably lasted about two years. It was an ill-conceived if high-minded project and never had a chance of achieving its major object—the abolition of ranks and distinctions in the medical profession.

Wakley, however, supported the establishment of the first British Medical Association in 1836 (not to be confused with the present one) and even suggested its name; and he supported it chiefly because he disliked the Provincial Medical and Surgical Association which, being provincial in origin, he was certain would fail.[48] This British Medical Association was founded by Dr George Webster (MRCS Edin. 1815, MD Edin. 1829) who was a general practitioner in Dulwich, and to avoid the confusion his association should be named Webster's Medical Association.[49] Its purpose was political in that it intended to instigate legislation to improve the state of general practice.

Much the most successful of all the medical associations of this kind was the Provincial Medical and Surgical Association founded by Charles Hastings (MD Edin. 1818), a Worcester physician, in 1832. It became the British Medical Association in 1855, the name having lapsed with the dissolution of Webster's association in 1845. The strength of the Provincial Medical and Surgical Association (PMSA) lay in three features. First it was a provincial initiative, and, in spite of Wakley's

[45] *Lancet* (1830–1), i, 821.

[46] Ibid. (1830–1), ii. 52, 178–83, 212–22, 248, 376, 822, and (1831–2), i. 456–7.

[47] Gloucestershire CRO, Gloucester, D 4018, F 14.

[48] *Lancet* (1836–7), i. 173: 'The Provincial Medical and Surgical Association under the auspices of a little knot of MDs and such insignificant personages as Mr Something Crosse of Norwich … its complete fall cannot be protracted to a distant period.' John Greene Crosse was anything but insignificant.

[49] *BFMR* 3 (1837), 289–90. 'H. S.' from Leighton Buzzard recommended support of the Association because the general practitioner suffered from the absence of 'a union', whereas physicians and surgeons congregated at hospitals because 'where the carcass is, there will the eagles be gathered together'. *Lancet* (1836–7), i. 363.

conviction that nothing which started in the provinces could ever succeed, it rapidly became a national success. Secondly, it attracted and admitted to its offices surgeons, physicians, and general practitioners on a basis of equality. Thirdly, it became an association which combined both scientific and political objectives. In fact, until the growth of postgraduate education in the second half of this century, it was almost the sole provider of postgraduate instruction for the mass of medical practitioners in Britain. The *Midland Medical and Surgical Reporter* (1828–32) was taken over as the *Transactions of the Provincial Medical and Surgical Association* (1833–53), and the transactions were mainly devoted to the publication of scientific papers. The *Provincial Medical and Surgical Journal* was established in 1840 and, incorporating the *London Journal of Medicine* in 1852, became the *Association Medical Journal* in 1853 and the *British Medical Journal* in 1857.[50]

Other and independent provincial medical associations were also established. For example, the North of England Medical Association, founded in Newcastle in November 1849, was 'forced into existence by the profound conviction, almost universal amongst medical men, of the necessity of an important change in the general economy and government of our profession'.[51] One of its self-appointed tasks was to draw up a scale of fees.[52] In Manchester a Medical Reform Committee was founded in the 1840s,[53] and local associations were founded, among other places, at Glasgow, Gloucester, South Devon, Cornwall, Taunton, and Nottingham.[54] A comprehensive history of medical societies and associations in the nineteenth century has yet to be written. Other more specialized societies played an important part in the diffusion of medical knowledge rather than the politics of the profession, such as the Society of Physicians of the United Kingdom,[55] established in 1824 to encourage the publication of scientific papers and books. It excluded anyone practising surgery, pharmacy, or midwifery.[56] The Obstetrical Society of London, established in 1825, faded out and was re-established in 1859 when it made important contributions to the science of obstetrics and gynaecology and had some influence on the teaching and examination

---

[50] W. R. LeFanu, *British Periodicals of Medicine, 1640–1899*, revised ed. (Oxford, 1984).
[51] 'Medical Reform', *BFMR* 9 (1840), 290.
[52] *Lancet* (1830–1), i. 536.
[53] *PMSJ* 9 (1845), 156–8.
[54] E. M. Little, *History of the British Medical Association, 1832–1932* (BMA, London, reissue, no date).
[55] *BFMR* 3 (1837), 290.
[56] *LMPJ* 52 (1824), 179–81.

Table 31   *The National Association of General Practitioners and the attempt to establish a College of General Practitioners: a chronological table*

Aug.	1840	The first Bill (Wakley and Warburton) for the regulation of the medical profession.
Sept.	1843	Charter of the Royal College of Surgeons in which the Fellowship of the College was introduced.
Dec. 7	1844	Meeting in Hanover Square at which The National Association of General Practitioners was founded.
Feb.	1845	The National Association petitions Sir James Graham, the Home Secretary.
Apr.	1845	Formation of the joint deputation by the Society of Apothecaries and the National Association of General Practitioners.
May	1845	Sir James Graham's Bill for the regulation of the medical profession was introduced, but dropped in July.
Feb.	1846	Sir James Graham refused to have any more to do with the plan for the incorporation of general practitioners.
May	1846	The National Institute of Medicine, Surgery, and Midwifery was established.
June	1846	Sir George Grey replaced Sir James Graham as Home Secretary.
Apr.	1847	Wakley introduced another Bill for medical reform resulting in the Select Committee on Medical Registration (1847 and 1847–8).
Aug.	1847	Council of the National Institute was established and Sir George Grey approached.
Jan. and Feb.	1848	A joint conference was held by the three medical corporations and the National Institute of Medicine, Surgery, and Midwifery. Agreement was reached but the Council of the College of Surgeons rejected the agreement.
July	1850	Mr Wyld introduced a Bill (the third attempt) for the incorporation of general practitioners, but no more was heard of it.
Nov. 19	1952	The present Royal College of General Practitioners was established as the College of General Practitioners; incorporated under the Companies Act of 1948 in 1961; allowed to use the prefix 'Royal' in May 1967, and granted a Royal Charter in 1972.

of students in obstetrics. These and similar associations, however, lie outside the scope of this book. The final association of importance in the development of general practice needs to be considered in some detail and forms the subject of the next section.

The attempt to establish a College of General Practitioners

Although the attempt to establish a separate college ended in failure, the events which took place in the attempt are important indicators of the power of the medical corporations and the medical press, the status of general practice, and the relationship between the State and the medical profession (see table 31).[57]

The first hint of the need for a separate institution devoted to general practice appears in the early proceedings of the Association of Apothecaries and Surgeon Apothecaries in 1812, where it was referred to as 'a fourth body', the other three, of course, being the Colleges of Physicians and Surgeons and the Society of Apothecaries. The idea was dropped, however, after opposition from the College of Physicians and lay dormant. There was no question of the Society of Apothecaries being able to fill the role; it was neither willing nor able, being content to administer the examination for the LSA (efficiently) and the penal clauses of the Apothecaries Act (reluctantly and inefficiently). General practitioners therefore pinned their hopes on the College of Surgeons accepting them as surgeons with full representation, although the College did nothing to encourage such a plan. When the College introduced its new charter in 1843, by which it became the Royal College of Surgeons of England instead of London—a logical opportunity for opening its doors to general practitioners if it was ever going to—general practitioners at last realized that they were to be permanently excluded. The new charter introduced the higher grade of Fellowship as the mark of the surgical specialist but the ordinary membership was left exactly where it always had been—excluded from any part in the running of the College and without the right to vote.

This creation of two divisions in the College was not the only source of annoyance to the general practitioner membership; what really infuriated them was the way in which a large number of honorary Fellowships were granted with the introduction of the new charter.[58]

[57] The main sources on which this chapter is based are as follows: *The Transactions of the National Association of General Practitioners* (1845–6), the most important parts of which are summarized in *Three reports by the joint deputation of the Society of Apothecaries and the National Association of General Practitioners* (London, 1846), and also in *An address by the Society of Apothecaries to the General Practitioners of England and Wales on the second report of the joint deputation* (London, 1845); *SCMR*, PP 1847, IX, and PP 1847–8, XV. Minutes of Council of the Royal College of Surgeons of England, for 1843–9, at the Royal College of Surgeons' Library, Lincoln's Inn, London; and certain periodicals, particularly the *Lancet*, and *Provincial Medical and Surgical Journal*, the *London Medical Gazette*, and the *Medico-Chirurgical Review*. See also Arvel B. Erickson, 'An Early Attempt at Medical Reform in England, 1844–5', *J. Hist. of Medicine*, 5 (1950), 144–55; and I. Waddington, *The Medical Profession in the Industrial Revolution* (1985).

[58] Three hundred honorary Fellowships were awarded. The list of recipients and details of the new charter can be found in *BFMR* 17 (1844), 279–85. In the immediate years following the honorary Fellowships, those who had passed the FRCS by examination generally wrote 'FRCS (by exam.)' after their names to dissociate themselves from the suspicions surrounding the honorary awards.

Most were awarded to men of some fame, but in some cases the choice of recipient seemed quite arbitrary, and it was suspected that this had been done to 'buy off' those who complained of their exclusion from the franchise. *The Medico-Chirurgical Review* remarked:

> The principle which has been followed in the selection [of Fellows of the College] is not to be discovered; for, although eminent names are necessarily included, others of not the slightest note are there to be found ... the governing powers of the *College of Surgeons* have come into an unfortunate, and what must be considered an alarming, collision with the great body of its members, just at the very period when unanimity and confidence are most required.[59]

Rejection by the College of Surgeons brought to a head the feeling amongst general practitioners that they were isolated from the centres of power in the profession. They alone, they said, had 'no head, no body', no college, hall, nor institution devoted to their interests.[60] This sense of isolation led to the establishment of the National Association of General Practitioners at a meeting held on 7 December 1844, called on the initiative of sixty-two general practitioners from the City of London and Marylebone. Seven hundred medical men attended including a large number from the provinces. It was decided that 'prior to the passing of any Bill for the regulation of the practice of medicine and surgery ... the general practitioners of medicine, surgery and midwifery should be legally recognised'.[61] By January 1845 a thousand members had enrolled in the National Association of General Practitioners of Medicine, Surgery, and Midwifery to give it its first official title; by April 1845 the membership had grown to about 4,000 members out of a total of about 14,000 general practitioners in England and Wales, and new members were joining at the rate of thirty to forty a day.[62] It was 'a larger number of medical practitioners than has ever previously combined for purposes of mutual protection'.[63]

The President of the National Association, Robert Rainey Pennington (1764–1849; MRCS 1787, Hon. FRCS 1843), was eighty years old when elected and claimed to be the oldest living member of the Royal College of Surgeons. He was familiar with the world of medical politics, having been active during the period 1812–15 when he was already

---

[59] *MCR*, NS I (1845), 285–6.
[60] *Lancet* (1842–3), i. 722; *PMSJ* 11 (1847), 76; *SCMR*, Q. 934–5.
[61] Evidence of James Bird in *SCMR*, Q. 934.
[62] *BFMR* 19 (1845), 614–15; and *Transactions of the National Association* for March 1845.
[63] *Address by the Society of Apothecaries* (1845), 5.

in his fifties. The Association was served by two honorary secretaries, James Bird (LSA 1821, MRCS 1825) Fellow of the Medico-Chirurgical Society, and Henry Ancell (LSA 1828, MRCS 1831) surgeon to the Western Dispensary and lecturer in medical jurisprudence at the medical school adjoining St George's Hospital. The Council of the Association were mainly London practitioners, many of whom were members of London medical societies including the Westminster Medical Society, the Royal Medico-Chirurgical Society, the Hunterian Society, and the London Medical Society. Dr Webster of Dulwich, the founder of the first British Medical Association, joined the National Association, bringing his members with him.

From the beginning the central purpose of the National Association was to petition Parliament for the incorporation of general practitioners into a college.[64] With this in mind the Home Secretary Sir James Graham was approached, and Sir James raised two possible objections when he understood that general practitioners wished to control their own medical education. First he wanted to be assured provincial practitioners held the same views as the London ones. The secretaries were able to reassure him on this after circulating a questionnaire to provincial medical associations. The Home Secretary's second objection consisted of a refusal to treat with the National Association alone, even if they were representative of general practitioner opinion as a whole. The plan for incorporation implied the repeal of the Apothecaries Act of 1815, and if they objected the Society of Apothecaries would have the power to veto the proposal. The Society reassured the Home Secretary that they were willing to relinquish their powers under the 1815 Act provided that a satisfactory alternative could be guaranteed. Indeed, they offered to form, together with the National Association, a joint deputation to deal with the whole business of incorporation.[65] This was agreed, and the deputation consisted of R. R. Pennington, James Bird,

---

[64] The earliest suggestions were for a college of general practitioners and not a royal college, see *Lancet* (1844), ii. 164, and report of the Act of Parliament Committee of the Society of Apothecaries for 15 Nov. 1844 (Guildhall MS 8212). However, by the spring of 1845 it was clear that opinion had come round to applying to the Crown for a royal charter, possibly in order to be closer in status to the other medical colleges. Other titles suggested for the College of General Practitioners were: the Institute of Medicine, the Faculty of Medicine, the Royal College of Medicine and Surgery of England, the Royal College of Physic Surgery and Midwifery, the College of Medicine and Surgery, the Royal National College of General Practitioners in Medicine and Surgery, the Royal College of Licentiates in Medicine and Surgery, the Royal College of Doctors, and the Medico-Chirurgical College. *Transactions of the National Association*, 2 June 1845.

[65] *Address by the Society of Apothecaries* (1845), 6, 7.

and Henry Ancell (the President and two secretaries of the National Association), and John Bacot and John Ridout as the representatives of the Society of Apothecaries. Robert B. Upton was the solicitor to the deputation.[66]

The joint deputation published three separate reports dated 12 May 1845, 5 August 1845, and 25 February 1846. In the preface to the first report they stated their view that the legislation of 1815 had been a 'great mistake'. It had·linked the general practitioner to the apothecary and failed to take account of his 'elevated status' in recent years. For this reason the connection between the Society of Apothecaries and the general practitioners should be severed, and an entirely new system should be introduced by which general practitioners would be able to exert 'a real influence and control over the education and examination of their own class'.

It was proposed that the College should be called 'The Royal College of General Practitioners in Medicine, Surgery and Midwifery', and that it alone would have the power to confer 'letters testimonial'[67] which would allow future candidates to register as general practitioners. Radical changes that would affect the whole of the medical profession were proposed. In future, it was suggested, all entrants to the profession should first undergo a preliminary examination in medicine and surgery at which the examiners would be physicians and surgeons. Then the candidate would decide in which branch of the profession he would practice and, after a due period of specified study, he would apply to the appropriate College (of Physicians, Surgeons, or General Practitioners) to take the final examination.[68] The minimum age of candidates for physic or surgery would be twenty-six and for general practice, twenty-two. Such a system would have gone a long way towards elevating the status of the general practitioner to a level similar to that of physicians and surgeons.

True to form, the Colleges of Physicians and Surgeons objected strongly to the proposals. Objections were also received from the London, Scottish, and Irish medical schools. The Home Secretary was about to find himself at the centre of a prolonged and bitter quarrel in which even he may not have anticipated the cantankerous nature of the participants and at a time when his own temper had been sorely tried. The physicians objected to the inclusion of the word 'medicine'

---

[66] *Reports of the Joint Deputation*, first report, 14.
[67] Ibid., 11.
[68] Ibid., 11–13.

in the title of the proposed college of general practitioners. They also objected that the proposals would favour the Scottish and Irish medical schools which would continue to hold a single examination for their candidates. Finally, they objected to a clause in the proposed Bill which stated that 'all medical and surgical posts' would be open to general practitioners.[69] The College of Surgeons found even more to fear in the proposals than the Physicians. The examination fee (£22 for provincial candidates and £32 for London) was the most important source of revenue for the College. Under the proposals of the joint deputation, the probability was that the number taking the Membership of the College would be reduced when the number applying to take the Fellowship was increasing. The College could become an institution which resembled an army which was not only poor, but consisted of officers and no other ranks. The *London Medical Gazette* remarked:

The granting of such a charter [to general practitioners] would be attended with the destruction of the Royal College of Surgeons. The membership of that College would be no longer sought for, and the Fellowship would be left to the few whose views might lead them to practise surgery alone. The College of Surgeons would therefore be limited to the Council and Fellows, its funds would decline, and its power over the profession as a Corporate Institution would cease.[70]

The conspicuous feature of the objections of the two Royal Colleges was their blatant display of self-interest. The Society of Apothecaries, however, which had been in the best position to monitor the changes in general practice since 1815, believed that general practitioners had been successful in their aim of elevating 'their social status' and the standard of 'their professional requirements', while the Colleges of Physicians and Surgeons 'had been indisposed to admit the necessity or even the expediency, of a high standard of qualification for members of that branch of the profession'. For this reason the joint deputation objected, with some reason, to entrusting the education and examination of future general practitioners to physicians and surgeons.[71] Sir James Graham had received a letter from Henry Robinson, the Master of the Society of Apothecaries, in 1842 on just this point.

As the General Practitioner practises all the branches of the Profession, his Examination should be confined chiefly to men of his own rank: for if it were conducted by a Board of which the General Practitioner formed only a small

---

[69] *Reports of the Joint Deputation*, second report, 16.
[70] *LMG*, NS 2 (1846), 780–1.
[71] *Address by the Society of Apothecaries* (1845), 9–11.

minority, ... they would on all occasions be subject to the control of physicians and surgeons; and there would be no security that General Practitioners could retain that position as well educated men, and that rank and station in their profession which they have acquired under the Act of 1815 and which it is important they retain, not for their own advantage, but for the benefit and security of the public health.[72]

However, the deputation, in the face of such opposition, decided that they had no choice but to compromise. They agreed to remove the words 'medicine' and 'surgery' from the title of the proposed College. The proposed College was to be simply the Royal College of General Practitioners. It was a minor concession, made without undermining the basic plans of the National Association. Addressing the Royal College of Surgeons, the joint deputation suggested that the fully qualified general practitioner should be allowed, if he wished, to become a member of the Royal College of Surgeons simply by payment of a fee and without further examination. He would then be entitled to use the title 'surgeon' and would have access by right to the library of the Royal College of Surgeons and the Hunterian Museum. At this stage, during the first seven months of 1845, the College of Physicians kept a watching brief but took little part in any negotiations. It was the Royal College of Surgeons which took up the cudgels against the general practitioners. On 13 March 1845 the Council of the College of Surgeons instructed the President (Sir Benjamin Collins Brodie), the Vice-President, and two members 'to watch the proceedings of the National Association with reference to a charter of incorporation of the General Practitioners and to report thereon from time to time'.[73] On 27 March 1845 it was reported that they had received a letter from the National Association. This letter, which was blunt and aggressive, consisted of four sections summarized as follows:

1. The National Association recorded its displeasure at the way honorary Fellowships had been granted under the new (1843) charter.
2. The letter demanded that ordinary members of the College should be given fair representation on the Council of the College.
3. The National Association asked whether the surgeons would co-operate in establishing a College of General Practitioners?
4. Finally, the Association asked whether the College of Surgeons would

---

[72] Guildhall Library, London, records of the Society of Apothecaries, letter dated 10 Feb. 1842, MS 8218.
[73] Library of the Royal College of Surgeons, London. Minute book for 1843–9.

receive a deputation to discuss how best to manage the establishment of such a new College?

Council considered these questions one by one. The first they ignored; the second, third, and fourth were answered in Council with an instant and uncompromising negative. These decisions were communicated to the National Association in a convoluted letter of extraordinary length (occupying pp. 266–73 of the minute book) that may well have been a source of confusion. But in essence the letter said 'no' three times on the grounds that the charters of the College were granted on the basis of its being a College of Surgeons; it was not, and never had been, a College of General Practitioners.

In June 1845 Council of the College of Surgeons held a special meeting to consider Sir James Graham's Bill for regulating the medical profession. Tempers were rising. They were angry at the suggestion of a College of General Practitioners that would be equal in rank with the Colleges of Physicians and Surgeons; it would not be 'beneficial to the community', and a title such as Fellow of the Royal College of General Practitioners 'would mislead the public'. A deputation of members of the Council was instructed to wait on Sir James Graham, and it is recorded that Sir James was dismayed at their objections and said 'he almost despaired of doing any good'.[74] On 5 July 1845 another special meeting was called and showed the hardening of the opposition of the Surgeons to the incorporation of general practitioners. At this meeting it was proposed that Council should approve the establishment of a College of General Practitioners with powers to conduct examinations; but it was insistent that passing this examination should not allow the candidate to qualify or to be registered when the new proposed Bill for medical registration was introduced. The purpose of the examination was to be no more than a preliminary that conferred on the candidate the right to sit for the examination conducted by physicians and surgeons; in addition, G. J. Guthrie proposed that the new College of General Practitioners should be forbidden to examine in surgery. This decision by the Council of the College of Surgeons was a resounding slap in the face of the general practitioners.[75] Possibly aware of the hurt they had inflicted, Council attempted to soften it by adding that the candidate, when he had passed the examination in which they were the examiners, would be allowed to call himself 'surgeon' and have the right to use the library

---

[74] Ibid. 296. The coment suggests that Sir James Graham had some sympathy with the aims of the National Association of General Practitioners.

[75] *Reports of the Joint Deputation,* second report, 25–7.

and the Hunterian Museum at their College. Sir James Graham was informed of these demands by the physicians and surgeons, and had to explain them and justify them to the joint deputation. This he did by saying to the general practitioners:

Educate your candidates, therefore, as highly as you think necessary; examine them in those branches of medical and general knowledge which you may deem essential as a qualification for general practice; no one shall be permitted to practise as a general practitioner without the sanction of your diploma; and the exercise of your discretion in these respects shall be unfettered. But although I have thus far modified my plan to remove all ground for apprehension on your part, I see no reason for exempting the general practitioner from an examination before a joint Board of Physicians and Surgeons—an examination they will be required to pass before the examining boards of their own Colleges. I am of the opinion that the connexion which will thus be established between the three branches of the profession will operate beneficially for the profession itself.[76]

Sir James, in other words, suggested a compromise which he hoped would pacify both general practitioners and the surgeons. The deputation agreed to the suggestion because it still preserved the idea of a Royal College of General Practitioners and an examination carried out by a board from that College. The *Medical Gazette* commented that the second report of the joint deputation was 'a sort of laboured apology for giving way to the Colleges of Physicians and Surgeons ... the deputation virtually surrendered'. They added 'we believe that the deputation acted throughout with good faith, [but] biased by their anxiety to secure a charter of incorporation for the general practitioners'.[77]

A Bill was printed, and the deputation were annoyed to find that it 'failed to carry out the terms of the agreement to which the deputation had assented'. There were discrepancies which were thought to be unintentional, and which, it was assumed, would be removed.[78] Instead, nothing happened at all, and when the joint deputation finally wrote to Sir James Graham they received a reply from his secretary that Sir James had received 'communications' in the Christmas recess which led him to abandon the whole plan for the incorporation of general practitioners because there was no general agreement in the profession

---

[76] *Address by the Society of Apothecaries* (1845), 12–13.
[77] *LMG*, NS 1 (1845), 786–7.
[78] *Reports of the Joint Deputation*, second report, 34.

on the issue.[79] The deputation protested, but in vain—they were defeated. To what extent was Sir James Graham responsible for the defeat of the general practitioner? He is described in the *Dictionary of National Biography* as: 'Tall and handsome, he had the manner of a dandy and his style was stiff and pompous.' His appointment as Home Secretary was 'scarcely well suited to one who was so little conciliatory in manner and so rash in utterance'. His character might well have been constitutionally unsympathetic to the lower echelons of the medical profession; and this is the impression that is gained from the accounts of the struggle to establish a College of General Practitioners. Moreover, this was the period when he was embittered by the personal attacks launched against him for the affair of secretly using his authority as Home Secretary to open and examine the post of his opponents, and by the lack of support or sympathy from members of his own party when exposed. Nevertheless, he had a deep interest in medical affairs, although his own troubles may have overshadowed the problems of a College of General Practitioners. His biographer wrote that medical reform

appeared to have a sort of fascination for him ... he was never tired of collecting or collating evidence ... [But] nobody else wanted to have done what he disinterestedly wanted to do. Though he had sometimes successfully shifted a hive of bees from a rickety stand to a safer spot, without caring much for a casual sting or two, he made up his mind never again to try the experiment of lifting three hives at once, or of concentrating them all under one glass. The medical Bill, which he spent no end of time and trouble putting together was praised and abused, debated and amended, committed and recommitted, during the session of 1845, till everybody except himself was weary of the endless controversy.[80]

The general practitioners were not, however, prepared to admit defeat. The same group formed another association—another in name only—in April 1846, when some seven hundred practitioners met in the Hanover Square rooms and established the 'National Institute of Medicine, Surgery and Midwifery'.[81] Once again it was headed by R. R. Pennington and the two secretaries were James Bird and Henry Ancell. It was established, like the National Association of General Practitioners,

---

[79] Ibid. 338.

[80] Torrens McCullagh Torrens, *The Life and Times of the Rt. Hon. Sir James Graham, Bart.* (London, 1863). See also A. B. Erickson, *Journal of the History of Medicine*, 5 (1950). There seems little doubt Sir James had a considerable interest in medical reform and medical education.

[81] *PMSJ* 10 (1846), 197–8.

with the purpose of obtaining a charter of incorporation for the general practitioners. Why they troubled to change the name is uncertain. There was one difference; now a subscription of one guinea was demanded from the membership. The membership of the National Institute fell promptly from the level achieved by the National Association of between four and five thousand, to a little over one thousand.[82] Some general practitioners said they could not afford the fee: others may have become bored, frustrated, or disheartened by the defeat of the National Association. But the low membership of the National Institute weakened its position for the negotiations that lay ahead.

In January 1847 the National Institute approached the Society of Apothecaries to ask if they would once again form a joint deputation with them, as they had with the National Association. The Society replied that they were reluctant, but in May 1847 they went independently to see the Home Secretary and explained their views.[83] In 1846 Sir George Grey replaced Sir James Graham as Home Secretary. In contrast to the haughty and sour-natured Graham, Grey was kindly and genial, and he suggested towards the end of 1847 that the problems of the general practitioners might be solved by a joint conference between representatives of the physicians, the surgeons, the apothecaries, and the National Institute, to be held at the College of Physicians.[84] This was agreed, and astonishingly the conference came rapidly to a unanimous decision to recommend the establishment of a Royal College of General Practitioners. The Presidents of the College of Physicians, the College of Surgeons, and the National Institute, and the Master of the Society of Apothecaries all signed the recommendation in February 1848. It was stated clearly in clause 1 'that a charter of incorporation should be granted to the Surgeon-Apothecaries of this country under the title of "The Royal College of General Practitioners of England" '.[85] It seemed to be victory at last.

In the event the signed agreement that was obtained at the joint conference held at the Royal College of Physicians came to nothing. The College of Surgeons refused to ratify it:

---

[82] *LMG*, third series 3 (1846), 1 August. Here the total membership of the National Institute is given as 1,337. James Bird in *SCMR*, Q. 1124, gave the total of 1,350, 865 in the provinces and 485 in London. 866 of the total membership were members of the Royal College of Surgeons.

[83] Guildhall Library, London. Records of the Society of Apothecaries, MS 8212.

[84] *Lancet* (1850), i. 456–63.

[85] *Lancet* (1848), i. 319.

all parties had pledged their concurrence and support. ... When the Government undertook to reduce the outline to a Bill that had been drawn up by the conference to legal shape, the Council of the College of Surgeons intimated their dissent to its principles, although formerly agreed to by their representatives, and raised objections to the unfettered power of examining candidates for its diploma, that had been conceded to the proposed College of General Practitioners.[86]

From the point of view of the general practitioners this was an act of pure treachery and they were furious.[87] The representatives of the College of Surgeons, including the President of the College, had agreed to the contents of the document at the joint conference, but Council of the College had turned it down.

Between 1845 and 1848 the attitude of the College of Surgeons to the general practitioners had softened perceptibly, so why did Council refuse to ratify the agreement of its representatives? The answer lay in the second clause of the fourth principle of the agreement. Council agreed without demur to the first principle which simply stated that a Royal College of General Practitioners should be established. The second clause of the fourth principle concerned the registration of surgeons in the context of the Bill then under consideration. Here it stated that 'surgeons who also dispensed medicine ... shall be required to enroll themselves in the College of General Practitioners and to be registered as Surgeons and General Practitioners.' Council had no objection to this suggestion; there was no dispute on this matter. It was the following sentence they could not accept. This sentence stated: 'After the passing of the Act, Members of the Royal College of Surgeons shall not be registered as Surgeons unless they be also admitted as Members of the Royal College of General Practitioners, and registered both as Surgeons and General Practitioners.' It is a mystery how this sentence was ever agreed to at the joint conference. It would be difficult to imagine a more inflammatory suggestion than this—that the Abernethys, Guthries, and Benjamin Brodies of the future who, from the beginning of their careers as students intended a career as pure hospital surgeons, should be forced at first to become registered as general practitioners and be entered as such in the register. I am inclined to believe that the inclusion of this sentence as it stood was a mistake, an oversight. This view is to a certain extent supported by the muddled evidence of James Bird before the Select Committee on Medical Registration.[88] If it was not a mistake then

---

[86] *Lancet* (1850), i. 457.
[87] Ibid. 251 and 456.
[88] *SCMR*, Q. 1075–1104.

it was an extraordinary tactless suggestion, the consequence of which should have been foreseen. Council's (of the Royal College of Surgeons) understandable refusal to accept this clause led to a crisis in the relationship between the surgeons and the general practitioners.[89] In their anger the surgeons resuscitated old matters of contention and refused to allow that if a new College was established it should be allowed to conduct any examination in surgery. This brief, inept, and ill-considered sentence, which was peripheral to the main issues, was a small matter. It should have been easy to discuss and to resolve it but for the enmity that had grown up between the surgeons and the general practitioners.

During this period—1849 and the first half of 1850—the subject of the College of General Practitioners was discussed at several large meetings and aired in the medical press. Essentially nothing new was said, but the College of Surgeons was repeatedly branded as the real villain, not only by the general practitioners but also by the provincial surgeons.[90] In the summer of 1850 another Bill for incorporation of general practitioners was drawn up by the Council of the National Institute and introduced into the House of Commons by Mr Wyld and Colonel Thompson.[91] Nothing more was heard of it, and the National Institute presumably died from inanition because there is no record of its being formally terminated. Sporadic letters concerning a College of General Practitioners appear during the remainder of 1850 and in 1851 in the context of the long series of Bills which ended finally in the Medical Act of 1858. But the plan for a College of General Practitioners died in the summer of 1850.

The ultimate failure of the plan for a College of General Practitioners can be attributed to a number of factors. One of great importance was the simultaneous movement to introduce a Bill for medical registration. This involved the whole profession and captured most of the attention of the politically minded section of the medical profession. This movement also received the lion's share of attention in the medical periodicals, whose power to influence medical opinion was considerable. Wakley's loathing of the College of Surgeons and his view of himself as a champion of the underdog should have made the *Lancet* a supporter of the National Association of General Practitioners. On the contrary,

[89] Library of the Royal College of Surgeons, London. Minutes of Council from 10 and 18 Feb. 1848.

[90] 'Medical Reform: Great Meeting of the Profession', *Lancet*, (1850) i. 450–463; see particularly speech by Mr Paget of Leicester, 460–1. Also *LMG*, NS 8 (1849), 782–7, 1112–15.

[91] *Lancet* (1850), ii. 177–8, and *LMG*, NS 11 (1850), 334–7.

Wakley was scornful of the whole idea of a College for general practitioners and he vilified the secretaries Bird and Ancell by constantly
referring to them as 'Snipe and Sneak'.[92] The reason seems to have
been that Wakley was intent on overcoming the rejection of general
practitioners by the College of Surgeons, and the plan for a separate
college weakened his attack. The two most influential journals in the
1840s were the *Lancet* and the *Provincial Medical and Surgical Journal*.[93]
From the start the latter, with its wide representation of general practitioners, was lukewarm towards the idea of a College of General Practitioners because the PMSA was engaged in canvassing Council of the
College of Surgeons for representation of provincial surgeons.[94] The
journal did not wish to associate itself with a proposal so firmly rejected
by the College they were trying to win over. But there was another
respect in which the PMSA found itself hesitant in supporting the plan
for the incorporation of general practitioners. The primary aim of the
PMSA was unity. Over the five years in which the general practitioners
were agitating for a College lukewarm support for the plan turned to
cold dislike, and the whole idea was condemned by the PMSA as
divisive when unity was needed. General practitioners were asking to
be totally divorced from the physicians and surgeons and to have
complete power over the training and the examination of the future
general practitioner.

It is because we are anxious to uphold the conditions of the provincial members
of the College of Surgeons that we desire to do all in our power to prevent their
incorporation into a third College of General Practitioners which would at once
separate the profession into *three* classes with well defined lines of demarcation
to the manifest loss of *status* and dignity by the lowest department.[95]

At just this time, the closing years of the 1840s, the PMSA believed
they were on the edge of obtaining their 'just demands from the College
of Surgeons'. In 1851 another editorial announced that there were
clear signs that the two Royal Colleges were 'in cordial and effective co-
operation'.[96] A memorial was sent by Charles Hastings, the President

---

[92] *Lancet* (1845), ii. 185–92, 544–6, 597–600, 624–7, 681–3, etc.
[93] Letters published on the subject of the College of General Practitioners between 1845
and 1850 were counted. A small majority of those published in the *Lancet* were favourable
to the idea, and the reverse was the case for the *PMSJ*. Those published in the *LMG*
tended to be neutral in tone.
[94] *PMSJ* 9 (1845), 52–4.
[95] Ibid. (1850), 6 March.
[96] Ibid. (1851), 30 April.

of the PMSA, to the Home Secretary, urging the introduction of the long awaited Bill for medical reform—but it was to be a Bill in which the issue of a Royal College of General Practitioners was dead and forgotten.

General practitioners who were members of the PMSA and of the Association of General Practitioners found themselves in a dilemma. A letter published in 1846 suggested that dual membership could even be interpreted as disloyalty to the PMSA.[97] This was going too far, but it was certainly true that the strength of the PMSA was the weakness of the Association of General Practitioners; and the lack of support from the PMSA was probably much more important as a contributory cause to the failure of the general practitioner's Association than the opposition of the *Lancet*, whose radicalism and raucous aggression created as many enemies as friends.

The National Association (and Institute) of General Practitioners had therefore attempted to push through its proposal for a College against the united opposition of the two medical colleges, the apathy of a majority of general practitioners, the hostility of Wakley, and the initial indifference and later hostility of the PMSA. The behaviour of the National Association suggested, more than once, political ineptness; and their president was too old for such an enterprise. And yet the plan very nearly succeeded. Had it done so the structure of the medical profession might have been very different, although it can certainly be argued that the existence of a College of General Practitioners would have been divisive when unity was needed, and that the plans for such a College to undertake the greater part of the medical education of future general practitioners were impractical. Had the Association been content to be what would now be called a postgraduate institution, acting as a meeting place for established general practitioners and providing the official representatives of their branch of the profession, it might have been successful. But postgraduate institutions in the modern sense were unknown at the time. It may not have escaped the reader that when a plan to found a College of General Practitioners was finally successful in 1952, it was, in fact, a postgraduate institution whose influence has grown steadily since it was founded.

[97] *PMSJ* 10 (1846), 235.

14

Postscript: The Medical Act of 1858

THE opportunity for radical changes in the structure of the medical profession was largely confined to the brief period from 1820 to 1850. The opportunity was created by the rise of the general practitioner and the belief in many quarters that the rise could continue, leading to substantial developments in the status of the general practitioner *vis-à-vis* the physician. This, as stressed in previous chapters, was not a conceit confined to certain over-ambitious general practitioners. In 1843 a senior London physician, Sir James Clark, believed Dr Barlow's view (chapter 6) was correct—that the general practitioner was the doctor of the future.[1] Clark even suggested a union of the Royal Colleges of Physicians and Surgeons (by implication into a joint college of consultants) because, to an ever-increasing extent, the work of physicians and surgeons had fallen into the hands of the general practitioners. Sir James Clark's view of such radical changes was based on his perception of the elevated status of the general practitioner; but he was also doubtless influenced by the effeteness of the medical colleges and the derisory state of medical education in the older universities.

With the defeat of the plan for a college of general practitioners, however, the opportunity for radical change disappeared. The Medical Act of 1858 had still to come; but in their conflict with the general practitioners the medical corporations had demonstrated not only their dislike of radical change but their ability to prevent it.

Meanwhile, the progress towards 'an Act to regulate the medical profession' ground slowly through fifteen unsuccessful Bills (the first in 1840) before the sixteenth received the royal assent.[2] The final result of the Medical Act of 1858 resembled the Apothecaries Act of 1815 in one important respect: to a majority of practitioners it was a bitter disappointment. At the very least the profession wanted a Bill which would outlaw quackery and control the druggists; and to achieve this

[1] Sir James Clark, *Remarks on Medical Reform* (London, 1843).
[2] For a detailed account of the passage of these Bills, see C. Newman, *The Evolution of Medical Education in the Nineteenth Century* (London, 1957).

they wanted a definition of medical qualification, a register of qualified doctors, a medical council which represented the profession as a whole, and a rationalization of the chaotic state of medical education and examinations. The advance of medical education, it was said, was hampered by the chaos of a multiplicity of medical institutions awarding licences, diplomas, and degrees; there were eighteen in the United Kingdom in the 1850s.[3] The alternative of a 'single portal of entry' was strongly supported. This would have been a state examination (similar to the nurses' today) to be held simultaneously in the capitals of each part of the Kingdom. What happened to these proposals?

The single portal of entry failed because none of the medical corporations would surrender their privileges, and the non-representative nature of the General Medical Council (heavily weighted by members of the corporations) ensured their continuation. The proposal to control druggists failed, as it had done between 1812 and 1815. The major disappointment, however, was the failure to outlaw quackery, although a substantial part of the profession realized it was impossible. In an age of *laisser-faire* it would have been hard enough to persuade Parliament to drive the blatantly fraudulent quack from the streets; to prosecute the numerous women of villages and backstreets who acted the part of nurse, healer, or midwife when there was no legally qualified alternative would have been unthinkable. A major flaw of the Act was the perpetuation of the partially qualified doctor. A practitioner could register on the basis of a single qualification in either medicine or surgery; compulsory examination of all students in medicine, surgery, and midwifery was only introduced in 1886.[4] For these and other reasons, the majority of the profession found the Act was less than perfect. What have modern historians to say about it?

Until quite recently the Medical Act has been applauded as one of the great landmarks in the advance of medicine whereby the medical education and ethical behaviour of medical practitioners came under firm control for the benefit of the public. It was an Act by which the profession put its house in order. Now, it is more usual to describe the Medical Act as a prime example of professional consolidation and monopolization based on motives of self-interest; which, of course, it was. But the two views are not incompatible, especially when considered

[3] W. Dale, *The Present State of the Medical Profession* (London, 1860).
[4] The Medical Act Amendment Act of 1886.

within the mid-nineteenth-century climate of opinion.[5] Then it was commonly agreed that a professional man's self-interest was the best guarantee of good public service. The efficient would prosper and the bad go to the wall. It was not the purpose of the state to interfere more than possible in social transactions between customer, client, or patient, and the provider of services. In medicine it was necessary only to ensure a minimum standard of competence—a belief which became enshrined in the concept of 'the safe general practitioner'. Such arguments concerning the state and the provisions of health care are still familiar today. Was the Act, therefore, of benefit to the public and the profession?

In the long term the answer must be in the affirmative, even if it is an affirmative with reservations. The disciplinary powers of the General Medical Council have a powerful deterrent effect on professional misbehaviour, even if the decisions of the disciplinary committee have sometimes appeared to be capricious. The primary purpose of the Act, the regulation of medical education, is clearly important although (except as a last resort) the Council only has power to advise, not to compel.[6] Until recently the method of appointing members of the Council was not representative, and the part played by the medical corporations was excessive. But the public is much better served and protected than it would have been if medicine had been totally free from the control of a Medical Council. Did the Act, however, confer immediate advantage on the profession?

Those who support the thesis that the Act was the triumphant product of a movement based purely on medical self-interest are forced to the logical conclusion that it was welcomed by the profession for the benefits it bestowed on them. They emphasise that, as a result of registration, outdated legal restrictions on medical practice were removed, and practitioners could sue for fees and apply for public service; but these were not important issues. It is also said, and is hard to deny, that registration conferred a certain psychological advantage on the registered practitioner, and it is certain that the medical cor-

---

[5] An illuminating account of the Medical Act of 1858 in the context of nineteenth-century liberalism, libertarianism, and *laisser-faire* can be found in J. L. Berlant, *Profession and Monopoly: A Study of Medicine in the United States and Great Britain* (Los Angeles, 1975), esp. pp. 145–65.

[6] The General Medical Council can refuse to recognize the licence diploma or degree of a medical institution whose educational standard has fallen to an unacceptable level; but this is an extreme measure that has rarely been used. The Council would, however, be able to refuse to recognize a new medical school if it chose to, and in this way has control over future medical educational institutions.

porations gained greatly by the passing of the Act; the Act virtually guaranteed their continued existence and rubber-stamped their authority. The suggestion that the Medical Act was responsible for introducing modern medical education is so wide of the mark that it needs only to be mentioned to be dismissed. Finally, it is sometimes suggested that, for all its failings, at least the Medical Act was responsible for unifying the profession; but this is nonsense, confusing causes with results. The Medical Act of 1858, like the Apothecaries Act of 1815, was the product, not the cause of changes in the profession. In any occupational group, unification is promoted by a common pathway of entry and an ethos which provides a sense of corporate identity, purpose, and pride. At best the Medical Act contributed to a very minor degree to these components of professional unity. But it would be hard to justify an assertion that, in the short term, the Act conferred material advantage on practitioners in terms of better education, more patients, higher fees, reduced competition from irregulars, greater respect from the public, or even greater ability to control the development of the profession. Certainly, neither the practice nor the position of physicians and surgeons was affected materially by the Act; nor, contrary to received opinion, did the general practitioners gain anything. Indeed, they lost the opportunity for social and professional mobility which, in the 1820s and 1830s was their source of optimism and vitality. The authentication of the corporations and medical qualifications had the effect of fossilizing the prospects of the general practitioner and ensuring that he remained as a subordinate grade. To this extent the general practitioners were disappointed people who had challenged the medical corporations and lost. Their views of the Act were forcibly expressed by a London practitioner, Edwin Lee, who wrote in 1863 that the Medical Act had added no advantages to medical men, had not altered medical education, and provided only a means of levying an extra tax.[7] Lee provided an impressive body of evidence from the press, lay and medical, deriding the Act as 'a very considerable failure'. 'Depend upon it,' wrote one practitioner, 'the Medical Council will make it their duty to serve only the interests of the medical corporations they represent.' Another complained, 'The Medical Council ... are supposed to be our rep-

---

[7] Edwin Lee, *The State of the Medical Profession further exemplified* ... (London, 1863), 8–18. The quotations which follow are taken from this work. W. Rivington, in *The Medical Profession* (Dublin, 1879), also held a low opinion of the Medical Act chiefly on the two grounds that it had failed to outlaw quackery, and allowed the continuation of the partly qualified doctor.

resentatives. What have they hitherto represented? The monopoly and exclusiveness of effete corporations.' A writer to the Dublin medical press complained that the Council was 'not accountable to those who compose the medical body politic' and the *Medical Circular* asserted that the Act, far from promoting unity, had 'increased the evil of multifarious qualifications ... [and] ... helped to exasperate the lamentable divisions that have made our profession the reproach of society'. 'We have got our protection,' wrote a Dr Wilks, 'we have obtained our registration at last; but as for advantage it may be of to the profession, I, for one, value it at a straw.'

Yet although the Act of 1858 conferred no advantage on general practitioners, the subsequent development of medicine at least provided them with occupational security. The growing tendency of physicians and surgeons to practise as consultants centred on hospitals depended on a solid base of general practitioner in the community. This symbiotic relationship was strengthened by the gradual acceptance of the peculiarly British principle of referral, introduced as an ethical principle in the late nineteenth century. Only slowly was it accepted that it should be a universally applied principle, but in practice it meant that, to an ever-increasing extent a patient could (with a few exceptions) obtain access to a physician or surgeon only by first consulting a general practitioner. In Rosemary Stevens's well-known phrase, 'The physician and surgeon retained the hospital but the general practitioner retained the patient'.[8] The exclusion of the general practitioner from hospitals (except, of course, the Cottage Hospitals and the new Community Hospitals), together with the application of the principle of referral, are the keys to understanding the medical profession in Britain. Neither applied in the United States of America and it is significant that it was in Britain that the general practitioner persisted and today is thriving.[9] His persistence was in the interests of the public and of all branches of the medical profession. The development of general practice after the mid-nineteenth century lies beyond the limits of this study; but the roots of present practice in this branch of the medical profession in Britain were firmly established by 1850.

[8] Rosemary Stevens, *Medical Practice in Modern England* (New Haven, 1966), 33.

[9] I. Loudon and R. Stevens, 'Primary Care and the Hospital', in J. Fry (ed.), *Primary Care* (London, 1980), chapter 7.

List of books bought by a medical student during his year in London attending the hospitals, 1811

6 vols. Benjamin Bell's *Surgery*
3 vols. *System of Anatomy*
2 vols. Burns on Inflammation
3 vols. Fyfe's *Anatomy*
2 vols. Charles Bell's *Operative Surgery*
2 vols. Cullen's *Practice of Physic*
Samuel Cooper's *Surgery*
John Pearson's *Principles of Surgery*
Abernethy on Local Diseases

James Brigg on the Eye
Hooper's Medical Dictionary
The Edinburgh Dispensatory
William Cheselden's *Anatomy*
Jones on Haemorrhage
John Innes on the Muscles
Townsend's *Vade Mecum*
Henry's *Chemistry*
Parkes' *Chemical Catechism.*

Source: Letters of Poyntz Adams, Northampton County Record Office, ref. ZA 6277, Box X 5508.

List of books and stationery bought by
G. Washburn Charleton of Gloucester, surgeon,
during his time as a student, 1826

	Price
British Medical Almanack	£0. 2s. 0d.
Swan on the nerves	£1. 11s. 0d.
Bell on the teeth	£0. 14s. 0d.
Hoblyn's Dictionary	£0. 9s. 0d.
Davis's Obstetrical Medicine, vols. 1 and 2	£0. 1s. 0d.
Copland's Medical Dictionary, vols. 1, 2, and 3	£1. 7s. 0d.
Manual of Auscultation, etc.	£0. 5s. 0d.
Beck's Medical Jurisprudence	£1. 1s. 0d.
12 sheets Rough Imperial	£0. 7s. 0d.
1 oz of red chalk	£0. 1s. 2d.
1 oz of Italian chalk	£0. 1s. 6d.

Source: Letters of George Charleton, Gloucester County Record Office, ref. D 4432/1

Glossary of terms used in pharmaceutical practice—Issues and setons—Measures used in pharmacy

Bolus—any medicine rolled round, about the size of a bean, and not too large to be swallowed whole. Often contained volatile salts so that it had to be taken while freshly made up.

Cataplasm—a poultice or a plaster, originally; later, a plaster.

Collyrium—eye lotion or powders insufflated into the eye.

Confection—originally a medicine consisting of dry ingredients, powdered and held together by honey. By the nineteenth century this included conserves and electuaries as there were insufficient grounds to separate them.

Decoction—a medicine prepared by boiling one or more ingredients in water. When cool, it was strained and allowed to stand until clear.

Draught—any liquid medicine to be taken all at once, or (less accurately) in two or three doses. Medicines for insomnia were prescribed in draughts.

Electuary—a Latin corruption of the Greek, Ekleiton, something to be licked. Similar to a bolus, but sweetened by preserves, honey, or sugar, either as a luxury or to disguise a bitter-tasting medicament.

Elixir—strictly a tincture drawn from several ingredients, where a tincture is drawn only from one. In the nineteenth century all such preparations were included under tinctures. Originally, perhaps, *the* medicine, the great panacea sought after by Arab chemists.

Emplastrum—a plaster ('plaister') consisting of medicaments for external application spread on linen cloth, silk, or leather.

Haustus—a draught.

Infusion—a medicine made by pouring hot or boiling water on finely divided ingredients and letting it stand: tea, for example.

Julep—a draught to which syrup was added to make it sweet, usually consisting of three or four doses. It was abandoned as a term in the nineteenth century when all such medicines were called mixtures. The term was used by the Arabs exclusively for clear sweet liquids.

Mixtures or 'Mistura'—any water-based medicine in which two or more ingredients were dissolved or suspended.

Ointment 'Unguentum'—an ointment, stiff ones being called pastes, and fluid ones creams.

Pill or 'Pilula'—a small, round, solid medicine the size of a pea. Originally used for medicines which operated in small dosage and were too nauseous to be taken in any other way.

Powders or 'Pulvis'—self-evident. Light powders were taken in thin fluids (milk or tea); heavy in syrup, jelly, or honey.

Sinapsim—a poultice made with vinegar and 'rendered warm' by the addition of mustard, horse-radish, or garlic. Was employed as a counter-irritant or to 'bring the blood and the spirits' to a weak part as in palsy or atrophy. It was intended to supersede the blister.

Tincture—a solution or liquid extract of any substance in alcohol.

An issue was an artificial ulcer caused by making an incision through the skin and keeping it open by the insertion of metal 'tents' or peas, to form a drain to carry off noxious humors. Originally they were sited as near as possible to the affected part, but later the preferred sites were the nape of the neck, the upper arm, the hollow above the inside of the knee or on either side of the spine on the back. Often used in fevers, and in the treatment of leg ulcers in which they formed an alternative drain for humors while the ulcer was being healed.

The seton consisted of pinching up a fold of skin and inserting through it a large cutting needle armed with several threads which were left through the skin and pulled back and forth to cause suppuration. The principle was the same as in an issue; the results usually more drastic, inflammatory and painful.

Apothecaries' measures

Pints		Fluid Ounces		Fluid Drachms		Minims
1	=	16	=	128	=	7680
		1	=	8	=	480
				1	=	60

CONVENTIONALLY
1 minim (꧝ ᛏ) = 1 drop
a drachm (ʒ ᛏ) = 1 teaspoonful
½ fluid ounce (ʒ ss) = 1 tablespoonful
1 fluid ounce (ʒ ᛏ) = 2 tablespoonsful

Sources: R. James, *Medical Dictionary*, 3 vols. (London, 1743); R. Morris and J. Kendrick, *Edinburgh Medical and Surgical Dictionary* (Edinburgh, 1807); R. Hooper, *Lexicon Medicum*, 4th edn. (London, 1820); R. Hoblyn, *Dictionary of Terms used in Medicine*, 9th edn. (London, 1868). Dr T. D. Whittet kindly supplied a great deal of the information on pharmaceutical terms.

Population and numbers of medical men in certain English counties: England and Wales, 1841

County	Population	Physicians	Surgeons, apothecaries, and medical students	All medical men	Ratio of population to each medical man
Berkshire	161,147	5	160	165	1:976
Bucks	155,983	4	94	98	1:1,591
Cambridge	164,459	11	117	128	1:1,284
Cornwall	341,279	13	229	242	1:1,410
Cumberland	178,038	18	134	152	1:1,171
Derby	272,217	7	107	204	1:1,381
Devon	533,640	46	551	597	1:893
Durham	324,284	16	337	353	1:918
Gloucester	431,383	46	444	490	1:880
Lancaster	1,667,054	76	1,246	1,322	1:1,261
Middlesex	1,576,636	324	3,592	3,916	1:402
Norfolk	412,664	17	299	316	1:1,305
Northumberland	250,278	17	258	275	1:910
Oxford	161,643	8	151	159	1:1,016
Somerset	435,982	33	445	478	1:912
Stafford	510,504	14	335	359	1:1,422
Suffolk	315,073	7	278	285	1:1,105
Wiltshire	258,783	9	177	186	1:1,391
Worcester	233,336	13	173	186	1:1,254
Yorks (West Riding)	1,154,101	56	805	861	1:1,340
Brecon	55,603	3	41	44	1:1,263
Cardigan	68,766	2	43	45	1:1,528
Carmathen [sic]	106,326	6	52	58	1:1,833
Flint	66,919	1	69	70	1:905
Glamorgan	171,188	6	113	119	1:1,438
Pembroke	88,044	2	44	46	1:1,914
Radnor	25,256	1	17	18	1:1,408

Source: 1841 Census: tables of occupation, Parliamentary Papers (1844), XXVII.

Population, numbers of medical men, nurses and midwives, chemists and druggists in selected towns in England and Wales, 1841

	Population	Physicians	Surg.-Apoth.	All medical men	Chemists and druggists	Ratio of population to each doctor	
						All medical men	GPs
England	15,000,154	1,063	15,422	16,485	9,648	910	1,185
Liverpool Borough	286,487	27	328	355	365	807	977
Manchester Borough	242,983	19	253	272	272	893	1,075
Birmingham	182,922	16	167	183	194	1,000	1,219
Leeds	152,084	14	137	151	138	1,006	1,246
Bristol	122,296	29	181	210	147	582	764
Norwich	62,344	7	66	73	77	854	1,056
Nottingham	53,091	7	46	53	90	1,000	1,294
Exeter	31,312	10	54	64	56	489	530
Oxford	23,834	4	40	44	27	541	662
Gloucester	14,152	2	24	26	28	544	673
Cardiff	10,077	2	12	14	12	719	959
Winchester	6,708	2	17	19	12	353	447

For the method of calculating the number of general practitioners see Table 19, n.[b].

Source: 1841 census. Parliamentary Papers (1844). XXVII.

Certain selected male occupations in England and Wales, 1841

Occupation	Number	% of total population
Total male population	7,961,244	100.00
Occupied	4,786,488	
Unoccupied	3,174,756	
The professions		
Clerical	20,450	0.25
Medical	17,666	0.22
Legal	14,155	0.17
Other pursuits requiring education	92,009	1.15
Government and civil service	13,559	0.16
Municipal and parochial offices	20,276	0.25
Domestic servants		
Male	253,805	3.20
(Female)	(765,519)	
Commerce, trade and manufacture	2,068,562	25.80
Agriculture	1,203,677	15.00
Army		
At home	36,673 ⎫	
Abroad and in Ireland	89,230 ⎭	1.60
Navy and merchant service, fishermen, etc.		
At home	95,193 ⎫	
Afloat	93,799 ⎭	2.40
Living on means	123,780	1.50
In institutions	92,975	1.20

Source: G. M. Young and W. D. Hancock, *English Historical Documents, 1833–1874* (London, 1956).

The ratio of medical practitioners to population in England and Wales 1841–1971

Year	Population in England and Wales	Number of medical practitioners	No. of medical practitioners per 100,000 population
1841	15,911,757	17,117	107
1851	17,927,609	19,190	107
1861	20,066,224	15,297	76
1871	22,712,266	16,292	72
1881	25,974,439	16,493	65
1891	29,002,525	19,037	66
1901	32,527,843	22,230	68
1911	36,070,492	23,469	65
1921	37,886,699	22,965	60
1931	43,952,377	25,669	64
1951	43,757,888	38,468	87
1971	48,854,000	47,049	96

Notes: The data in the final column are calculated to the nearest whole number. Exact comparisons based on the decennial census are difficult because of changes in methods of classification of medical practitioners. For example, in 1841 they were classified as (1) physicians, (2) surgeons, apothecaries, and medical students. In 1851 this was altered to (1) physicians, (2) surgeons, (3) other medical men; and in 1861 to (1) physicians, (2) surgeons and apothecaries, (3) medical students and assistants; and in 1881 to (1) physicians, surgeons, and general practitioners, (2) medical students and assistants. In 1951 and 1971 retired medical practitioners were excluded, while data for the number of retired before 1931 are not available. The source for this table was the decennial census, with the exception of 1971 when the data were derived from the Health and Social Services Statistics for England (DHSS, 1975).

Brief Biographical Notes

These notes are intended briefly to provide, or to supplement, the biographies of some of the practitioners whose records or publications are mentioned in the text. The majority, being surgeon-apothecaries or general practitioners, are not usually well known, and biographical data are often scanty. Others whose names are familiar to historians of medicine have been included because of their contributions to the debates on medical reform and the role of the general practitioner in the medical profession. Short references are included as a guide to the main sources for biographical data; they are not necessarily complete.

BARLOW, Edward (1779–1844), MD (Edin.) 1803. Born in County Meath, Ireland, son of a medical practitioner. Practised in Dublin as a surgeon, and then moved to Bath and practised as a physician; was appointed physician to the City Infirmary and the General Hospital. 'He loved science and disliked the trade of medicine' and did not cultivate a large practice. He wrote extensively on medical and pathological subjects, but his favourite theme was medical reform. His papers on medical reform from 1807 to 1820 were published anonymously, no doubt because he was highly critical of the Royal College of Physicians and a strong supporter of the general practitioner. In 1838–9 he was President of the Provincial Medical and Surgical Association, and he took part in the foundation of the Association. He was also an advocate of 'The Science of Phrenology'.

PMSJ (1844).

BAYNTON, Thomas (1761–1820). Surgeon-apothecary of Bristol who insisted on being called a 'surgeon'. He cultivated a successful practice amongst the upper classes in Kingswood, leaving his shop in the old market to his partner. He was vain and tight-fisted, and practised midwifery extensively believing it paid well. He considered himself an adept surgeon, but no one else did. Disappointed at not being appointed to the Bristol Infirmary, he nevertheless acquired fame through the invention of a genuinely effective method of treating leg ulcers which brought him patients from far and wide. He earned a large income, speculated in land successfully, and died a wealthy man allowing his son to lead a leisurely life as a country gentleman.

DNB; BIBM 2; *Proceedings of the Royal Society of Medicine*, 8 (2), 95–102.

BRODERIP, William (died *c.* 1824). Apothecary in Bristol. He was apprenticed to Joseph Shapland, apothecary of Bristol, who took him into partnership in 1775. Broderip was a prime example of the way that apothecaries in the late eighteenth century could thrive and make very high incomes from dispensing vast quantities of medicine. He lived well, owning a town and country house, but when the golden age of the apothecary came to an end at the beginning of the nineteenth century he lost almost all his possessions and practice, and died in penury. he was considered a 'dull stick' by most of his colleagues and was shunned by the physicians of Bristol, partly because he was a mere apothecary, and partly because of his skill in persuading patients to stay under his care rather than that of a physician.

BIBM 2.

BURROWS, George Man (1776–1846), MRCS LSA, MD St Andrews, LRCP, FRCP. Born at Chalk near Gravesend. Educated at King's School, Canterbury, apprenticed to a surgeon-apothecary in Rochester, and then trained at Guy's and St Thomas's Hospital medical school. Practised in London as a general practitioner and was the first chairman of the Association of Apothecaries and Surgeon-Apothecaries, an association of which was undoubtedly the main driving force. He has sometimes been called the 'father of general practice'. His views on the Apothecaries Act are described in chapter 7. They led to his resignation not only from the Association he had dominated and from the Society of Apothecaries, but also from general practice, and he subsequently practised as a physician with a special interest in insanity. Sadly, his reputation was gravely damaged when he ordered the detention of a young man who was thought to be violently and dangerously insane. Burrows was an honourable man and acted in good faith, but gave the order to detain the patient without ever having seen him. There are certain parallels between the career of Burrows and that of A. T. Thomson (q.v.). Thomson was more successful in his lifetime, but in the end Burrows had the greatest influence on the development of the medical profession.

F. Tubbs, 'Centenary of the Death of G. M. Burrows', *British Medical Bulletin*, 5 (1947), 83; Memoir, *LMG* (11 Dec. 1846); *Gazette of Health*, 14 (1829), 781.

CARR, William. Four generations of the Carr family, all medical practitioners, are known to have practised medicine in the eighteenth and nineteenth centuries. William Carr I (b. 1715) lived in Settle in Yorks. William Carr II (1745–1821) was apothecary to Leeds Infirmary from 1774 to 1781, and practised thereafter as a surgeon-apothecary in Elland, near Leeds, Yorks. William Carr III (1785–1861) (no formal qualifications, having been in practice pre-1815) also practised near Leeds at Gomersal. William Carr IV (1828–1905), FRCS, became a consultant surgeon. Quotations in this study are largely from the diaries of William Carr II.

Wellcome MS 5203–7.

CHAMBERLAINE, William (1749–1822). General practitioner of Aylesbury St. Clerkenwell. Secretary to the Society for the Relief of Widows and Orphans of Medical Men in London, of which he was one of the founders. Author of a few medical tracts, including one of historical interest on apprenticeship (see chapter 2).

LMPJ 48 (1822), 279.

CLARK, Sir James, Bart. (1788–1870). Physician, LRCS (Edin.) 1809, MD (Edin.) 1817, LRCP (London) 1826, FRS 1832. Born in Banffshire, he started as a writer to the signet (lawyer) in Scotland, and soon turned to medicine, his first post being that of assistant surgeon in the Navy. He came to London in 1826, and soon became a fashionable physician and medical attendant to royalty. His practice increased steadily until he became involved in the case of Lady Flora Hastings, whose fatal abdominal tumour he is reputed to have mistaken for a pregnancy, thus appearing to confirm the unjust slur on the lady's character. At all events the blame was placed on his shoulders and the affair had an immediate effect on his practice which took some years to pass off; but it did not affect his part in medical and university politics, and he was mainly responsible for creating the medical side of the University of London. His importance in this study lies in his sensible and influential views, clearly expressed, on medical reform and the role of the general practitioner in medicine.

DNB; Munk's Roll.

CLEGG, James (1679–1755), MD (Aberdeen) 1729. Presbyterian minister in Chapel-en-Frith. He married Ann Champion from Edale who bore him nine children. Needing to supplement his income, he farmed and then practised medicine, having learnt the rudiments from Dr Adam Holland, a physician in Macclesfield. He practised at first amongst the poor, but by 1722 (aged forty-three) he had a large practice amongst the well-to-do as well. Threatened by the Anglican clergy with prosecution in the ecclesiastical courts for misusing his position as a minister to obtain patients, and for practising without a licence, he applied first to Edinburgh and then, successfully, to Aberdeen, buying an MD on the recommendation of three physicians, two of whom were dissenting ministers. He practised solely as a physician, doing the minimum of surgery and, as far as one can determine, no obstetrics; but, like many provincial physicians of the time, he dispensed drugs for his patients, having his own elaborate pharmacopoeia. His work as a physician was known and respected as far as Manchester and Sheffield. His diary has survived.

'Diary of James Clegg', *Derbyshire Record Society* (1978,1979, 1981); H. Kirke, *Extracts from the Diary . . . of James Clegg* (1899).

CROSSE, John Green (1790–1850) of Norwich, FRS 1834, FRCS 1843. The son of a Suffolk yeoman, he was apprenticed to a surgeon-apothecary, studied at St George's Hospital and the Windmill St. school of anatomy in London, and then, after a spell in Paris, went to the Dublin medical school as demonstrator in anatomy. In 1815 he settled in Norwich where he became known locally and nationally as an exceptionally able surgeon and accoucheur. By the 1840s he was earning £2,500 p.a. from (to use his own words) 'a large general practice in medicine, surgery, and midwifery, consulting practice from 80–100 doctors a year, senior surgeon to the [Norfolk and Norwich] Hospital, surgeon to the Magdalen Hospital and much vaccination, 30–40 weekly at my home.' In this respect his practice was typical of the successful provincial surgeons of his time.

DNB; V. Mary Crosse, *A Surgeon in the Early Nineteenth Century* (1968); the midwifery notebooks of John Greene Crosse, Wellcome MS 1916–17.

DENMAN, Thomas (1733–1815), MD (Aberdeen) 1764, physician-accoucheur in London. His texts and teaching were a major influence on the practice of midwifery at all levels in the late eighteenth and early nineteenth century. His descriptions of the mechanism and conduct of normal labours were clear and accurate and he advised a very conservative approach in the practice of midwifery—probably too conservative. He acquired an extensive practice amongst the wealthy and aristocracy, occupying 'the first position in midwifery' after the death of William Hunter in 1783. He handed on his practice to his son-in-law, Richard (later Sir Richard) Croft who was present at, and blamed for, the death in labour of Princess Charlotte and her baby.

H. R. Spencer, *The History of British Midwifery from 1650 to 1800* (1927).

FLINDERS, Matthew (1755–1802), surgeon of Donington, Lincolnshire. Son of John Flinders, surgeon (1713–76), and grandson of John Flinders (1682–1741), farmer and grazier of Nottinghamshire and then of Lincolnshire. His first wife bore him eight children (including premature stillborn twins and a boy who died aged two months) and the oldest son, also Matthew, (b. 16 March 1774) became a captain in the Navy and the famous explorer and cartographer of Southern Australia. Flinders' first wife died of malaria but he married again, and his second wife bore him another daughter. Matthew Flinders suffered numerous bouts of malaria (treating himself with 'the bark') and finally died aged 52, probably of carcinoma of the stomach. Further details of his life are included in chapter 5.

Notebooks, Lincoln Archives Office.

GOOD, John Mason (1764–1827), FRS 1805, MD (Marischal College, Aberdeen) 1820, LRCP 1822. Played an active part in the General Pharmaceutical Association of 1794 writing, at the request of friends, *A History of Medicine so far as it relates to the Profession of the Apothecary* (1795), see chapter 6. Practised in London from 1793 to 1820 as a surgeon-apothecary/general practitioner and, after a bad start, gained a high reputation by his writing. From 1820 he practised as a physician. Was known as a scholar who was familiar with 'Hebrew, Spanish, Portuguese, Russian, Arabic, Sanskrit, Chinese and other languages'; but his published works, including his *Study of Medicine* in four volumes, proved to be disappointing. He was religious and benevolent, possessing exceptional powers of acquiring knowledge but no creative ability, so that he produced works of great erudition but no permanent value.

DNB; London Medical Repository and Review, NS 4.

GREEN, Joseph Henry (1791–1863), MRCS 1815, PRCS 1850, Surgeon of St Thomas's Hospital and Professor of Surgery at King's College, London, elected in 1830. In 1834, when his father died and left him a large fortune, Green gave up practice and his chair at King's College, intending to devote his time to the publication of the philosophical views of his close friend Coleridge who died in 1834 and named Green as his literary executor. Green's contributions on medical reform, which were moderate in tone (e.g. *Distinction without Separation: A Letter to the President of the College of Surgeons*, 1831), were widely quoted in the medical periodicals. Although his work may now seem humdrum, he was regarded as one of the most thoughtful writers in the field of medical politics in his time.

DNB; Z. Cope, *History of the Royal College of Surgeons* (1959).

GUTHRIE, George James (1785–1856). Obtained the diploma MRCS at the age of fifteen. He served as an army surgeon, and saw service in the Peninsular War and at Waterloo. He was appointed surgeon to the Westminster Hospital and President of the Royal College of Surgeons in 1833, 1841, and 1854. A strong individualist whose views, always forcible and often wittily expressed, showed an unpredictable mixture of liberalism, bigotry, and common sense. A terror to the lazy student, and a great believer in surgery as a specialty to be practised by 'pure surgeons', he was an early exponent of the view that general practitioners were of necessity members of an inferior branch—'General practitioners of nothing' he called them—and he was the main force behind the College of Surgeons when it succeeded in preventing the establishment of a College of General Practitioners in the 1840s.

Lancet (1850), i. 728–36.

HARRISON, Edward (1766–1838), physician, MD (Edin.) 1784. Studied medicine in London, Paris, and Edinburgh. Settled in Lincolnshire in the early 1780s, first at Louth and then at Horncastle. Founded the Horncastle Dispensary, the Horncastle General Book Club, and the Lincolnshire Medical Benevolent Society of which he was the first president. His efforts to introduce reforms in the medical profession are recounted in chapter 6. They left him embittered by the behaviour of the London College of Physicians who were unwise enough to prosecute him (unsuccessfully) in 1828 for practising in London without the licence of the College. With remarkable incompetence, the College chose a case which Harrison had treated which was clearly surgical, and the case was dismissed, depriving Harrison of his longed-for opportunity to challenge the College's jurisdiction in open court. He died a wealthy but disappointed man. Not only were his attempts at medical reform unsuccessful, but his views on spinal disease (one of his great interests) were labelled by his contemporaries as 'peculiar'; as, indeed, they were.

BFMR 6 (1838); *Gazette of Health*, 15 (1830).

HARRISON, Job (1753–89), apothecary of Chester. His father was a yeoman holding small leasehold properties near Alford. One son (William), a grocer and ironfounder, was mayor of Chester in 1795–6; the second son was Job who was apprenticed in 1786 to John Crowe, apothecary of Chester, for seven years at a premium of £105. In October 1774 Job Harrison went to Edinburgh as a medical student staying until April 1776 when he left without any formal qualification to enter into partnership with his former master. The partnership agreement gave Harrison a one-third share for the first five years, and bound him to visit all the patients outside Chester and attend all calls between 10 p.m. and 8 a.m. Harrison, who was a friend of Currie of Liverpool and Haygarth of Chester, had an extensive practice amongst the middle and professional classes. It was said that 'his abilities and humane disposition obtained him the countenance, encouragement and preference of a respectable part of the inhabitants', and he was noted for 'his moderate use of medicine and moderate bills'.

Chester Record Office, the Harrison papers, G/HS/72–106.

KAY, Richard (1716–51), practitioner of Baldingstone near Bury, Lancashire. Apprenticed to his father, Robert Kay (1684–1750). Initially uncertain whether to enter the ministry, or become a medical practitioner, at the age of twenty-seven he settled for medicine and went to London as pupil to Mr Steade, the apothecary to Guy's Hospital where he attended lectures on surgery and two courses of midwifery under William Smellie. He returned to practice in partnership with his father. A deeply religious and humane man, he left a diary which provides a vivid picture of day-to-day medical practice in the provinces. He and most of his family died in an outbreak of fever (probably typhus) in 1751. It is impossible to read this diary and not feel a warm regard for this man and for his devotion to his patients.

'Diary of Richard Kay', *Chetham Society*, 16 (1968).

KERRISON, Robert Masters (1776–1847), MRCS, MD (Edin.) 1820, LRCP 1820, FRS. Practised for many years in London as a general practitioner before becoming a physician. He was a member of the committee of the Association of Apothecaries and Surgeon-Apothecaries from 1812 to 1815, and his two publications *An Inquiry into the Present State of the Medical Profession* (1814) and *Observations on a Bill for the Better Regulating of the Medical Profession* (1815) were influential. He was one of that small but important group of London general practitioners in the early decades of the nineteenth-century who were often successful and wealthy, who took part in medical politics, wrote short books or pamphlets on medical reform, and sometimes after many years of general practice acquired an MD (nearly always from Scotland) and practised as physicians.

Munk's Roll; obit., *Medical Directory* (1848).

LEE, William (d. 1780), surgeon-apothecary and farmer of Odiham, Hants. A ledger of his survives, but nothing more is known of him.

Wellcome MS 3974.

MCCULLOCH, John (1757–1853), MRCS, surgeon of Liverpool. Gained some early medical experience on slave ships before training in Edinburgh. After early but unremunerative practice in Saddleworth, West Riding, McCulloch settled in Liverpool about 1790. He held no hospital appointments but had an exceptionally active and long practice in obstetrics, especially amongst the poor and those of modest income in Liverpool. His obituaries portray a humane, skilful, and greatly respected man. A surviving account book records details of over 4,800 deliveries. He survived three sons to one of whom, Samuel (1792–1853), he had passed his practice in about 1830.

London and Provincial Medical Directory (1854), 821–2. My grateful thanks to Dr Paul Laxton of Liverpool for this biographical note.

MAURICE, Thelwall (1767–1830), surgeon-apothecary of Marlborough, Wilts. Attended St Thomas's Hospital, and then settled in Marlborough at the age of twenty-five in partnership with Dr Pinckney. Members of the Maurice family have continued to practise in Marlborough ever since, and the practice claims to be the oldest group practice in the country. Some early records of the practice have survived.

BMJ, 12 June 1982, 1756.

PARKINSON, James (1755–1824), MRCS. Surgeon/general practitioner, palaeontologist, and member of the Geological Society of London. Practised in succession to his father (John Parkinson, surgeon), in Hoxton Square, East London, and was a founder member of the committee of the Association of

Apothecaries and Surgeon-Apothecaries of which he was the chairman from 1817 to 1819/20, immediately after the resignation of George Man Burrows. He was a member of the radical London Corresponding Society and in 1794 was examined under oath before the Privy Council in connection with the 'pop-gun' plot to assassinate George III. He wrote a variety of books, including a number of works on domestic medicine. His famous 'Essay on the shaking palsy', from which the disease Parkinsonism derives its name, was published in 1817, but its importance was not recognized in the author's lifetime. He is often described as a physician, or even as a neurologist; he was in fact a London general practitioner working in an area which was not as poor then as it was later. Although he was a reformer, publishing a pamphlet in 1794 entitled 'Revolutions without Bloodshed . . .', and was closely involved in the Association of Apothecaries, he appears to have written nothing on medical reform.

DNB; L. G. Rowntree, *Bulletin of the Johns Hopkins Hospital*, 23 (1912), 33.

PAXTON, Richard, of Maldon in Essex, practised as a surgeon-apothecary and man-midwife from about 1755 to 1799 with a partner (name unknown). Finally sold his practice, weakly and reluctantly, to a young man who was clearly a rogue, if not an imposter. The account of this affair and of a number of his surgical and obstetric cases survive in a memoir of his time in practice which he wrote at the end of his career.

Wellcome MS 3820.

PEART, Henry (1808–67), LSA 1829, MRCS 1830, general practitioner, Feckenham, Worcs. Born in York into a Roman Catholic family. His parents appear to have been landowning farmers in Pocklington. He spent a brief period attending medical lectures in Liverpool from 1827–8 before going to London to study and qualify in medicine. He then went to Paris for three months to attend medical lectures and anatomical dissections. He probably practised briefly in Wolverhampton but had settled in Feckenham by 1835 if not earlier where he was appointed Poor Law surgeon to the Feckenham district of the Alcester Union. There he married, had two children, and continued in practice until his death. He seems to have led a quiet and undistinguished life so that his records may be regarded as those of the average medical student and general practitioner of his time.

Warwick RO 'A Doctor's Cash Book', CR1840, Wellcome MS 5263.

PENNINGTON, Robert Rainey (1764–1849), MRCS 1787. General practitioner in London with a large practice amongst the wealthy which allowed him to accumulate a very large fortune. He once boasted that he had attended every member of the Cabinet and every judge upon the bench. He was 'a great physicker', making sure whenever possible that his patients continued endlessly with the medicine he had prescribed. In this he resembled William Broderip (*q.v.*). Although sociable and hospitable, he never attended societies and never wrote or published. It seems he was not considered by his colleagues to be a particularly able doctor. Such was his reputation for success, however, that while in his eighties he was elected President of the National Association of General Practitioners (see chapter 13). His greatest gift was probably his ability to work with the minimum of sleep, visiting his 'town' patients in the daytime and his 'country' patients in the night.

J. F. Clarke, *Autobiographical Recollections* (1874).

PULSFORD, Benjamin and William, surgeons in partnership at Wells, Somerset. Benjamin (1716–84), who was the uncle of William (1737–65), had previously been in partnership with his uncle, Christopher Lucas (*c.*1676–1756), surgeon of Wells and friend of the physician Claver Morris, MD (1659–1756). Following the premature death of William, Benjamin Pulsford took his son Lucas (1750–1819) into partnership and the family partnership seems to have died out with the latter's death. Benjamin Pulsford owned property and land and counted amongst his friends lawyers, clergy, and farmers. His interests, shared by his nephew, seem to have lain in the direction of horses and outdoor sports such as shooting. William Pulsford earned the accolade of a memorial tablet in the cloisters of Wells Cathedral, although a modest one compared to the memorial of Claver Morris. The unusually comprehensive ledger kept by William Pulsford from 1757 to the mid-1760s, exceptionally rich in clinical, social, and economic detail, has survived.

Somerset CRO, Taunton: doctor's journal, 1757–65. DD/FS Box 48.

RIVINGTON, Walter (1835–97), MRCS 1859, LSA 1860, MB (London) 1863, FRCS 1863, MS (London) 1864, surgeon to the London Hospital and author of *The Medical Profession* (Dublin 1879), for which he is chiefly remembered. He possessed a wonderful memory, was regarded as the best amateur chess player in England, and could deliver a long lecture without notes which was word-perfect to his printed text. He was dean of the Medical School and 'the bent of his mind was essentially literary'. He was not noted for surgical ability. Died of typhoid contracted from eating oysters.

Lancet (1897), i. 1380; *BMJ* (1897), i. 1255; *London Hospital Gazette* (June 1897), 23.

RUMSEY, Henry Wyldbore (1809–76), MRCS (1831), FRCS (by examination), MD Dublin (Hon.) 1867, FRS (1874). Studied medicine at Nottingham and St George's Hospital, London; surgeon to Gloucester Infirmary, then left to practise in Cheltenham. In 1835 he was appointed Honorary Secretary to the Poor Law Committee of the Provincial Medical and Surgical Association. Through this appointment he acquired a wide knowledge and deep interest in the care of the sick poor and state medicine. 'To him State Medicine was not a word; it was the central idea of his life', and he was instrumental in the appointment of the Sanitary Committee in 1862, leading to the Public Health Act of 1872. His best known work is 'Essays in State Medicine' (1857).

BMJ (1876) and *Medical Times* (1876).

SIMPSON, John (1793–1867), physician, MD (Edin.) 1821. Born into a medical family in Knaresborough, he settled in Bradford in 1822 where he practised as a physician until 1825 when his uncle died and left his estate to John Simpson. A manuscript journal for the year 1825 has survived and been published. In 1827 Simpson married, and when his wife, who came from the old Cumberland family of Hudleston, inherited property from her grandfather both John Simpson and his wife adopted the name of Hudleston. Simpson's account of practice in Bradford in 1825 shows that there was an excess of medical practitioners, especially physicians, in that part of Yorkshire. Simpson was able to live in reasonable style, one assumes, because of private sources of income.

E. Wilmot (ed.), *The Journal of Dr John Simpson of Bradford* (Bradford, 1981).

SMITH, Richard, junior (1772–1843), surgeon of Bristol and surgeon to the Infirmary from 1796. His father, also a surgeon, likewise held an appointment at the Infirmary. Richard junior was apprenticed to his father until the latter died suddenly in 1791. He was then 'turned over' to Mr Godfrey Lowe, the senior surgeon to the Infirmary, and it was while he was a student that he discovered the old records of the Bristol Infirmary (founded in 1737) were being destroyed, and took them home to preserve them. This began his life-long collection of a vast amount of material about medicine in Bristol and the West Country interlaced with numerous letters, memoirs, anecdotes and, most of all, his own inimitable biographies of medical men, and comments on medicine in the city. These were bound in fourteen large volumes, now known as the Bristol Infirmary Biographical Memoirs, a source of the greatest interest to historians of medicine, for he was a superb natural writer and a brilliant biographer. By temperament Smith was convivial and cheerful; and he was an enthusiastic freemason. He married Anne Eugenia, daughter of Henry Creswick in 1802. They had no children.

BIBM; A. L. Eyre-Brook, 'Richard Smith junior and his Life and Times, *Bristol Medical Chirurgical Journal*, 84 (1) (1969).

SOLOMON, Samuel, of Liverpool (d. 1819). He regarded himself as a physician and claimed to possess an MD from Aberdeen. He was in fact a highly successful proprietor of patent medicines and quack remedies who accumulated a fortune as 'The inventor and sole proprieter of the "Cordial Balm of Gilead", "Ante

Impetigenes", "Abstergent Lotion", "Detergent Ointment" and "Boerhaave's Red Pills Nos. 1 and 2".' But his fame rested on the Cordial Balm (said to be chiefly spirits of wine), which was 'celebrated in every newspaper in England' as he spent thousands of pounds on advertising. He also published *A Guide to Health; or, Advice to Both Sexes, with an Essay on a Certain Disease, Seminal Weakness, and a Destructive Habit of a Private Nature, Also an Address to Parents, Tutors and Guardians of Youth* (1796) which, not surprisingly with such a promising title, went into many editions. He lived at Gilead House, and left his business in his will to his sons Abraham and John and his clerk Ebenezer Daniell. 'Sensible of the odium of quackery and advertisements, Dr Solomon gave his son a proper education, and he entered the world as a regular physician.' But it seems that the son was ostracized and, failing to obtain practice either as a physician or surgeon, 'he was obliged to return to Liverpool and sell balm of Gilead.'

Wellcome MS 14,314. Further details from *Williamson's Liverpool Advertiser* and other local sources were kindly supplied by Adrian Allan, Assistant Archivist to Liverpool University.

THOMSON, Anthony Todd (1778–1849), MD (Edin.), MRCS, FRCP. Born and educated in Edinburgh. Shortly after graduation he came to London to set up in Sloane Street as a general practitioner where he rapidly became exceptionally successful, earning £3,000 a year. He lectured on medical botany and wrote extensively on therapeutics. All through his life, until his seventies, he rose at 5 a.m., wrote for three hours, spent the whole day visiting patients or lecturing, returned late for dinner and then worked until two or three in the morning, never allowing himself more than three or four hours' sleep. In 1814 he joined George Man Burrows (q.v.) and Mr Royston as joint editor of the *London Medical Repository* with the intention of making it the voice of the Association of Apothecaries and Surgeon-Apothecaries. He played a major part in the affairs of that association and in the introduction of the Apothecaries Act. In 1826 he became a licentiate of the Royal College of Physicians, played a major part in the foundation of the University of London and was appointed there as the first professor of Materia Medica and Therapeutics. In 1832 he was appointed to the chair of Medical Jurisprudence as well.

Memoir, *Medical Times*, 20 (1849).

TRYE, Charles Brandon (d. 1811), FRS, surgeon of Gloucester, and senior surgeon to the Gloucester Infirmary. Trained in London under John Hunter and at the Westminster Infirmary. He was remembered as a good surgeon and an especially kind and considerate master to his apprentices and pupils.

MPJ 26 (1811).

WAKLEY, Thomas (1795–1862), MRCS 1817, general practitioner in London (1818–23), founder (in 1823) and editor of the *Lancet*. Elected MP for Finsbury in 1835 and coroner in 1839. The son of a Tory Devon farmer who admired his son's success but hated his radicalism; he was strongly built, athletic, and a boxer in his youth. Apprenticed to an apothecary in Taunton at the age of fifteen, he left early to become assistant to a well-known surgeon in Henley-on-Thames. In 1815 he enrolled as a pupil at the Borough Hospitals and attended the Webb private medical school of anatomy. His early years in practice were marred by severe injuries inflicted during a murderous attack which nearly killed him (the culprits were never discovered), by the loss of his house and furniture in a fire and a false accusation of arson by the insurance company, and by his wife's dislike of the neighbourhood in which he practised and his status as a general practitioner. As editor of the *Lancet* he was obsessed by hatred of the medical corporations and the nepotism amongst the honorary staff of the London Hospitals. His attacks were written in violent and intemperate language (initially entertaining but soon tedious) which should not detract from the reality of the evils he exposed or the excellence of the *Lancet* as one of the leading medical periodicals in both scientific and political fields. Wakley was never afraid of publishing views contrary to his own. His friendship with William Cobbett stimulated a radicalism which was in tune with his pugilistic nature, but his greatest successes as a reformer were achieved as a Member of Parliament and coroner, where he expressed himself forcibly and effectively in more moderate language than he used in the leading articles in the *Lancet*. Although he always protested that he was the friend of the general practitioner, his ambivalent attitude to general practice (due in part to his unhappy early experiences in practice, and in part to his hatred of the term 'general practitioner' rather than 'surgeon'), meant that his support was less than wholehearted. Although traditionally described as a great medical reformer, his achievements in medical reform were hampered by prickly prejudices, by the ridiculous use of nicknames (hospital surgeons were 'bats', Scotch doctors 'dubs', the joint secretaries of the National Association of General Practitioners 'snipe' and 'sneak') and by personal attacks which were often gratuitously offensive. His use of ridicule and satire was that of a crude bruiser rather than a polished fencer. Towards the end of his life he recognized and regretted this use of a style which did less than justice to his considerable energy, intelligence, and ability.

DNB; S. Squire Sprigge, *Life and Times of Thomas Wakley* (1899); J. F. Clarke, *Autobiographical Recollections* (1874).

WARD, Danvers, MRCS 1787. Practised in Bristol in the late eighteenth and early nineteenth century. As a surgeon he had ambitions to hold an honorary appointment at the Bristol Infirmary and tried twice, in 1783 and 1791, but failed to get elected. He practised mainly as an accoucheur and acquired a large obstetric practice, enjoying the exercise of his considerable obstetric skills.

BIBM 3 and 4; G. Munro Smith, *A History of the Bristol Royal Infirmary* (Bristol, 1917).

YEATMAN, John Charleton (1790–c.1841), MRCS (1809), surgeon-apothecary. Born in Bristol, his father was the apothecary and his uncle one of the surgeons to the Bristol Infirmary. He embarked for America at the age of five where it was intended he should become a merchant; but he returned, served an apprenticeship with his father, and became a pupil at the Infirmary in 1807. In 1808 he went to St George's Hospital in London and in 1809 became an army surgeon, seeing service in the Peninsular War and resigning at the peace of Amiens. He had intended to settle in Bristol on the promise of his uncle that he could succeed to his practice, but in the event his uncle's own son changed his mind about his career and decided on surgery, displacing the disappointed nephew. Instead, John Yeatman settled in Frome in Somerset where, against all expectations because the competition was formidable, he succeeded, published a number of papers, and, unusually for a surgeon-apothecary, took pupils as well as apprentices—'the former for one year or more, the latter for five years with liberty to leave at four.' For this he was accused of presumptuousness by his medical colleagues, but he defended himself vigorously and successfully. He became a successful West Country practitioner and Surgeon Extraordinary to the Duke of Gloucester. His publications suggest an energetic, intelligent, observant, and thoughtful man, who contributed to the reform of his branch of the medical profession.

BIBM 8, 281.

Select Bibliography

PARLIAMENTARY PAPERS

Report of the Select Committee on Medical Education, PP 1834 (602, I, II, and III), XIII

Report of the Royal Commission for Inquiring into the Administration and Operation of the Poor Laws, PP 1834 (44), XXVII–XXXIX

Reports from the Select Committee to Inquire into the Administration of the Relief of the Poor under the Provisions of the Poor Law Amendment Act, PP 1837, XVII, Parts I and II

Report from the Select Committee on the Health of Towns, PP 1840 (384), XI

Reports on the Sanitary Condition of the Labouring Population, PP 1842 (HL.–), XXVI, 1842 (HL.–), XXVII

First, second and third Reports from the Select Committee on Medical Poor Relief, PP 1844 (312, 387, 531), IX

First Report of the Royal Commission on the State of Large Towns and Populous Districts, PP 1844 (572), XVII

Reports of the Select Committee on Medical Registration, PP 1847 (620), IX, and PP 1847–8 (210 and 702), XV

Reports of the Royal Commission on the Health of the Metropolis, PP 1847–8 (888), XXXII

Report from the Select Committee on Medical Poor Relief, PP 1854 (348), XII

PERIODICALS (arranged chronologically by date of first publication)

Medical Observations and Inquiries (1757–84)

London (The) Medical Journal (1781–90), which continued as *Medical Facts and Observations* (1791–1800), cont. as *Medical and Physical Journal* (1799–1814), cont. as *London Medical and Physical Journal* (1815–33), cont. as *Medical Quarterly Review* (1833–5), cont. as *British and Foreign Medical Review* (1836–47), cont. as *British and Foreign Medico-Chirurgical Review* (1848–77)

Medical Facts and Observations (1791–1800)

Medical (The) and Chirurgical Review (1794–1808)

Medical (The) and Physical Journal (1799–1814)

Edinburgh (The) Medical and Surgical Journal (1805–55), cont. as *The Edinburgh Medical Journal* (1855–)

London (The) Medical and Surgical Spectator (1808–9)

Medico-Chirurgical Transactions (1809–1907), cont. as *Proceedings of the Royal Society of Medicine* (1907–1977), cont. as *The Journal of the Royal Society of Medicine* (1978–)

London (The) Medical, Surgical and Pharmaceutical Repository (1814), cont. as *London Medical Repository: Monthly Journal and Review* (1814–28), cont. as *London Medical and Surgical Journal* (1828–37)

London (The) Medical Repository: Monthly Journal and Review (1814–28)

London (The) Medical and Physical Journal (1815–33)

Gazette of Health (The Monthly) (1816–31)

Medico-Chirurgical (The) Journal (1818–20) cont. as *Medico-Chirurgical Review and Journal of Medical Science* (1820–24) cont. as *Medico-Chirurgical Review* (1824–7), and joined with the *British and Foreign Medical Review* (q.v.) to become the *British and Foreign Medico-Chirurgical Review* (1848–77)

Medico-Chirurgical Review and Journal of Medical Science (1820–24)

Transactions of the Associated Apothecaries and Surgeon-Apothecaries of England and Wales (1823)

Lancet (The) (1823–)

Medico-Chirurgical Review (1824–47)

London (The) Medical Gazette (1827–51) joined with the *Medical Times* to become *The Medical Times and Gazette* (1852–85)

Midland (The) Medical and Surgical Reporter (1828–32), cont. as *Transactions of the Provincial Medical and Surgical Association* (1833–53)

London (The) Medical and Surgical Journal (1828–37)

Glasgow (The) Medical Journal (1828–)

North (The) of England Medical and Surgical Journal (1830–1)

Doctor (The): A Medical Penny Magazine (1832–7)

Medical (The) Quarterly Review (1833–5)

British (The) and Foreign Medical Review (1836–47)

Medical (The) Times (1839–51) joined with the *London Medical Gazette* to become the *Medical Times and Gazette* (1852–85)

Provincial Medical and Surgical Journal (1840–52), cont. as *Association Medical Journal* (1853–6), cont. as *British Medical Journal* (1857–)

Transactions of the National Association of General Practitioners in Medicine, Surgery and Midwifery (1845–6)

British (The) and Foreign Medico-Chirurgical Review (1848–77)

Medical (The) Times and Gazette (1852–85)

Association (The) Medical Journal (1853–6)

Edinburgh (The) Medical Journal (1855–)

British Medical Journal (1857–)

St Bartholomew's Hospital Reports (1865–)

London Medical Press and Circular (1866), cont. as *Medical Press and Circular* (1866–)

MANUSCRIPT SOURCES (and published diaries)

Bedfordshire County Record Office, Bedford
Samuel Whitbread correspondence, late eighteenth and early nineteenth century, concerning parish surgeons and an account of an outbreak of fever at Langford, 1801–2.

Bristol Record Office, The Council House, Bristol
Bristol Infirmary Biographical Memoirs (the papers of Richard Smith junior (1772–1843)), 14 vols.

Cheshire County Record Office, Chester
Letters, etc. of Job Harrison of Chester, apothecary. The Harrison papers, G/HS/72–106.

Dorset County Record Office, Dorchester
Medical notebook of J. Chaplin (1667–1715); 15 PHI.
Records of Robert Battiscombe, Apothecary-in-Ordinary to King George III (1781–4), D/239.

Herefordshire County Record Office, Hereford
Case histories recorded by Dr Martin Dunne, Gatley collection, F/76/IV/67–242.

Gloucestershire County Record Office, Gloucester
Correspondence of George Charleton, surgeon (1826–34), D.4432/1–4.
Correspondence of C. B. Trye, surgeon (1787), D.303 C1.
Records of Ann Stanley, female quack (1784) PC 1159.
Account book of Danvers Ward, surgeon-accoucheur (1786–7), D.1928 A3.

Lincoln Archives Office
The diaries/ledgers of Matthew Flinders, surgeon of Donington, Lincs. (1755–1802).

LONDON

British Library
Orders to Mr Fentham, apothecary of Nottingham (*c.*1740), MS 34, 769, ff. 116–53.

Guildhall Library
Records of the Society of Apothecaries.

Public Record Office, Kew
Diaries of W. Gillespie, naval surgeon, ADM 101.102/1.

Royal College of General Practitioners Library
Case-book of unidentified practitioner (1726–8), no. 711.
Day-book of a medical practitioner near Leeds (1702–10).

Royal College of Surgeons of England Library
Minutes of Council (1845–8).
Case-books of Camberwell general practitioner (1831–6).

Royal Society of Medicine Library
Student notebooks of John Greene Crosse, 285.g.11.
St Thomas's Hospital Medical School Library
Correspondence of Richard Weekes and Hampton Weekes (1801–2), surgeon-apothecary and medical student.

Wellcome Institute for the History of Medicine: manuscript collection
Letters of William Budd, physician (1840s).
Diaries of John Dixon, general practitioner of Bermondsey (1859–62), MS 2141–3.
J. Haighton, syllabus of lectures on midwifery (1808 and 1814), MS 2665–6.
Medical practitioner's day-book (catalogued as pharmaceutical chemist), Charles Heygate, Northants. (1852–70), MS 2833.
Account book of T. H. Holberton, apothecary/general practitioner of Hampton Court (1829–33), MS 2862.
William Jenner of Berkeley, Glos., diary of visits and fees received, etc. (1794), MS 3018.
Account book of Thomas Mister, surgeon-apothecary of Shipton-on-Stour (1776–81), MS 3584.
Medical case-book of Alexander Morgan, surgeon of Bristol (1714–47), MS 3631.
Case-book of Richard Paxton, surgeon, of Maldon, Essex (1753–99), MS 3820.
Account book of J. L. Petit, physician of London (1751–9), MS 3855.
Account book of 'unidentified apothecary' (1774–80), MS 3974. Now identified as Mr Lee, surgeon-apothecary of Odiham, Hants.
Professional memoranda, London (c.1820), MS 4008.
Account books of Thomas Roots, medical practitioner of Kingston-upon-Thames (1749–56), MS 4254–5.
Visiting lists and diaries of Buxton Shillitoe, general practitioner (1851–83), MS 4528–63.
Medical notes and prescriptions of F. P. Smith, general practitioner of Aylsham, Norfolk (1818–35), MS 4633.
Account book of James Steedman, medical practitioner of Kinross (1758–60), MS 4702.
Apprentice's case-notes by 'W. W.' (1755), MS 4958.
Notebooks of the Carr family, surgeons near Leeds (1780–1853), MS 5203–7.
The obstetric notebooks of John Greene Crosse of Norwich (1816–43), MS 1916–17.

Northampton Record Office
Letters of Poyntz Adams, medical student and practitioner, to his uncle and patron, the Revd Mr Thomas of Farndon, ZA 6227–93.
Ledgers of Mr Sabin, surgeon of Towcester, Northants. (1797–1831), misc. ledger 687–8, YZ 1770.

Overseer's Accounts and Private Medical Bills, (various)—at most record offices listed here.

Sheffield Public Library, local collection
Ledger of William Elmhirst, surgeon of Leeds (1768–73), FH/13, 63398.

Somerset County Record Office, Taunton
Ledger of William Pulsford, surgeon of Wells (1757–64), catalogued as 'Doctor's journal—? Benjamin Pulsford', DD/FS Box 48.

Warwick Record Office
Cash-book of Henry Peart, general practitioner of Feckenham, Worcs. (1821–31), CR 1840.

Wiltshire County Record Office, Trowbridge
Overseer's accounts (1756–1820).

Privately Possessed Records
Student's notebook, unknown authorship (c.1846) in the possession of Mr Philip Awdry, FRCS, of Oxford.
Records of the Maurice family, surgeon-apothecaries and general practitioners in Marlborough, Wilts., from the late eighteenth century to the present, in the possession of Dr Dick Maurice of Marlborough.

Published Diaries
W. Brockbank and F. Kenworthy (eds.), 'The Diary of Richard Kay (1716–51) of Baldingstone near Bury', *The Chetham Society*, 16 (1968).
B. Cozens Hardy (ed.), *The Diary of Silas Neville, 1767–88* (Oxford, 1950).
Vanessa S. Doe (ed.), 'The Diary of James Clegg of Chapel-en-Frith, 1708–55', *Derbyshire Record Society*, 3 vols. (1978, 1979, and 1981).
James Greig (ed.), *The Farington Diary, 1793–1821*, 8 vols. (London, 1922–8).
E. Hobhouse (ed.), *The Diary of a West-Country Physician* (London, 1934).
E. Willmot (ed.), *The Journal of Dr John Simpson of Bradford* (Bradford, 1981).

PRINTED PRIMARY SOURCES (pre-1900)

In the first half of the nineteenth century the volume of printed sources on the subject of medical reform published in the medical periodicals was immense. Here, a small selection is given of those letters, leading articles, and reports, etc. which seemed of most historical importance.

ADAMS, N., *Man-Midwifery Exposed: Or what it is and what it ought to be, with broad hints to new married people and young men and women* (London, 1830).
ALCOCK, THOMAS, 'An Essay on the Education and Duties of the General Practitioner in Medicine and Surgery', *Transactions of the Associated Apothecaries and Surgeon-Apothecaries*, 1 (1823), 1–135.
'ALEXIPHARMICUS', *A General Exposition of the Present State of the Medical Profession in the Metropolis especially with a Plan for its Ameloriation, embracing*

the Question relating to the Removal of the existing Obstructions to the Study of Human Anatomy (London, 1829).

ALLARTON, GEORGE, *Mysteries of Medical Life* (London, 1856).

ALLISON, W. P., *Remarks on the Poor Laws of Scotland* (London, 1844).

Anon., *The Present State of Physick and Surgery in London* (London, 1701).

Anon., *The Present Ill State of the Practice of Physick in this Nation Truly Represented: And Some Remedies thereof Humbly Proposed to the Two Houses of Parliament. By a Member of the College of Physicians* (London, 1702).

Anon., *A General Description of all Trades* (London, 1747).

Anon., *An Address to the Public on the Propriety of Midwives instead of Surgeons practising Midwifery* (London, 1826).

Anon., *An Exposition of the State of the Medical Profession ... and of the injurious effects of the monopoly by usurpation, of the Royal College of Physicians in London* (London, 1826).

Anon., 'A plea for Physicians', *Fraser's Town and Country Magazine*, (Mar., 1848), 286–98.

Anon., *Whom to consult: Or a Book of Reference for Invalids* (London, 1865).

Apothecaries, Society of, *An Address by the Society ... to the General Practitioners of England and Wales on the Provisions of the Bill for the Better Regulation of Medical Practice throughout the United Kingdom* (London, 1844).

——, *A Statement by the Society ... on the Subject of their Administration of the Apothecaries Act* (London, 1844).

——, *An Address by the Society of Apothecaries to the General Practitioners of England and Wales on the Second Report of the Joint Deputation* (London, 1845).

——, *Three Reports by the Joint Deputation of the Society of Apothecaries and the National Association of General Practitioners Appointed to Confer with the Secretary of State on the Subject of the Incorporation of General Practitioners in Medicine, Surgery and Midwifery* (London, 1846).

Apprenticeships: 'On Medical Apprenticeships', leading article, *The London Medical Repository*, 15 (1821), 89–101.

ASHE, ISAAC, *Medical Education and Medical Interests*, Carmichael prize essay for 1868 (Dublin, 1868).

AVELING, J.H., *English Midwives* (London, 1872), reprinted with biographical sketch of the author by J. L. Thornton (London, 1967).

BARLOW, E., published under 'A Disinterested Physician', letter to the *The Medical and Physical Journal*, 30 (1813), 265–96.

——, [published anonymously], 'An Attempt to develop the Fundamental Principles which should guide the Legislature in Regulating the Profession of Physic', *Edinburgh Medical and Surgical Journal*, 14 (1818), 1–26.

——, [published anonymously], 'Exposition of the Present State of the Profession of Physic, and of the Laws enacted for its Government', *Edinburgh Medical and Surgical Journal*, 16 (1820), 479–509.

——, 'An Essay on the Medical Profession ...', *Edinburgh Medical and Surgical Journal*, 28 (1827), 332–56.

——, 'An Essay on Medical Reform', *London Medical Gazette*, 12 (1833–4), 899–905, 936–43.

BARON J., *The Life of Edward Jenner*, 2 vols. (London, 1827–38).

BARRETT, C. R. B., *History of the Society of Apothecaries* (London, 1905).

BATEMAN, THOMAS, *Reports on the Diseases of London* (London, 1819).

BELL, JACOB, *Historical Sketch of the Progress of Pharmacy* (London, 1843).

——, and Redwood, T., *Historical Sketch of the Progress of Pharmacy in Great Britain* (London, 1880).

BELL, JOHN, *Principles of Surgery*, 2 vols. (Edinburgh, 1801).

BELLARS, JOHN, *An Essay towards the Improvement of Physic* (London, 1714).

BLACK, J., 'On the Medical Profession and its Reform', *Provincial Medical and Surgical Journal*, 1 (1840–1), 147–9, 161–3.

BLAND, R., 'Midwifery Reports of the Westminster General Dispensary', *Philosophical Transactions*, 71 (1781), 355 ff.

BLANE, GILBERT, *Select Dissertations* (London, 1822).

BLUNT, JOHN, *Man-Midwifery Dissected* (London, 1793). [John Blunt was the pseudonym of the bookseller S. W. Fores.]

'British Medical Association' [Dr Webster's association], *British and Foreign Medical Review*, 3 (1837), 289–90.

BRODIE, SIR BENJAMIN, *Introductory Discourse on the Duties and Conduct of Medical Students and Practitioners* (London, 1843).

BROWN, JOHN, *Rab and his Friends and Other Essays* (first published 1858, Everyman ed. undated).

BROWN, JOHN TAYLOR, *Dr John Brown: A Biography and Criticism* (London, 1903).

BURROWS, GEORGE MAN, *A Statement of Circumstances connected with the Apothecaries Act and its Administration* (London, 1817).

CAMPBELL, R., *The London Tradesman: Being a Compendious View of all the Trades, Professions, Arts, both Liberal and Mechanic, now practised in the Cities of London and Westminster* (London, 1747).

CHAMBERLAINE, W., *Tirocinium Medicum: Or a Dissertation on the Duties of Youth apprenticed to the Medical Profession* (London, 1813).

CHAMPNEY, T., *Medical and Chirurgical Reform proposed from a Review of the Healing Art throughout Europe* (London, 1797).

CHAPMAN, J., *The Medical Institutions of the United Kingdom: A History exemplifying the Evils of Over-Legislation* (London, 1870).

CLARK, SIR JAMES, BART., *Remarks on Medical Reform in a Letter addressed to the Right Hon. Sir James Graham, Bart.* (London, 1843).

——, *Remarks on Medical Reform: In a Second Letter addressed to the Right Hon. Sir James Graham, Bart.* (London, 1843).

CLARKE, J. F., *Autobiographical Recollections* (London, 1874)

(College of General Practitioners), 'The Proposed College of General Practitioners', leading article, *Provincial Medical and Surgical Journal*, 14 (1850), 124–6.

COLTHEART, P., *The Quacks Unmasked* (London, 1727).

COOKE, W., *Separation without Dissension: Observations addressed to General Practitioners, on the best means of maintaining their Privileges and Respectability* (London, 1831).

CORRY, J., *The Detector of Quackery* (London, 1802).

COWAN, CHARLES, 'Report of Private Medical Practice for 1840', *Lancet* (1841), ii. 358–61, 395–401, 433–9.

——, *On the Danger, Irrationality and Evils of Medical Quackery* (London, 1839).

CURRIE, J., *Medical Reports on the Effects of Water as a Remedy for Fevers* (London, 1805).

DALE, WILLIAM, *The Present State of the Medical Profession* (London, 1860).

DAVENANT, F., *What shall my Son be?* (London, 1870).

DAVIES, JOHN, *An Exposition of the Laws which relate to the Medical Profession in England* (London, 1844).

DENHAM, W. HEMPSON, *Verba Consilia, or Hints to Parents who intend to bring up their Sons to the Medical Profession* (London, 1837).

DENMAN, T., *An Essay on Natural Labours* (London, 1786).

——, *An Introduction to the Practice of Midwifery*, 5th edn. (London, 1805).

DE STYRAP, JUKES, *The Young Practitioner* (London, 1890).

DICKINSON, N., 'On the State of the Medical Profession', *Medical and Physical Journal*, 44 (1820), 470.

Directory, The Medical, 2 vols. (London, 1847), vol. i; London; vol. ii, Provincial.

DUNN, J., 'Suggestions for the Relief of the Sick Poor', *London Medical Repository*, 11 (1818), 235–6.

EDWARDS, D. O., 'Thoughts on the Real and Imaginary Grievances of the Medical Profession', *Lancet* (1841–2), ii. 510–14, 606–14, 742–7, 776–83.

EVANS, DAVID, 'A Series of Cases of Bad Practice in Midwifery and Surgery illustrative of the Evils which result from Uneducated Persons being allowed to practise those branches of the Medical Profession', *Transactions of the Associated Apothecaries and Surgeon-Apothecaries of England and Wales*, 1 (1823), 201–7.

'Evils which beset the Profession', leading article, *Provincial Medical and Surgical Journal*, 1 (1840–1), 64–7.

'Faculty of Medicine', leading article, *Lancet* (1833–4), i. 526–31.

FELDMANN, J. E., *Quacks and Quackery unmasked, or Strictures upon the Medical Art as now practised by Physicians, Surgeons and Apothecaries; with Regulations as to its Reform* (London, 1842).

FERRIAR, J., *Medical Histories and Medical Reflections*, 2 vols. (London, 1810).

FORBES, J., 'On the Patronage of Quacks and Imposters by the Upper Classes of Society', *British and Foreign Medical Review*, 21 (1846), 533–40.

General practitioner, (H), 'Sage Advice to Medical Practitioners', *London Medical and Surgical Journal*, 1 (1828), 53–4.

GISBORNE, THOMAS, *An Enquiry into the Duties of Men in the higher and middle classes of Society in Great Britain resulting from their respective Stations, Professions and Employment*, 2 vols., 3rd edn. (London, 1795).

GLAISTER, JOHN, *Dr. William Smellie and his Contemporaries* (Glasgow, 1894).

GOOD, JOHN MASON, *The History of Medicine so far as it relates to the Profession of the Apothecary* (London, 1796).

GRANVILLE, A. B., *A Report on the Practice of Midwifery at the Westminster General Dispensary during 1818* (London, 1819).

——, *Autobiography*, 2 vols. (London, 1874).

GREEN, JOSEPH HENRY, *Distinction without Separation: A Letter to the President of the College of Surgeons* (London, 1831).

——, *The Touchstone of Medical Reform in Three Letters addressed to Sir Robert Harry Inglis, Bart.* (London, 1841).

GREENHILL, W. A., *Address to a Medical Student* (London, 1843).

GREGORY, J., *Lectures on the Duties and Qualifications of a Physician* (London, 1772).

GRIFFIN, R., *The Grievances of the Poor Law Medical Officers further elucidated in the Report of the Proceedings of the Deputation to the Poor Law Board, Feb. 24 1859* (Weymouth, 1859).

GUTHRIE, G. J., 'Introductory Lecture to Medical Students, October 3, 1831', *London Medical and Physical Journal*, NS 11 (1831), 444–7.

GUYBON, F., *An Essay concerning the Growth of Empiricism or the Encouragement of Quacks* (London, 1712).

HARRISON, EDWARD, *Remarks on the Ineffective State of the Practice of Physic in Great Britain* (London, 1806).

——, *An Address to the Lincolnshire Benevolent Medical Society* (London, 1810).

HILLARY, W., *A Practical Essay on the Small-Pox, to which is added an account of the principal variations of the Weather and the concomitant Epidemic Diseases as they appeared in Rippon ... from 1726–1734*, 2nd edn. (London, 1740).

——, *An Enquiry into the Means of improving Medical Knowledge* (London, 1761).

HODGKIN, THOMAS, *Medical Reform: An Address read to the Harverian Society, Oct 2, 1847* (London, 1847).

HORN, T., *Important Hints connected with the present Medical Practice on real Quackery and the Necessity and Commencement of Medical Reform* (Newcastle, 1834).

HUDSON, J. C., *The Parent's Handbook* (London, 1842).

HULL, ROBERT, 'On the Division of Medical Labour: The Apothecary', *London Medical Gazette*, NS 2 (1841–2), 70–3.

——: 'The Man-midwife', ibid., 473–5.

——: 'The General Practitioner', ibid., 917–19.

——: 'The Hospital Surgeon', ibid., NS 1 (1842–3), 520–3.

'IETROS', 'Of Quacks and Empiricism', *Medical and Physical Journal*, 12 (1804), 137–40, 212–16, 423–6.

JEFFREYS, HENRY, *Cases in Surgery* (London, 1820).

JENKINS, J., *Observations on the Present State of the Profession and Trade of Medicine* (London, 1810).

JONES, J., *Observations on the Self-Supporting Dispensaries* (London, 1844).

KEETLEY, C. B., *Student's Guide to the Medical Profession*, 2nd edn. (London, 1885).

KENNEDY, JAMES, *A Sketch of the Medical Monopolies, with a Plan of Reform. Addressed to the Rt. Hon. Lord John Russell, His Majesty's Secretary of State for the Home Department* (London, 1836).

KERRISON, ROBERT MASTERS, *An Inquiry into the Present State of the Medical Profession in England* (London, 1814).

——, *Observations and Reflections on the Bill now in progress through the House of Commons* (London, 1815).

——, 'State of the Medical Profession', *London Medical Gazette*, NS 1 (1841–2), 122–3.

KIDD, J., *Observations on Medical Reform* (London, 1841).

——, *Further Observations on Medical Reform* (London, 1842).

LEAKE, JOHN, *Lecture Introductory to the Theory and Practice of Midwifery* (London, 1773).

——, *A Syllabus of the Lectures on the Theory and Practice of Midwifery* (London, 1776).

LEE, EDWIN, *The State of the Medical Profession further exemplified in a fourth series of notes* (London, 1863).

LEFEVRE, SIR GEORGE, *The Life of a Travelling Physician* (London, 1843).

LETTSOM, J. C., *Medical Memoirs of the General Dispensary in London for part of the years 1773–1774* (London, 1774).

'Licentiate of the Royal College of Physicians of London', *Observations on the Present System of Medical Education, with a view to Medical Reform* (London, 1834).

LIND, JAMES, *A Treatise on Scurvy* (London, 1753).

(The) London College of Medicine, *Lancet* (1830–1), i. 797, 821, 846, and ii. 178–83, 212–22, 248, 376, 502, 822; (1831–2), i. 456–7, ii. 822.

LUCAS, JAMES, *A Candid Inquiry into the Education, Qualifications and Offices of a Surgeon-Apothecary* (Bath, 1800).

MANN, J. L., *Recollections of my Early and Professional Life* (London, 1887).

MAPOTHER, E. D., *The Medical Profession and its Education and Licensing Bodies*, the Carmichael prize essay for 1868 (Dublin, 1868).

MARRYAT, T., *Therapeutics: Or the Art of Healing*, 7th edn. (Birmingham, 1785, first published Dublin, 1764).

MARSHALL, W. B., *An Essay on Medical Education* (London, 1827).

MAUBRAY, JOHN, *The Female Physician* (London, 1724).

Medical and Chirurgical Review, 13 (1806), preface. Letters to Dr Edward Harrison in reply to his questionnaire on the nature of regular and irregular practice in Britain.

Medical Institutions 'The History and Condition of our Medical Institutions', *Lancet* (1842–3), i. 719–22.

'Medical Legislation', *Lancet* (1826–7), ii. 514–17.

'Medical Protection Assembly', *Lancet* (1844), i. 49–51.

'Medical Reform', *Quarterly Review*, 67 (1840), 53–79. Unsigned, but author was Sir Benjamin Brodie.

'Medical Reform', leading article, *British and Foreign Medical Review*, 9 (1840), 281–9.

'Medical Reform', (Anon.), *Remarks on Medical Reform* (Edinburgh, 1841).

'Medical Reform', *Medico-Chirurgical Review*, NS 34 (1841), 585–90.

'Medical Reform: Conferences On', *Provincial Medical and Surgical Journal*, 2 (1841), 17–19, 37–40, 54–8, 77–80, 97–9, 119–20.

'Medical Reform', leading article in *London Medical Gazette*, NS 1 (1841–2), 117–20.

'Medical Reform: A New Bill', *Edinburgh Medical and Surgical Journal*, 63 (1845), 159–257.

'Medical Reform', leading article in *Medico-Chirurgical Review*, NS 1 (1845), 277–91.

'Medical Reform', *Edinburgh Review*, 81 (1845), 235–72.

'Medical Reform: Great Meeting of the Profession', leading article *Lancet* (1850), i. 456–63.

'MEDICO-CHIRURGUS', *A Letter addressed to the Medical Profession on the Encroachments on the Practice of the Surgeon-Apothecary by a New Set of Physicians* (London, 1826).

'MEDICUS', 'On Practitioners', *Gazette of Health*, 11 (1817), 603–5.

MERRETT, C., *A Short History of the Frauds and Abuses committed by the Apothecaries* (London, 1670).

——, *The Accomplisht Physician, the Honest Apothecary and the Skilful Chyrurgeon* (London, 1676).

MOLYNEUX, E., *Recollections of William Stewart Irvine, MD FRCSE* (Edinburgh, 1896).

MOORE, JOHN, *Medical Sketches* (London, 1786).

MUNK, W., *The Roll of the Royal College of Physicians of London*, vol. ii, 1701–1800, vol. iii, 1801–25 (London, 1878).

MURCHISON, C., *A Treatise on the Continued Fevers of Great Britain*, 2nd edn. (London, 1873).

'National Association of General Practitioners', *Provincial Medical and Surgical Journal*, 10 (1846), 197–8.

'(The) New Medical Bill', leading article, in *British and Foreign Medical Review*, 19 (1845), 193–232.

OGLE, W., *Professional Grievances* (presidential address, Midland branch of the British Medical Association, 8 June 1871). (Printed for private circulation 1871.)

OGLE, W., 'Statistics of Mortality in the Medical Profession', *Transactions of the Medico-Chirurgical Association*, 69, 217–37.

'Overcrowding of the Profession', leading article, *Lancet* (1841–2), i. 795–8.

PAGET, JAMES, *The Motives to Industry in the Study of Medicine*, an address delivered at St Bartholomew's Hospital (London, 1846).

PARKINSON, JAMES, *Medical Admonitions to Families Respecting the preservation of Health and the Treatment of the Sick* (London, 1801).

——, *The Villager's Friend and Physician, or a Familiar Address on the Preservation of Health* (London, 1804).

PEDDIE, ALEXANDER, *Recollections of Dr John Brown* (London, 1893).

PERCIVAL, THOMAS, *Medical Ethics* (Manchester, 1803).

PITT, R., [published anon.], *The Calamities of all the English in Sickness and the Sufferings of the Apothecaries from their Unbounded Increase* (London, 1707).

'Poor Law Committee of the Provincial Medical and Surgical Association', report of *Provincial Medical and Surgical Journal*, 1 (1840), 166–8, 184–6, 197–9, 212–14, 228–30, and 2 (1841), 266–71, 292–5, 304–10, 354–7, 372–4.

POWER, D'ARCY, 'The Medical Institutions of London: The Rise and Fall of the Private Medical Schools in London', *British Medical Journal* 1 (1895), 1388–91, 1451–3.

PRACTITIONER (A), *Is the Practice of Medicine in 1850 a Degenerate Pursuit?* (London, 1850).

'PRACTITIONER' (AN OLD)', *The Public and the Medical Profession* (London, 1844).

'PROPRIETAS', *An Address to the Public on the Propriety of Midwives instead of Surgeons practising Midwifery*, 2nd edn. (London, 1826).

'Report of a Committee on the new Poor Law Amendment Act, appointed by the Provincial Medical and Surgical Association', *Medico-Chirurgical Review*, 25 (1836), 325–33.

REYNOLDS, SIR RUSSELL, *Essays and Observations* (London, 1896).

RIVINGTON, W., *The Medical Profession*, the Carmichael Prize Essay for 1879 (2nd edn. Dublin, 1888; first published 1879).

SANKEY, W. H. O., 'Medical Reform', *London Medical Gazette*, NS 2 (1842–3), 395–6, 428–30.

Scale of charges suggested by Mr Greenhow of Newcastle-on-Tyne, *Lancet* (1830–1), i. 536–7.

'Scotch Doctors', editorial, *Lancet* (1827–8), ii. 211–12.

'SCRUTATOR', *The Medical Charities of Birmingham* (Birmingham, 1863).

[SIMMONS, SAMUEL FOART], *The Medical Register* (London, 1779; new edns., 1780, 1783).

SMITH, ADAM, *Wealth of Nations* (London, 1776).

SOUTH, J. F., *Memorials of the Craft of Surgery* (London, 1886).

SPILSBURY, F., *Free Thoughts on Quacks and their Medicines* (London, 1776).

SPRIGGE, SAMUEL SQUIRE, *The Life and Times of Thomas Wakley* (London, 1897).

——, *Medicine and the Public* (London, 1905).

——, *Physic and Fiction* (London, 1921).

STANSFIELD, GEORGE, 'Statistical Analysis of the Medical Profession in England and Wales', *Association Medical Journal* (29 March 1856), 258.

'State of Medicine in Great Britain', *Gazette of Health*, 5 (1821), 545–52.

STEVENS, J., *Man Midwifery Exposed* (London, 1849).

STONE, SARAH, *A Complete Practice of Midwifery* (London, 1737).

'SURGEON SNIPE', *Remarks on Physicians, Surgeons, Druggists and Quacks* (London, 1842).

Surgeons, 'Important to Surgeons', *Medico-Chirurgical Review*, NS 14 (1831), 570–1.

SYME, JAMES, *Open Letter to the Right Hon. Viscount Palmerston on Medical Reforms* (undated, c.1855).

'T', *Lancet* (1829–30), i. 476–7.

TAYLOR, A. S., 'On the Numerical Relation of the Medical Profession to the Population of Great Britain', *London Medical Gazette*, NS 1 (1844–5), 497–503.

THOMPSON, H. B., *The Choice of a Profession* (London, 1857).

'T.L.', 'Confessions of a Half-ruined Man', *Lancet* (1828–9), ii. 683–4.

TOOGOOD, JONATHAN, 'On the Practice of Midwifery, with Remarks', *Provincial Medical and Surgical Journal*, 7 (1844), 103–8.

Trades: *The Book of English Trades and Library of Useful Arts* (London, 1818).

Transactions of the Associated Apothecaries and Surgeon-Apothecaries, 1 (1823), i–clxv, 'Introductory Essay: Comprising an Account of the Origin of the Associated Apothecaries and Surgeon-Apothecaries, and other Objects'.

[WARDROP, JAMES], 'Intercepted Letters' (published anonymously), *Lancet*, 'On the Duties of a Young Physician, etc.' (1833–4), i. 562–3, 647–8, 724–6, 797–9, 870–2.

WEST, CHARLES, *An Address delivered at St Bartholomew's Hospital* (London, 1850).

WILLAN, R., *Reports on the Diseases of London* (London, 1801).

WILLOCK, W., *The Laws relating to the Medical Profession: With an Account of the Rise and Progress of its Various Orders* (London, 1830).

WILLIAMS, C. J. B., *Memoirs of Life and Work* (London, 1884).

WINSLOW, F. B., *Physic and Physicians*, 2 vols., new edn. (London, 1842).

YOUNG, ARTHUR, *A Six Weeks Tour through the Southern Counties of England and Wales* (London, 1768).

YEATMAN, JOHN C., 'Remarks on the Profession of Medicine in Sicily; and Exposition of the Principal Evils to which it is subject in Great Britain; and Observations on Medical Reform', *Medical and Physical Journal*, 34 (1815), 187–93.

YEATMAN, JOHN C., 'Remarks showing the Expediency of some Legislative Enactment to insure Competent Medical and Surgical Aid to Sick and Hurt Poor', *Medical and Physical Journal*, 38 (1817), 364–6.

X.Y.Z.', 'Physician's Per-centage System', *Lancet* (1828–9), ii. 591.

SECONDARY SOURCES (post-1900)

ABEL-SMITH, BRIAN, *The Hospitals, 1800–1948* (London, 1964).

ACKERKNECHT, E. H., 'Aspects of the History of Therapeutics', *Bulletin of the History of Medicine*, 36 (1962), 389–419.

——, *A Short History of Medicine* (revised edn., Baltimore and London, 1982).

ADAMI, J. G., *Charles White of Manchester (1728–1813) and the Arrest of Puerperal Fever* (London, 1922).

ANNING, S. T., *The History of Medicine in Leeds* (Leeds, 1980).

——, and WALLS, W. K. J., *A History of the Leeds School of Medicine* (Leeds University Press, 1982).

BARNSLEY, R. E., 'Cost of Medicine, 1811', *British Medical Journal*, 2 (1956), 156.

BATTEN, LINDSEY W., 'The Medical Adviser', the seventh James Mackenzie lecture of the Royal College of General Practitioners for 1960, *Practitioner*, 186 (1961), 102–12.

BATTY SHAW, A., 'Benjamin Gooch: Eighteenth-century Norfolk Surgeon', *Medical History*, 16 (1972), 40–50.

BERGER, J and MOHR, J., *A Fortunate Man: The Story of a Country Doctor* (London, 1967).

BERLANT, J. L., *Profession and Monopoly: A Study of Medicine in the United States and Britain* (Los Angeles, London, 1975).

BERRIDGE, V. and EDWARDS, G., *Opium and the People: Opiate Use in Nineteenth-century England* (London, 1981).

BICKERTON, T. H., *A Medical History of Liverpool from the Earliest Days to the Year 1920* (London, 1936).

BISHOP, W. J., 'The Evolution of the General Practitioner in England', in E. Ashworth Underwood (ed.), *Science, Medicine and History*, 2 vols. (London, 1953) ii. 351–7.

BLOOR, D. U., 'The Rise of the General Practitioner in the Nineteenth Century', *Journal of the Royal College of General Practitioners*, 28 (1978), 288–91.

BRANCA, P. (ed.), *The Medicine Show, Patients, Physicians and the Perplexities of the Health Revolution in Modern Society* (New York, 1977).

BRIGHT, PAMELA, *Dr Richard Bright: 1789–1858* (London, 1983).

BROCKBANK, W. and KAY, M. I., 'Extracts from the Diary of Richard Kay of Baldingstone, Bury, Surgeon (1737–1751)', *Medical History*, 3 (1959), 58–68.

BUER, M. C., *Health, Wealth and Population in the Early Days of the Industrial Revolution* (London, 1926).

BURNBY, J. V. L., *A Study of the English Apothecary from 1660–1760* (London, Wellcome Institute for the History of Medicine, *Medical History*, supplement no. 3, 1983).

CARR-SAUNDERS, A. M. and WILSON, P. A., *The Professions* (new edn. London, 1964, first published 1933).

CARTWRIGHT, ANN, *Patients and their Doctors: A Study of General Practice* (London, 1967).

CHAPLIN, ARNOLD, *Medicine in the Reign of George III* (London, 1919).

CHRISTIE, A. B., *Infectious Diseases: Epidemiology and Clinical Practice* (2nd edn. London, 1974).

CLARK, SIR GEORGE, *A History of the Royal College of Physicians of London*, vols. i–ii (Oxford, 1964 and 1966).

COLLINGS, J., 'General Practice Today: A Reconnaisance', *Lancet* (1950), i. 555–85.

COOKE, A. M., *A History of the Royal College of Physicians of London*, vol. iii (Oxford, 1972).

COPE, Z. Sir, *Some Famous General Practitioners and Other Essays* (London, 1961).

——, 'The Private Medical Schools of London (1746–1914)', in Poynter, F. N. L. (ed.), *The Evolution of Medical Education in Britain* (London, 1966).

——, *The Royal College of Surgeons of England: A History* (London, 1959).

COWEN, D. L., 'Liberty, Laissez-Faire and Licensure in Nineteenth-Century Britain', *Bulletin of the History of Medicine*, 43 (1969), 30–40.

CROSSE, V. MARY, *A Surgeon in the Early Nineteenth century: The Life and Times of John Greene Crosse, MD FRCS FRS 1790–1850* (London, 1968).

CROWTHER, M. A., 'Paupers or Patients? Obstacles to Professionalisation in the Poor Law Medical Services before 1914', *Journal of the History of Medicine and Allied Sciences*, 60 (1984), 33–54.

CULE, JOHN, 'William Price of Llantrisant, 1800–1893', *British Medical Journal*, 284 (1982), 483–4.

DAICHES, D., 'George Eliot's Dr Lydgate', *Proceedings of the Royal Society of Medicine*, 64 (1971), 13–14.

DONNISON, JEAN, *Midwives and Medical Men* (London, 1977).

DUREY, MICHAEL, 'Medical Élites: The General Practitioner and Patient Power in Britain during the Cholera Epidemic of 1831–2', in Inkster, I. and Morrell, J. (eds), *Metropolis and Province: Science in British Culture, 1780–1850* (London, 1983).

ERICKSON, ARVEL B., 'An Early Attempt at Medical Reform in England, 1844–1845', *Journal of the History of Medicine*, 5 (1950), 144–55.

FISK, DOROTHY, *Dr Jenner of Berkeley* (London, 1959).

FLEXNER, ABRAHAM, *Medical Education in Europe*, a report for the Carnegie Foundation for the advancement of teaching (New York, 1912).

——, *Medical Education: A Comparative Study* (New York, 1925).

FLINN, M. W., 'Medical Services under the New Poor Law', in D. Fraser (ed.), *The New Poor Law in the Nineteenth Century* (London, 1984).

FOSTER, W. D., 'Dr William Henry Cook: The Finances of a Victorian General Practitioner', *Proceedings of the Royal Society of Medicine*, 66 (1973), 46–50.

FREIDSON, ELIOT, *Profession of Medicine* (New York, 1972).

——, *Professional Dominance* (New York, 1970).

FULLER, MARGARET, *West Country Friendly Societies* (Reading, 1964).

GARRISON, F. H., *An Introduction to the History of Medicine*, 4th edn. (Philadelphia, 1929).

GELFAND, T., 'The Decline of the Ordinary Practitioner and the Rise of a Modern Medical Profession', in Staum, S. and Larsen, D. E., *Doctors, Patients and Society: Power and Authority in Medical Care* (Ontario, 1981).

GEORGE, M. DOROTHY, *London Life in the Eighteenth Century* (Penguin edn. 1976).

GIBSON, SIR RONALD, *The Family Doctor* (London, 1981).

GRAY, ERNEST A., *By Candlelight: The Life of Arthur Hill Hassall, 1817–1894* (London, 1983).

HADFIELD, STEPHEN, 'A Field Survey of General Practice', *British Medical Journal*, 2 (1953), 683–706.

HAMILTON, BERNICE, 'The Medical Professions in the Eighteenth Century', *Economic History Review*, second series, 4(2) (1951), 141–69.

HAMILTON, D., *The Healers: A History of Medicine in Scotland* (Edinburgh, 1981).

HANS, NICHOLAS, *New Trends in Education in the Eighteenth Century* (London, 1951).

HIMMELFARB, G., *The Idea of Poverty: England in the Early Industrial Age* (London, 1984).

HODGKINSON, R., *Origins of the National Health Service: Medical Services of the New Poor Law, 1834–1871* (London, 1967).

HOLLOWAY, S. W. F., 'Medical Education in England, 1830–1858', *History*, 49 (1964), 299–324.

——, 'The Apothecaries Act 1815', part I, 'The Origins of the Act', *Medical History*, 10(2) (1966), 107–29; part II, 'The Consequences of the Act', *Medical History*, 10(3) (1966), 221–36.

HOLMES, GEOFFREY, *Augustan England: Professions, State and Society, 1680–1730* (London, 1982).

HONIGSBAUM, FRANK, *The Division in British Medicine: A History of the Separation of General Practice from Hospital Care, 1911–1968* (London, 1979).

HORNER, N. G., *The Growth of the General Practitioner of Medicine in England* (London, 1922).

JEWSON, N. D., 'The Disappearance of the Sick-man from Medical Cosmology, 1770–1870', *Sociology*, 10(2) (1976), 225–44.

——, 'Medical Knowledge and the Patronage System in Eighteenth-century England', *Sociology*, 8 (1974), 369–85.

KERR, J. M. MUNRO, JOHNSTONE, R. W. and PHILLIPS, M. H., (eds.), *Historical Review of British Obstetrics and Gynaecology* (London, 1954).

KETT, JOSEPH F., 'Provincial Medical Practice in England, 1730–1815', *Journal of the History of Medicine* (Jan. 1964), 17–29.

KING, LESTER S., *The Medical World of the Eighteenth Century* (Chicago, 1958).

LANE, JOAN, 'The Provincial Practitioner and his Services to the Poor, 1750–1800', *Bulletin of the Society for the Social History of Medicine*, 28 (1981), 10–14.

——, 'The Medical Practitioners of Provincial England', *Medical History*, 28 (1984), 353–71.

LEFANU, W. R., *British Periodicals of Medicine: A Chronological List*, revised edn. (Oxford, Wellcome Unit for the History of Medicine, 1984).

LLOYD, C. and COULTER, J. L. S., *Medicine and the Navy, 1700–1900*, 4 vols. (London, 1961).

LOUDON, I. S. L., 'Historical Importance of Out-patients', *British Medical Journal*, 1 (1978), 974–7.

——, 'Leg Ulcers in the Eighteenth and Early Nineteenth Centuries', *Journal of the Royal College of General Practitioners*, Part I: 31 (1981), 263–73; Part II: 'Treatment', 32 (1982), 301–9.

——, 'The Origin of the General Practitioner', the James Mackenzie lecture of the Royal College of General Practitioners for 1982, *Journal of the Royal College of General Practitioners*, 33 (1983), 13–18.

——, 'A Doctor's Cash-book: The Economy of General Practice in the 1830s', *Medical History*, 27 (1983), 249–68.

——, 'The Concept of the Family Doctor', *Bulletin of the History of Medicine*, 58 (1984), 347–62.

——, 'Two Thousand Medical Men in 1847', *Bulletin of the Society for the Social History of Medicine*, 33 (1983), 4–8.

——, 'The Nature of Provincial Medical Practice in Eighteenth-century England', *Medical History*, 29 (1985), 1–32.

——, 'Deaths in Childbed from the Eighteenth Century to 1935', *Medical History*, 30 (1986) 1–41.

——, and STEVENS, R., 'Primary Care and the Hospital', in Fry, J. (ed.), *Primary Care* (London, 1980).

MCKENDRICK, N., BREWER, J., and PLUMB, J. H., *The Birth of a Consumer Society* (London, 1982).

MCMENEMEY, W. H., 'Education and the Medical Reform Movement', in Poynter, F. N. L. (ed.), *The Evolution of Medical Education in Britain* (London, 1966), 135–54.

MAIR, ALEX, *Sir James Mackenzie, MD, 1853–1925, General Practitioner* (Edinburgh and London, 1973).

MAURICE, DICK, 'Six Generations in Wiltshire', *British Medical Journal*, 284 (1982), 1756–9.

MILLER, JONATHAN, 'A Gower Street Scandal', the Samuel Gee lecture, 1982,

Journal of the Royal College of Physicians of London, 17(4) (1983), 181–91.

MITCHELL, B. R. and DEANE, P., *Abstract of British Historical Statistics* (Cambridge, 1962).

MORRIS, R. J., *Class and Class Consciousness in the Industrial Revolution 1780–1850,* studies in economic and society history (London, 1979).

MUSGROVE, F., 'Middle-class Education and Employment in the Nineteenth Century', *Economic History Review,* NS 12 (1959–60), 99–111.

NEWMAN, CHARLES, *The Evolution of Medical Education in the Nineteenth Century* (London, 1957).

OSLER, SIR WILLIAM, *A Way of Life and Selected Writings of Sir William Osler* (London, 1951).

PARRY, N. and PARRY, J., *The Rise of the Medical Profession* (London, 1976).

PEACHEY, G. C., *A Memoir of W. and J. Hunter* (Plymouth, 1924).

PEARSE, JAMES, MD, 'A Personal Retrospect of General Practice', *Lancet* (1919), i. 129–33.

PERKIN, HAROLD, *The Origins of Modern English Society, 1780–1880* (London, paperback edn. 1972).

PETERSON, M. JEANNE, *The Medical Profession in Mid-Victorian London* (Berkeley, Calif., 1978).

——, 'Gentlemen and Medical Men: The Problem of Professional Recruitment', *Bulletin of the History of Medicine,* 58 (1984), 457–73.

PICKSTONE, J. V., 'The Professionalisation of Medicine in England and Europe: The State, the Market and Industrial Society', *Journal of the Japan Society of Medical History,* 25(4) (1979), 550–520.

——, 'Medical Botany', *Memoirs of the Manchester Literary and Philosophical Society,* 119 (1976–7), 85–95.

——, *Medicine and Industrial Society: A History of Hospital Development in Manchester and its Region, 1752–1946* (Manchester, 1985).

PORTER, R., *English Society in the Eighteenth Century* (Penguin Books, Harmondsworth, 1982).

POYNTER, F. N. L., *The Evolution of Medical Education in Britain* (London, 1966).

—— and BISHOP, W. J., 'A Seventeenth-century Doctor and his Patients, John Symcotts, 1592?–1662', *Bedfordshire Historical Record Society,* 31 (1951).

READER, W. J., *Professional Men* (London, 1966).

REISER, S. J., *Medicine and the Reign of Technology* (Cambridge, 1978).

RHODES, P., *Doctor John Leake's Hospital* (London, 1977).

ROBERTS, R. S., 'The Personnel and Practice of Medicine in Tudor and Stuart England', Part 1: 'The Provinces', *Medical History,* 6 (1962), 363–82; Part 2: 'London', *Medical History,* 8 (1964), 217–34.

ROLLESTON, SIR HUMPHREY, 'The Early History of the Teaching of 1. Human Anatomy in London, 2. Morbid Anatomy and Pathology in Great Britain', *Annals of Medical History,* 3rd series, 1 (1939), 202–38.

ROOK, ARTHUR, 'General Practice, 1793–1803, the transactions of a Huntingdonshire Medical Society, *Medical History',* 4 (1960), 236–53, 330–47.

ROSEN, G., 'Fees and Fee Bills', *Bulletin of the History of Medicine*, supplement No. 6 (1946).

——, 'An Eighteenth-century Plan for a National Health Service', *Bulletin of the History of Medicine*, 16 (1944), 429–36.

ROWE, E. J. (ed.), 'London Radicalism, 1830–43', *London Record Society* (1970).

ROWLANDS J., 'Annals of a Teeside Practice, 1793–1969', *Medical History*, 16 (1972), 387–403.

ROWNTREE, L. G., 'James Parkinson', *Bulletin of the Johns Hopkins Hospital*, 23 (1912), 33–45.

SHEPHERD, J. A., 'The Evolution of the Provincial Medical Schools in England', *Transactions of the Liverpool Medical Institution* (1981–2), 14–39.

SHORTER, E., *A History of Women's Bodies* (London, 1983).

SHRYOCK, R., 'Public Relations of the Medical Profession in Great Britain and the United States, 1600–1870', *Annals of Medical History*, NS 2 (1930), 308–45.

——, *The Development of Modern Medicine: An Interpretation of the Social and Scientific Factors Involved*, new edn. (Madison, Wisconsin, 1979).

SIGSWORTH, E. M. and SWAN, P., 'An Eighteenth-century Surgeon and Apothecary: William Elmhirst (1721–1773)', *Medical History*, 26 (1982), 191–8.

SINGER, C. and HOLLOWAY, S. W. F., 'Early Medical Education in England in relation to the pre-history of London University', *Medical History*, 4 (1960), 1–17.

SMITH, G. MUNRO, *A History of the Bristol Royal Infirmary* (Bristol, 1917).

SPENCER, H. R., *The History of British Midwifery from 1650 to 1800*, being the Fitz-Patrick lectures for 1927 delivered before the Royal College of Physicians of London (London, 1927).

STEVENS, ROSEMARY, *Medical Practice in Modern England* (New Haven, 1966).

TAIT, H. P., 'A Gifted Country Practitioner: Francis Adams of Banchory', *Practitioner*, 186 (Feb. 1961), 252–5.

THORNTON, J. L., *Medical Books, Libraries and Collectors* (London, 1949, revised edn. 1966), chapter 8, 'Growth of Medical Periodical Literature'.

TILDESLEY, N. W., 'Richard Wilkes of Willenhall, Staffs: An Eighteenth-century Doctor', *Transactions of the Lichfield and South Staffs Archaeological and Historical Society*, 7 (1965–6), 1–10.

VAN ZWANENBERG, DAVID, 'The Training and Careers of those Apprenticed to Apothecaries in Suffolk, 1815–1858', *Medical History*, 27 (1983), 139–50.

——, 'GEORGE STEBBING, 1749–1825', *British Medical Journal*, 283 (1981), 1517–18.

WADDINGTON, I., 'The Struggle to Reform the Royal College of Physicians, 1767–1771: A Sociological Analysis', *Medical History*, 17 (1973), 107–26.

——, 'The Development of Medical Ethics: A Sociological Analysis', *Medical History*, 19 (1975), 36–51.

WADDINGTON, I.,'Competition and Monopoly in a Profession: The Campaign for Medical Registration in Britain', *Amsterdams Sociologisch Tijdschrift.* be jaargang, No. 2 (Oct. 1979), 288–321.

——, *The Medical Profession in the Industrial Revolution* (Dublin, 1984).

WALL, C., CAMERON, H. C. and UNDERWOOD, E. A., *A History of the Worshipful Society of Apothecaries of London* (London, 1963).

WHITTET, T. D., 'The Apothecary in Provincial Gilds', *Medical History*, 8(3) (1964), 245–73.

WILLIAMS, W., *Deaths in Childbed: A Preventable Mortality*, the Milroy lectures delivered at the Royal College of Physicians, 1904 (London, 1904).

——, 'Puerperal Mortality', *Transactions of the Epidemiological Society of London*, 15 (1895–6), 100–33.

WOODS, R. and WOODWARD, J. (eds.), *Urban Disease and Mortality in Nineteenth-century England* (London and New York, 1984).

Index